Essential Primary Care

SIMO
MB, Ch
General ... *xford*

KEN
BSc., MB,
General Practitioner, The Health Centre, Thame, Oxfordshire

FOREWORD BY

MICHAEL DRURY
MB, ChB, MRCS, FRCGP
Professor of General Practice,
University of Birmingham and
President of the Royal College of
General Practitioners

Blackwell Scientific Publications

OXFORD LONDON EDINBURGH

BOSTON PALO ALTO MELBOURNE

Editorial offices:
Osney Mead, Oxford, OX2 0EL
(*Orders*: Tel. 0865 240201)
8 John Street, London, WC1N 2ES
23 Ainslie Place, Edinburgh, EH3 6AJ
52 Beacon Street, Boston
Massachusetts 02108, USA
667 Lytton Avenue, Palo Alto
California 94301, USA
107 Barry Street, Carlton
Victoria 3053, Australia

First published 1987

Set by Spire Print Services Ltd., Salisbury, Wiltshire
Printed and bound in Great Britain by
Butler & Tanner Ltd, Frome and London

DISTRIBUTORS

USA
Year Book Medical Publishers
35 East Wacker Drive
Chicago, Illinois 60601
(*Orders*: Tel. 312 726-9733)

Canada
The C.V. Mosby Company
5240 Finch Avenue East
Scarborough, Ontario
(*Orders*: Tel. 416-298-1588)

Australia
Blackwell Scientific Publications
(Australia) Pty Ltd
107 Barry Street
Carlton, Victoria 3053
(*Orders*: Tel. (03) 347 0300)

British Library
Cataloguing in Publication Data

Essential primary care.
1. Pathology 2. Wounds and injuries
I. Street, S. H. II. Burch, K. W.
616 RB111

ISBN 0-632-00993-4

Contents

2 Maternity Care

Foreword

One of the more bewildering aspects of general practice to those unfamiliar with it is the range and variety of problems presented. There is, unlike the hospital or specialized clinic, very little indication of the nature of the problem to be addressed and thus little time to develop an appropriate drill. In a gynaecological or cardiovascular clinic, for example, the doctor is likely to be able to work within a fairly well-defined conceptual framework. The mental agility required to adjust, as patients present, to problems affecting any system and containing usually large social and psychological components has lead people to design a variety of flow-charts and *aide-mémoires*. These do not in any way supplant judgement or replace critical thinking, but they do attempt to highlight the important factors that might be considered and thus make their omission less likely. As our range of clinical activity embraces more anticipatory and continuing care their relevance increases.

It is, therefore, a great pleasure to introduce this book. It is written by two practising clinicians and will serve more often on the desktop than on the library shelf. The authors have aimed it at the new entrant to our discipline, but I suspect the experienced physician will welcome it equally and will look forward to new editions.

Michael Drury, PRCGP

Introduction

Patients present with symptoms, doctors pursue diagnoses. This is the central transaction of primary care. Health education, and prevention of illness, continuing and supportive care are its wider dimensions. This book aims to reduce these broad complexities into manageable essentials.

The book is designed as an *aide-mémoire*; aiming to remind rather than inform. It is written specifically for doctors emerging from hospital training and entering general practice. Students may find it helpful in their introduction to clinical medicine, housemen may value it when called upon to give primary care for problems outside their speciality, and it may have some use for established doctors making a referral for a specialist opinion.

The book is written in a concise and consistent format for easy reference. For each topic, the content is limited to the primary assessment, the options for management and the referral criteria. Only seldom is there explicit reference to underlying physiology and pathology. There is no discussion of clinical management beyond the scope of a generalists' knowledge or expertise.

Acknowledgements

We acknowledge and appreciate the influence of our vocational training in the initial planning of this text. Similarly, our partners and colleagues have helped to shape our ideas for its later development.

At an early stage the manuscript was read critically by our friends and colleagues Martyn Agass, Charles Chubb, Shirley Elliott, Stuart Frankum, Keith Hawton, Nigel Henderson, Tony Hillier, Ian MacKenzie, Neil MacLennon, Ann MacPherson, Tony Randall, Peter Sandercock, Doreen Shewan and Bernard Way. The proof copy was read by Judy Green and Andrew Farmer, we are indebted to them all for their clear and helpful comments.

Throughout the preparation we have greatly valued the encouragement and remarkable patience of our publisher, Peter Saugman. Deborah Thompson, the editor, coped with our linguistic ineptitudes with great good humour.

Karen Quarterman has undertaken the translation of all our illegible manuscripts into her elegant typescript.

Our families have tolerated undecorated stairways and unmended toys, late nights and early mornings; their forebearance and their support for this book is immeasurable.

Abbreviations

For convenience and out of sheer habit, abbreviations are used extensively in the text.

ACTH	Adrenocorticotrophic hormone
ADL	Activities of daily living
AF	Atrial fibrillation
AFP	Alpha feto protein
AI	Aortic incompetence
AIDS	Acquired immune deficiency syndrome
ANF	Antinuclear factor
APH	Ante partum haemorrhage
AS	Aortic stenosis
ASO	Antistreptolysin titre
BMI	Body mass index
BP	Blood pressure
BPD	Biparietal diameter
CCF	Chronic congestive failure
CDH	Congenital dislocation of the hip
CFS	Cerebro-spinal fluid
CHD	Congenital heart disease
CNS	Central nervous system
COAD	Chronic obstructive airways disease
CPK	Creatine phosphokinase
CVA	Cerebrovascular accident
CVS	Cardiovascular system
CXR	Chest X-ray
D & C	Dilatation and curettage
DVT	Deep vein thrombosis
ECG	Electrocardiogram
ECT	Electroconvulsive therapy
EDD	Expected date of delivery
EEG	Electroencephalogram
EMG	Electromyography
ENT	Ear, nose and throat
ESR	Erythrocyte sedimentation rate
FB	Foreign body
FBC	Full blood count
FHR	Fetal heart rate
FSH	Follicle stimulating hormone
GC	Gonococcal arthritis
γGT	Glutamyl transferase

GI	Gastrointestinal
GPI	General paralysis of the insane
GTN	Glyceryl trinitrate
GTT	Glucose tolerance test
Hb	Haemoglobin
HCG	Human chorionogonadotrophin
HEC	Health Education Council
HIV	Human Immunodeficiency Virus
HRT	Hormone replacement therapy
HVS	High vaginal swab
IHD	Ischaemic heart disease
i.m.	Intra muscular
i.v.	Intra venous
IVP	Intravenous pyelogram
IUCD	Intra-uterine contraceptive device
JVP	Jugular venous pressure
LAP	Lymphadenopathy
LE	Lupus erythematosus
LFT	Liver function tests
LH	Leutenizing hormone
LICS	Left intercostal space
LMP	Last menstrual period
LVF	Left ventricular failure
LVH	Left ventricular hypertrophy
MAOI	Monoamine oxidase inhibitor
MCHC	Mean corpuscular haemoglobin concentration
MCL	Mid-clavicular line
MCV	Mean corpuscular volume
MI	Myocardial infarction
MS	Multiple sclerosis
MSH	Melanocyte stimulating hormone
MSU	Midstream specimen of urine
NAIC	Non-accidental injury to children
NSAID	Non-steroidal anti-inflammatory drugs
NSU	Non-specific urethritis
5NT	5-Nucleotidase
OC Pill	Oral contraceptive pill (combined)
O.T.	Occupational therapist

PAN	Polyarteritis nodosum
PEF	Peak expiratory flow
PET	Pre-eclamptic toxaemia
PKU	Phenylketonuria
PND	Paroxysmal nocturnal dyspnoea
PO Pill	Progesterone-only pill
PPH	Post-partum haemorrhage
P.R.	Per rectum
PTT	Prothrombin time
PUO	Pyrexia of unknown origin
P.V.	Per vaginum
RA	Rheumatoid arthritis
RICS	Right intercostal space
RIF	Right iliac fossa
RTA	Road traffic accident
SBE	Sub-acute bacterial endocarditis
s.c	Subcutaneous
SDH	Sub-dural haematoma
SLE	Systemic lupus erythematosus
SMR	Sub-mucous resection
SOB	Shortness of breath
STD	Sexually transmitted disease
TB	Tuberculosis
TIA	Transient ischaemic attack
TIBC	Total iron binding capacity
TRH	Thyroid releasing hormone
TSH	Thyroid stimulating hormone
T/S	Throat swab
U & E	Urea and electrolytes
URTI	Upper respiratory tract infection
USS	Ultrasonic scan
UTI	Urinary tract infection
UVL	Ultraviolet light
VMA	Vanillylmandelic acid
WBC	White blood cell
WCC	White cell count

1 Symptoms and Signs

Abdominal pain

Pain in the abdomen is a commonly presenting symptom in general practice. Most cases seen are of a benign or self-limiting nature such as

dietary indiscretion
gastroenteritis or gastritis
indigestion
muscle strain.

Occasionally the condition presented is more serious and each case must be considered carefully to avoid disasters. Few of the following conditions can be adequately excluded over the telephone.

Causes

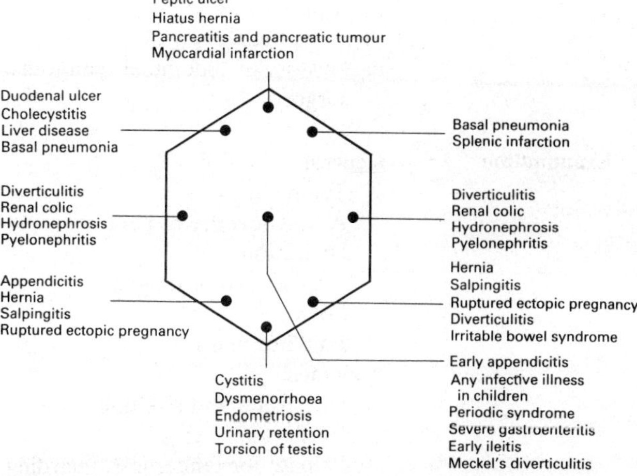

Fig. 1.1

Other causes

Intestinal obstruction
Irritable bowel syndrome
Mesenteric adenitis
Peritonitis
Intra-abdominal cancers
Mesenteric ischaemia
Herpes zoster (pre-rash)
Ruptured abdominal aorta
Porphyria
Sickle cell disease
Henoch–Schönlein purpura

Munchausen's syndrome
Hypercalcaemia
Food allergy

History

Pain
- onset and timing
- character
- site and radiation
- exacerbating and relieving factors

Associated features
- fever
- weight loss
- reduced appetite
- nausea and vomiting
- bowel habit
- micturition
- rashes

Menstrual history

Past history of abdominal symptoms, abdominal disease or surgery

Examination

General
- Temperature
- Assess severity of pain
- Hydration
- Appearance of tongue
- Foetor
- Jaundice and rashes

Abdomen
- Distension and swelling
- Hernias and scars
- Palpate for tenderness, guarding, rigidity and masses
- Percuss for ascites
- Auscultate for bowel sounds
- Check testes
- Vaginal and rectal examination

CVS
- Pulse
- BP
- Femoral pulses

Chest
- Auscultate lung bases

Investigation

- FBC
- ESR
- U & E
- LFT

Amylase
Plasma calcium
Blood sugar
MSU
Pregnancy test
Vaginal swabs
Stool culture and occult blood
Contrast radiography
Ultrasound

Options

Urgent referral – initial assessment must consider the severity of the acute abdomen

Reassurance – the majority of cases seen are of a benign, self-limiting nature. 'Masterly inactivity' with careful observation is the order of the day.

Specific treatment – depends on the underlying cause. Many of the conditions are discussed elsewhere (see below).

Referral

Acute surgical emergencies require urgent referral to hospital
appendicitis
intestinal obstruction
perforated peptic ulcer
suspected peritonitis
ruptured ectopic pregnancy
ruptured abdominal aorta
severe abdominal pain in pregnancy

Doubtful diagnoses in obviously ill patients are best observed and investigated in hospital.

See also:

Abdominal swellings (p. 4)
Anal bleeding (p. 8)
Ascites (p. 14)
Blisters (p. 29)
Chest pain – myocardial infarction (p. 46)
Enlarged liver (p. 85)
Food allergy (p. 113)
Hypochondriasis (p. 153)
Imported disease (p. 157)
Indigestion (p. 163)
Oliguria and anuria (p. 229)
Painful periods (p. 230)
Vomiting blood (p. 331)
Disorders of pregnancy (p. 357)
Common infectious disease in children (p. 402)

Abdominal swelling

The commonest cause of abdominal swelling is obesity and as such it constitutes a problem of considerable social and psychological significance.

Abdominal swelling is primarily a clinical sign and can be demonstrated in the absence of significant symptoms. The converse is also true and, in association with 'flatulence' and 'bloatedness', abdominal swelling may be a feature of indigestion, irritable bowel syndrome or premenstrual syndrome.

Some other less common causes of abdominal swelling constitute problems of pathological significance that must be considered in clinical assessment.

Causes

Gas
- malabsorption syndrome
- intestinal obstruction

Fat
- obesity (see p. 224)
- Cushing's syndrome
- high dose steroid treatment

Solid
- enlarged kidneys
- enlarged liver (see p. 85)
- enlarged spleen (see p. 91)
- uterine enlargement – pregnancy
fibroids
tumour
- constipated colon (see p. 55)
- polycystic kidneys
- retroperitoneal tumours
- gastrointestinal tumours

Fluid
- ascites (see p. 14)
- enlarged bladder
- ovarian cysts
- pancreatic cysts

History

Duration and mode of onset

Associated symptoms
- Pain
- Relationship to eating
- Weight loss
- Vomiting
- Bowel habit

Problems with micturition
Change in the nature of the stool

Menstrual history
Past medical history
Medication
Alcohol intake

Examination

Abdominal examination
- size, distribution and consistency of swelling
- skin striae
- herniae
- visible peristalsis
- resonance to percussion
- bowel sounds
- tenderness and guarding
- 'shifting dullness'
- bimanual examination (vaginal and rectal)

General check for
- enlarged lymph nodes
- anaemia
- congestive cardiac failure
- jaundice
- spider naevi
- cushinoid features

Investigations

FBC
ESR
LFT
Amylase
Cortisol level
Stool – occult blood and/or fat content
Chest X-ray
Abdominal X-ray
Contrast radiography
Ultrasound examination

Options

Treat the underlying cause
Advise on diet and life-style.

Referral

For further investigation and management of the rarer and more sinister causes.

See also:

Abdominal pain (p. 1)
Anal bleeding (p. 8)
Ascites (p. 14)
Constipation (p. 55)

Enlarged liver (p. 85)
Enlarged spleen (p. 91)
Indigestion (p. 163)
Malnutrition and malabsorption (p. 195)
Obesity (p. 224)
Premenstrual syndrome (p. 257)

Adolescent problems

Many adolescent problems never present in primary medical care. In most of those that do the family doctor is well placed to anticipate, recognize or prevent the symptoms and to support the adolescent and his family. However, certain cases are more appropriately managed by other agencies.

Patterns of presentation

Psychological
- Depression
- Psychosis
- Self-poisoning
- Problem drinking
- Obsessional states
- Anorexia nervosa
- Anxiety
- Moodiness
- Introversion

Psychosexual
- Contraceptive problems
- Fear of pregnancy
- Fear of sexually transmitted disease
- Promiscuity
- Homosexuality
- Jealousies
- Impotence

Psychosomatic
- 'Minor illness'
- Hypochondriasis
- Headache
- Insomnia
- Dysmenorrhoea
- Dissatisfaction with body image
- Acne

Delinquent behaviour
- Defiant trouble-making

Shows little affection
Truancy
Aggressiveness
Unpopularity
Social and emotional deprivation
Family history of delinquency or crime
Under-achievement
Drug abuse and glue sniffing
Delinquent behaviour independent from any peer group is an adverse prognostic feature

Risk factors

Family
- sibling rivalry
- neglect
- parental jealousy
- exacerbations of previous family disruptions
- overprotection

Environmental and cultural differences
- unemployment
- language barriers
- inappropriate estimation of IQ, dyslexia, etc.

Assessment

Physical and psychological assessment of all presenting symptoms
Peer group attitudes
Parental attitudes
Sibling attitudes
Exclude psychiatric problems in the patient and his family
Check for persistent and handicapping symptoms

Prevention

Anticipation of life events in the family
Support and counselling during life events
Advice and information to parents on infant welfare and school clinics
Early recognition of presentation of adolescent problems
Maintaining 'at-risk' registers

Options

Counselling and psychotherapy respecting the adolescent's confidence and facilitating 'face-saving' manoeuvres. Treating the whole family.

Unnecessary prescribing might inappropriately 'medicalize' a delinquent problem.

Co-operation with
- Health visitors

School nurses
Teachers
Educational psychologists
Social workers
Probation officers
Counsellors
Community physicians.

Referral All psychiatric disorders
Violent adolescents
Recidivist delinquents.

See also:

Anorexia (p. 12)
Depression (p. 63)
Headache (p. 133)
Hypochondriases (p. 153)
Insomnia (p. 170)
Obsessions (p. 227)
Painful periods (p. 230)
Problem drinking (p. 261)
Spots (p. 294)
STD (p. 301)
Stress and anxiety (p. 303)
Contraception (p. 446)
Overdose and self-poisoning (p. 530)

Anal bleeding

Anal bleeding is a common symptom presented in primary care. It is usually attributed to 'piles'. However, the more serious causes must be considered in every case, as the two conditions can co-exist, especially in the older patient with chronic or recurrent bleeding.

The majority of cases are self-treated or ignored and never presented to the doctor.

The bleeding can occur at any age and is usually painless. The amount may vary from a small streak in the stool and on the toilet paper to a large life-threatening haemorrhage.

Causes Piles
Perianal fissure and skin lesions
Proctitis
Trauma
Diverticulosis

Colorectal tumours
Ulcerative colitis
Crohn's disease
Intussusception in a child
Massive upper gastrointestinal bleed

History

Amount, duration and character of the bleeding (exclude vaginal bleeding in females)
Timing – before, after or mixed with the stool
Presence of mucus or pus with the stool
Associated symptoms
- Diarrhoea or constipation
- Change in bowel habit
- Anal pain or irritation
- Abdominal pain
- Weight loss
- Change in general health

History of bleeding diathesis
Drugs, e.g. indomethacin suppositories, anticoagulants
Patient's health beliefs and fears.

Examination

Weight
Anaemia, jaundice or bruising
Palpate abdomen for
- masses
- tenderness
- enlarged liver or spleen

Ano-rectal examination
- digital
- proctoscopy

Investigation

FBC
ESR
Liver function tests
Barium enema
Sigmoidoscopy

Options

Suggest a high roughage diet for piles, anal fissures, diverticulosis and inflammatory bowel disease
Local soothing creams for piles, anal-fissures and proctitis
Ice packs can relieve the pain of prolapsed, thrombosed piles
Salazopyrine 1 g 12 hourly is used in the prophylaxis and treatment of acute inflammatory bowel disease
Steroids used systematically and via enamas can control acute inflammatory bowel disease

Antacids H_2 antagonists can be used after major bleeding from a peptic ulcer.

Referral

For surgical assessment and treatment of suspected colorectal tumour if patient is over 25 years old, or if bleeding is recurrent
For surgical treatment of persistent local anal conditions
For the control of acute inflammatory bowel disease
Urgent referral is indicated if a large amount of bleeding is involved.

See also:

Annal irritation (p. 10)
Constipation (p. 55)
Diarrhoea (p. 68)
Imported disease (p. 157)
Piles (p. 249)

Anal irritation

This is a distressing set of symptoms which may include itching, burning and pain on defaecation.

The vast majority of causes are benign, but may be recurrent. A full assessment is necessary to exclude the rare but more serious causes.

Causes

Idiopathic pruritis ani
Piles
Threadworms
Fungal infection
Diabetes
Anal fissure/fistula
Pilonidal sinus
Proctitis
Crohn's disease
Ulcerative colitis
Venereal infection
Post-irradiation
Irritant suppositories (e.g. indomethacin)

History

Duration and timing of symptoms
Pain on defaecation
Change in bowel habit
Soiling
Visible worms in the stool

Blood or mucus in the stool
Urinary symptoms
Psychological factors

Examination

Local inspection
- Redness
- Bleeding
- Excoriation
- Fissure/fistula
- Pilonidal sinus
- Skin tags at the anal margin

Proctoscopy and digital examination

Investigation

Urine for sugar
Anal swab/skin scrapings for mycology
Sellotape slide for worms
Stool sample for
- ova and parasites
- occult blood

Barium enema
Sigmoidoscopy

Options

Diet

Suggest increased roughage in the diet, particularly in the presence of piles, fissures and inflammatory bowel diseases.

Local toilet

Clean around the anus carefully after defaecation using simple soaps – avoid astringent antiseptics

Loose cotton underwear is more absorbent and comfortable to wear.

Laxatives

For constipation, particularly stool softners, e.g. liquid paraffin.

Local soothing creams
- Zinc and castor oil ointment
- Local antiseptic creams with or without steroid or local anaesthetic
- Antifungal agents (e.g. Whifield ointment or miconazole cream)

(The long term use of local anaesthetic preparations may exacerbate the irritation by sensitization).

Antihelminthic drugs

May be used for threadworms. Dosage depends on age and may be repeated in 14 days

It is wise to treat the whole household if infestations are

recurrent, e.g. Pripsen (dosage varies with age of the patient).

Referral

Investigation of protitis
For surgical correction of
- piles
- fissures
- fistulas
- pilonidal sinus.

See also:

Anal bleeding (p. 8)
Localized rash (p. 185)
Piles (p. 249)
STD (p. 301)
Worms (p. 339)
Diabetes (p. 457)

Anorexia

Anorexia, or the loss of appetite, is a presenting symptom of several conditions. It seldom occurs in isolation and usually the associated symptoms are more significant in reaching a diagnosis.

Causes

Anorexia nervosa
Depression
Disorders of taste
Cardiac failure
Liver disease
Gastrointestinal disorders
Uraemia
Chronic illness
Malignant disease

Anorexia nervosa

Anorexia is the primary symptom in the syndrome anorexia nervosa. This syndrome occurs in both sexes and at any age but it most commonly affects teenage girls. Psychological factors are probably the only causes but the subsequent physiological effects result in a mortality of 2–5%.

Assessment

Psychological factors
- Loss of appetite
- Dysphagia
- Revulsion of certain foods
- Preoccupation with food and cooking for others

Guilt after eating
Distorted perception of body image
Loss of libido
Conflict in social relationships
Overactivity

Physiological effects
Loss of weight
Malnutrition
Constipation
Amenorrhoea
Lanugo hair
Peripheral cyanosis
Low blood pressure
Low pulse rate
Low metabolic rate
Long term effects on bone

History

Associated symptoms to exclude other causes
Weight
present weight
previous maximum weight
previous fluctuations
Height
Diet
Drugs
Laxative abuse, vomiting and 'binge-eating'
Depressive symptoms
Family expectations, attitudes and conflicts

Examination

Record
Height and weight
Check for
Cranial nerve lesions
Cardiac failure
Liver and kidney disease
Signs of malnutrition
Cancer

Options

Patient
Encourage acceptance of help despite any denial of an abnormality
Referral to, or co-operation with, a psychiatrist to increase weight in a controlled environment, to supervise drugs and commence psychotherapy
Maintain a consistent approach and follow up.
Family
Avoid implication of blame

Check for depressive symptoms within the family
Counsel the family towards resolution of any conflicts.

See also:

Adolescent problems (p. 6)
Depression (p. 63)
Enlarged liver (p. 85)
Malnutrition and malabsorption (p. 195)
Weight loss (p. 337)
Heart failure (p. 469)

Ascites

Ascites presents as abdominal swelling with the characteristic sign of 'shifting dullness' due to excess fluid in the peritoneal cavity. It is always a sign of serious pathology.

Differential diagnosis

Free blood in abdomen
Free air in abdomen
Distension of small or large bowel
Ovarian cyst
Pregnancy
Surgical complications, e.g. ileus

Causes

Transudate
- Cirrhosis
- Portal hypertension
- Congestive cardiac failure
- Nephrotic syndrome

Exudate
- Tuberculosis
- Carcinomatosis

Other causes

Malabsorption
Constrictive pericarditis
Hepatic vein obstruction/Budd–Chiari syndrome
Sodium retention
Chylous ascites

History

Onset and duration of symptoms
Weight change
Diet and alcohol intake
Associated symptoms
- Shortness of breath
- Cough
- Haemoptysis
- Oedema
- Urinary symptoms

Examination

Abdominal inspection, superficial oedema, everted umbilicus, prominent veins

Abdominal palpatation – 'shifting dullness' fluid thrill, abdominal girth, renal mass, enlarged liver, ovarian mass
Bimanual pelvic examination
Cardiovascular status including peripheral pulses
Signs of peripheral neuropathy
Encephalopathy.

Investigation

FBC
ESR
U & E + creatinine
LFT
Plasma proteins

Options

Refer for diagnostic drainage of ascites
Investigate for primary neoplasm
Treat any congestive cardiac failure (see p. 469)
Salt restriction diet
Potassium supplements, e.g. 'Slow-K' 600 mg 1–2 hourly
Multi-vitamin supplements
Stop alcohol
Spironolactone as diuretic, e.g. 50 mg 12 hourly.

Referral

All cases for drainage of ascites and investigation.

See also:

Abdominal swellings (p. 4)
Malnutrition and malabsorption (p. 195)
Heart failure (p. 469)
Hypertension (p. 475)
Pulmonary tuberculosis (p. 492)

Asthma and wheezing

Several types of wheezing are recognized
- classical asthma
- bronchitis with wheeze in adults
- wheezy bronchitis in children
- bronchial obstruction with tumour or foreign body
- cardiac asthma of LVF.

Asthma is a condition of variable and reversible narrowing of the airways. The narrowing has three components
- bronchial muscle constriction
- mucosal oedema
- intraluminal mucus.

It is a depressing observation that while the introduction of potent anti-asthma therapy has reduced morbidity there has been little change in the mortality levels over the last thirty years – about 1,500 deaths per year. Many of these deaths are attributable to an under employment of steroids, and further a lack of the available aerosol bronchodilators. Most cases lack an objective measurement of airways obstruction.

Associated and precipitating factors

Allergy
Inherited predisposition
Psychological factors
Male predominance
Infection
Exercise
Respiratory irritants (smoking)
Drugs (aspirin and β-blockers)
LVF
Foreign body
Carcinoma

History

Onset and duration of wheezing attacks
Presence of cough and sputum
Associated factors
- any known allergies
- hay fever
- eczema
- urticaria
- relationship to season
- smoking
- pets
- occupation
- stress levels

Precipitating factors
- infection
- dust contact with allergens
- drugs
- exercise

Recent history of choking attack from inhalation of foreign body
Past history of respiratory or cardiac disease
Family history of wheezing
Health beliefs and fears

Examination

Inspect the chest for deformity, poor expansion, hyperinflation and use of accessory muscles of respiration. Auscultate for expiratory wheeze and localizing signs. The wheeze is typically widespread in asthma. If localized consider bronchostenosis, carcinoma or inhaled foreign body.

Record pulse rate and character (pulsus paradoxus)
Examine CVS for evidence of cardiac failure

Investigation

Peak expiratory flow rate – if the wheeze is due to asthma this should increase at least 15% after inhalation of a bronchodilator
Chest X-ray – to exclude other pathology
Sputum and blood eosinophilia
Skin allergy testing – this is unreliable except as a measure of atopy

Emergency treatment of asthma

Assess severity
Pulse > 120/min
PEF < 100 litres/min
Inability to talk because of breathlessness
Cyanosis

Options

Nebulized bronchodilator, e.g. salbutamol 0.5% solution
Subcutaneous or intravenous bronchodilator, e.g. Ventolin s.c. 500 μg (8 μg/kg body weight); i.v. 250 μg (4 μg/kg body weight)
Aminophylline (i.v. 250–500 mg) i.v. slowly over 10 mins
Hydrocortisone (100–200 mg) i.v. (may take several hours to exert its effect)
Oxygen therapy
If there is no definite improvement with a measured increase in PEF after half to one hour, hospital admission should be arranged.

Long term management

Education about nature of disease and purpose of treatment
Instruction in breathing exercises and avoidance of allergens
Bronchodilators: salbutamol, terbutaline, or xanthine preferably by aerosol or rotahaler where possible. Ipratropium bromide inhaler may be a helpful bronchodilator, especially in chronic bronchitics
Disodium cromoglycate – especially of value in asthma of allergic origin. Even small children can be trained to use a spinhaler with the aid of a whistle attachment. May need to be given up to 6 times a day
Steroids
Aerosol (best to avoid side effects), e.g. Becotide
'Short sharp' courses (60 mg prednisolone), tailing off dosage over one week

Long term treatment dosage should be kept below 10 mg/day to avoid side effects and given in the morning to reduce adrenal suppression
Antibiotics, if indicated for co-existing bacterial infection

Follow-up

Acute — as often as required until stabilized
Chronic — 3 monthly checks recording PEF and associated symptoms

Failure to control

Poor compliance and faulty technique with aerosols
Co-existing infection
Aspergillosis
Misdiagnosis
- inhaled foreign body
- cardiac asthma
- fibrosing alveolitis
- chronic bronchitis

Review drugs (e.g. β-blockers)

Referral

Acute severe asthma unrelieved by emergency measures
Unexplained deterioration in PEF
Failure to control symptoms
For assessment of allergy.

See also:

Food allergy (p. 113)
Nasal obstruction (p. 214)
Chronic bronchitis (p. 440)
Respiratory distress – asthma (p. 536)

Backache

Backache is a commonly presented symptom and many working days are lost with much discomfort as a result of this condition.

In a large number of cases the symptoms are vaguely described by the patient making the diagnosis difficult to define. To this group equally vague diagnostic labels are applied such as 'postural back' 'chronic ligamentous strain', 'muscular strain' 'lumbago' and 'sciatica'.

In those cases in which a firm diagnosis can be made the cause may be intrinsic to the spine itself or extrinsic, i.e. referred from other sites.

Table 1.1. Causes of backache

	Intrinsic	**Extrinsic**
Inflammatory	Ankylosing spondylitis Rheumatoid arthritis Sacro-iliitis Osteochondritis	Pleurisy Pulmonary infarct Peptic ulcer Pancreatitis Polymyalgia rheumatica
Infective	Osteomyelitis Tuberculosis	Pleurisy Herpes zoster Urinary tract infection Pelvic inflammatory disease
Traumatic	Prolapsed intervertebral disc Facet joint disturbance Fractured vertebral body Fracture of transverse process Pathological fracture Coccidynia	
Metabolic	Osteoporosis Osteomalacia Paget's disease	Pregnancy Menopause Renal disease
Neoplastic	Metastasis from thyroid breast lung kidney prostate Meningioma Neuroma Myeloma	Carcinoma cervix uterus ovary rectum
Degenerative	Osteoarthritis Post-traumatic	
Congenital	Scoliosis Spondylolisthesis Transitional vertebrae Spina bifida	
Other	Chronic ligamentous strain Sacroiliac strain	Acute myocardial infarction Dissecting aneurysm Blood dyscrasias Dysmenorrhoea Psychological factors

History

Onset, duration and severity of pain
Site and radiation of pain
Exacerbating and relieving factors
- lifting
- coughing
- bending
- straining

Associated symptoms
- sensory loss (especially in L1-S1 distribution)
- loss of sphincter control or sensation
- weight loss
- sleep disturbance
- incapacity for work

History of trauma
Medical history
- previous therapy
- previous cancer

Examination

Inspect gait, posture and symmetry in spine and pelvis (erect and flexed)

Palpate
- Site of maximal pain
- Muscle tone
- Peripheral pulses

Assess
- Range of movements
- Real and apparent leg length
- Femoral stretch test
- Straight leg raise

Check for
- Hip disease
- Loss of power, sensation or reflexes in the legs
- Muscle wasting
- (Carcinoma of breast, prostate or rectum)

Investigation

When backache is severe or persistent
- FBC
- ESR
- acid phosphatase
- alkaline phosphatase, calcium and phosphate
- protein electrophoresis
- X-ray spine, pelvis and sacro-iliac joints (when indicated)
- chest X-ray

Prevention

Posture; standing straight or lying on a firm flat surface
Avoid lifting and bending or sitting with an arched back

Lumbosacral belt to maintain a slight lordosis
Exercise, especially swimming, to maintain muscle tone

Options

Rest on a firm flat surface
Analgesia (see p. 495)
Local heat with infra-red lamp, hot water bottles, baths or 'rubifascients'
Muscle relaxants, e.g. diazepam 5 mg 8 hourly
Manipulation, after excluding
- Neurological deficit
- Fever
- Anticoagulant therapy
- Referred pain
- Fracture
- Spinal neoplasm.

Referral

Traction
Epidural anaesthesia
Laminectomy
Spinal decompression
'Back Pain Association' for information and advice.

Patterns of presentation

Ankylosing spondylitis

This is an inflammatory condition of the spine and sacroiliac joints. The hip joints may also be affected. It usually occurs in young men. The patient complains of pain and stiffness. On examination there is loss of range of movement, particularly flexion and extension of the spine. Chest expansion may also be reduced. X-ray changes occur in the sacroiliac joints and there is bony ankylosis of the vertebral bodies (bamboo spine).

There is a variable prognosis from minor discomfort to crippling deformities with a rigid spine. Immobilization tends to make the condition worse. Regular daily activities and exercise should be encouraged with the use of adequate analgesia (e.g. naproxen 250–500 mg 8–12 hourly).

Osteochondritis

This is a condition of adolescence with osteochondritis of the vertebral body epiphysis. The patient complains of pain in the dorsal or lumbar spine possibly with kyphosis and paraspinal muscle spasm. Neurological signs are absent. X-ray changes are diagnostic. The cause is unknown although it is occasionally related to trauma.

Treatment is with rest and, in more severe cases, with

immobilization in a plastic jacket or brace. Swimming and postural exercises may aid subsequent mobility.

Prolapsed intervertebral disc

The intervertebral discs degenerate with age and may become liable to injury and damage from even minor trauma. This leads to mechanical inefficiency and sometimes pain. If the peripheral anulus is ruptured the softer core may herniate. Posterolateral protrusion may impinge upon the nerve roots leading to pain referred in the distribution of the sensory nerve and sometimes loss of function with more serious damage to the nerve root (sciatica). If the protrusion compresses the cauda equina, bladder symptoms may develop.

Treatment, initially, is by bed rest, adequate analgesia and muscle relaxants. Epidural analgesia is occasionally used with some success. When the acute pain subsides physiotherapy may help to strengthen the paraspinal muscles for future support. Some patients with chronic pain find a lumbosacral corset helpful.

If the pain does not settle with conservative treatment then referral may be necessary or a consideration of laminectomy. This is particularly important in the presence of marked nerve root signs. If bladder symptoms are evident then urgent referral is indicated.

Facet joint disturbance

Some patients describe a definite 'click' in the back on bending with the sudden onset of pain. If the pain is persistent manipulation may speed recovery. The disturbance is considered by some to represent subluxation of the facet joints in the spine; however pathological fractures should be excluded before manipulation is undertaken.

Fracture of vertebral body

A fracture, and the concomitant risk of paraplegia, must be suspected in all cases of painful acute flexion or hyperextension injury of the spine.

Any movement of the patient must be well supported and into a supine position for immediate transfer to an accident unit. In addition to other supports a cervical collar should be applied.

Check for

- power in all limbs
- fine movement in hands and feet
- sensation and areas of anaesthesia.

Fracture of the transverse process

Though painful, this fracture does not carry the same risk of paraplegia and management is usually conservative and home-based with rest and analgesia. Haematuria must be checked for to exclude associated renal damage with injuries in the loin area.

Coccidynia

Trauma is a common antecedent to persistent pain around the coccyx. The pain can be associated with child-birth, falls onto the bottom, congenital deformity, infection, arthritis and tumours.

Management includes explanation of the condition, adequate analgesia, local heat, special cushions and, occasionally, steroid injections. Manual reduction of a displaced fracture may be appropriate in the acute phase.

Osteoperosis and osteomalacia

Osteoporosis is classically a condition of older women. There is general loss of the bone substance and crush fractures may occur. It leads to a chronic and persistent but ill-defined backache. X-ray changes rarely show fractures of the bone. Treatment is unsatisfactory but various regimens have been tried using anabolic steroids, calcium fluoride and vitamin D supplements. Activity should be maintained if at all possible.

Patients with osteomalacia may have similar radiological changes but in addition show a low/normal serum calcium and raised alkaline phosphatase. It is due to vitamin D deficiency and treatment is with vitamin D and calcium supplements after exclusion of the underlying cause.

Paget's disease

This is a condition of the elderly. It can affect the spine, pelvis, limbs and skull. The affected bone architecture is disturbed by neovascularization, and pathological fractures may occur. If the condition is extensive circulatory 'shunting' occurs with possible subsequent heart failure. X-ray changes are characteristic and there may be an increase in serum alkaline phosphatase.

Bone pain is usually treated with analgesics and sometimes calcitonin. Pathological fractures are difficult to manage.

This is a pre-malignant condition, osteosarcoma being more prevalent in Paget's disease.

Chronic ligamentous strain

This is a rather vague diagnosis of poorly-defined back pain with few or no accompanying physical signs. It may occur as a result of excessive load or exercise, variance of leg length or congenital anomaly of the spine.

The patient complains of pain when bending, lying down or sitting for long periods.

Treatment in the initial stages is with rest on a firm bed, simple analgesics and local heat. As the pain subsides normal activity is gradually resumed. Some patients undoubtedly find that manipulation eases symptoms more rapidly.

Sacroiliac strain

There is a small amount of movement in the sacroiliac joint and as such it may be susceptible to derangement, with pain over the joint. Treatment is with rest, pain relief and occasionally manipulation.

Other causes of similar pain may be ankylosing spondylitis or pain referred from the lumbar spine.

Spondylolisthesis

In this condition a lumbar vertebra may slip forwards on the one immediately below. It typically affects the 4th and 5th lumbar vertebrae. The X-ray changes are evident but the degree of displacement may not correspond with symptoms. Major displacement tends to occur in adolescents.

On examination there may be a palpable 'step' in the lumbar spine with increased lordosis. If the displacement is severe there may be irritation of the nerve roots with sciatica.

In some cases a period of observation, to exclude progression, and physiotherapy may be all that is required. If symptoms persist then a surgical corset or operative stabilization may become necessary.

Scoliosis

Scoliosis is curvature of the spine to one side, associated with a degree of rotation. A postural or compensatory scoliosis can be abolished by forward flexion of the spine while a structural scoliosis is exaggerated by this manoeuvre.

Kyphosis and lordosis are the curvatures convex to the back and front respectively.

Backache, respiratory and cardiovascular displacement, and social disadvantage are the eventual complications of scoliosis and can often be avoided by early and effective intervention.

Case finding, at every opportunity, is by inspection of the spinal contour both erect and flexed. All primary relatives of patients with structural scoliosis should be similarly inspected.

All cases of structural scoliosis should be referred for

orthopaedic assessment. A compensatory scoliosis should be referred for assessment of the primary cause when appropriate.

See also:

Blisters (p. 29)
Chest pain
- dissecting aneurysm (p. 45)
- myocardial infarction (p. 46)

Menopause (p. 199)
Painful periods (p. 230)
Symptoms in pregnancy (p. 352)
Osteoarthritis (p. 485)
Pulmonary tuberculosis (p. 492)
Rheumatoid arthritis (p. 493)
Back injury (p. 512)

Bad breath

Bad breath or 'halitosis', as a presenting complaint is seldom of medical significance. It may have disproportionate social significance. The main benefit of a limited medical assessment may be reassurance, often more for the family than the affected patient.

Causes

Mouth breathing
Smoking
Dentures
Poor oral hygiene
Stomatitis
Dental sepsis
Tonsillitis
Sinusitis
Nasopharyngeal tumour
Retained FB in child
Bronchiectasis
Lung abscess
Pharyngeal pouch
Oesophageal pouch
Gastro-oesophageal reflux
Diet
Misapprehension
Anxiety

History

ENT and dental history
Oral hygiene

Diet
Social and psychological factors

Examination

Smell the breath
Temperature and LAP
Examination of
- nose
- throat
- chest

Investigation

FBC
ESR
Throat swabs
Barium swallow and meal
Chest X-ray

Options

Discussion of mechanism and range of normal oral hygiene
Dietary advice
Stop smoking
Dental care
Antibiotics
Decongestants
Reassurance.

See also:

Mouth symptoms (p. 207)
Sinusitis (p. 287)
Stress and anxiety (p. 303)

Bites and stings

The majority of bites and stings are never presented to a doctor. Stings are seen only with complications, and bites can range from mosquito bites to horse bites. Management may therefore range from advice or self-care through to surgical debridement, and the administration of specific anti-venoms after snake bites.

Causes

Stings
- Bee
- Wasp
- Hornet
- Horse Fly
- Nettle
- Poison ivy, etc.

Bites
- Mammals

Snakes
Mosquitoes and flies
Fleas
Scabies
Head lice
Pubic lice
Body lice

History

Details of the bites or stings
Previous reactions to stings
fever
anaphylaxis
arthritis
nephritis
LAP
Social factors, e.g. self-neglect

Examination

Check for
Visible lice and nits or scabies burrows
Visible bee sting
Local and systemic reactions
LAP
allergic or infective
immediate or delayed onset
bullae or urticaria

Emergency care

Anaphylaxis see p. 511

Options

Advice on first-aid
Advice on self-care – calamine and cold compresses
Antihistamines, e.g. chlorpheniramine 4 mg/8 hourly
Antibiotics for mammalian bites for secondary infection
Steroids for severe bullous reactions or for immediate prophylaxis with history of severe reactions
Sterile dressing for bullae – punctured or intact
Anti-tetanus toxin when appropriate
Avoid outdoor activities in summer if hypersensitive to stings
Avoid scents and colours attractive to insects
Adrenaline and antihistamines for self-administration in cases with risk of anaphylaxis.

Referral

Imported diseases
Snake bites for anti-venoms
Mammalian bites for surgical care.

Patterns of presentation

Fleas

Ctenocephalides canis

C. felis

Carried by dogs, cats, hedgehogs and other mammals. These fleas are active in late summer or in centrally heated buildings. Life cycle of 18 days to 18 months.

Allergic reactions to fleas: saliva gives a pruritic papule.

Avoid by regular dusting of pets and/or utilization of 'Vapona' or 'Mafu' impregnated strips in an unventilated room for 48 hours.

Scabies

Acarus scabiei (see also p. 188)

Transmitted by handling infected bedding.

Incubation time is six weeks.

Characteristically intensely itchy rash with skin burrows terminating in vesicles. These are found in finger clefts, wrists and ankles, buttocks and groin. The face is spared.

Treatment with gamma benzene hexachloride (steroids exacerbate the infestation).

Head lice

Pediculoris humanus capitis

Transmission is by direct contact, epidemics in schools are not uncommon and all socio-economic groups may be affected.

Nits are visible as adherent 0.5 mm scales on the hair shafts. May also find associated scalp irritation, and local LAP.

Treatment according to local DHA recommendations with malathion, carbaryl or gamma benzene hexachloride.

Pubic lice

Pediculoris pubis

A sexually transmitted disease. Crab-like lice are visible and nits may also be present. Check for other sites of infestation.

Treat with malathion.

Body lice

Vectors for typhus and relapsing fever.

Thrives on the neglected body, with multiple bites resulting in malaise – hence 'lousy'.

Treatment with malathion dust and normal laundry (clothes), and gamma benzene hexachloride to body.

See also:

Fever (p. 106)
Imported disease (p. 157)
Infections and parasites from pets (p. 165)

Localized rash (p. 185)
Anaphylactic shock (p. 511)

Blisters

These are discrete skin lesions which contain free fluid. Large blisters are known as bullae while smaller ones, less than 3 mm, are known as vesicles. The fluid may be serum, blood or pus.

Normal skin will blister if subjected to friction, trauma or burns. These conditions will not be described here.

Viruses of the herpes and coxsackie groups characteristically cause a vesicular eruption.

Herpes simplex

This virus commonly causes the 'cold sore' on the lips (Type I virus) but can affect other sites on the skin and mucous membranes. Patients with atopic eczema may suffer a generalized eruption. A different strain of the virus (Type II) may infect the genitalia.

Skin lesions

Small blisters become pustules in a few days with surrounding erythema and induration
Crusting then develops
Healing takes place within two weeks
On mucous membranes the lesions appear as white plaques on a red base, with subsequent ulceration.

Options

Idoxuridine in dimethyl sulphoxide solution or acyclovir cream can be applied to the early blister with partial success
Topical antibiotics can be used for secondary bacterial infection
Barrier creams may help to prevent lesions induced by sunlight.

Herpes zoster

Otherwise known as shingles. The same virus can cause chickenpox. The skin lesions develop in the distribution of a single sensory nerve root notably the opthalmic division of the trigeminal nerve. In a small number of cases a few lesions become more generalized. The condition can be extremely painful; the pain may precede the rash and then continue for some months after the lesions have disappeared. Occasionally shingles may develop in patients with depressed immunity, this then may require further investigation.

Distressing post-herpetic neuralgia may develop particularly in the elderly.

Skin lesions

Distributed along the area of a unilateral dermatone

Small blisters on a red base develop over a few days (these may be haemorrhagic)

Crusting then develops

The lesions clear within two weeks

Scarring usually occurs.

Options

Idoxuridine paint may help if applied within 48 hours of the appearance of the rash while the virus is still replicating

Acyclovir may be considered an alternative to idoxuridine

'Nobecutane' spray provides a protective layer to prevent secondary infection

Analgesics for pain

Antibiotics for secondary bacterial infection

Hypromellose drugs may improve lubrication when the eye is involved

Referral to ophthalmologist for care of eye complications.

Chickenpox (See p. 404)

Hand, foot and mouth disease (See p. 405)

Pemphigus

Pemphigus is a superficial skin disease in which the epidermal cells separate and form blisters which easily rupture. It affects the skin and mucous membranes. It is more common in the middle-aged and elderly. If untreated it can be fatal.

Skin lesions

Flaccid blisters of varying size but usually 1–2 cm diameter

They easily rupture to leave red exudative patches

Very superficial lesions may simply cause scaling and crusting without blister formation

Healing is slow and new lesions continue to appear

On mucous membranes red erosive lesions develop.

Options

Consider a biopsy to confirm the diagnosis

Long term follow-up should be arranged in consultation with a dermatologist

It may be necessary to administer oral steroids in high doses over long periods

Immunosuppressive drugs (methotrexate, azothiaprine) are occasionally successful

Antiseptic mouth wash and careful oral hygiene for mouth lesions.

Pemphigoid

Despite its name this condition is clinically different from pemphigus. It occurs in the elderly, and although it runs a chronic course the illness is less likely to be fatal. The blisters form lower down in the skin between the dermis and epidermis. The mucous membranes are less commonly affected than in pemphigus.

Skin lesions

Tense blisters of varying size (3 mm to 3 cm)
The fluid may be haemorrhagic
Commonly affects the limbs but may be widespread
There may be separate urticarial and erythematous patches.

Options

Consider a biopsy to confirm the diagnosis
Drain blisters
Topical antibiotics to treat secondary infection
Steroids in high doses
Immunosuppressive drugs are occasionally helpful.

Dermatitis herpetiformis

This is an immunological disorder found in patients with a gluten enteropathy, although the latter may not be overt. The blistering is sub-epidermal. Usually the lesions are grouped in defined areas but occasionally become more generalized. The lesions are intensely irritating. It is a persistent condition which develops in adult life.

Skin lesions

Small blisters (< 1 cm) on a raised red base, distributed over elbows, knees, buttocks, upper back and pressure points
Itching leaves erythematous papules and excoriation occurs.

Options

Advise a gluten-free diet
Folate and iron supplements may be necessary
Dapsone
Sulphapyridine initially 3–4 g daily, reducing to 0.5–1 g maintenance dose
Consider referral to a gastroenterologist for further investigation.

Toxic epidermal necrolysis

In children this condition is usually due to a staphylococcal skin infection. In adults it is a severe form of drug reaction which is often fatal in a matter of days. The drugs most commonly implicated are barbiturates, phenylbutazone and sulphonamides. The patient is febrile and acutely ill.

Skin lesions

Widespread erythema

Vesicles and bullae develop

Large areas of epidermis are shed, and the overall appearance resembles scalded skin.

Referral

Urgent referral to hospital is required on suspicion of this condition.

Other blistering conditions

Blisters occur in many other conditions particularly early in the development of the disease process. Many of these conditions are discussed elsewhere.

- Eczema
- Impetigo
- Insect bites
- Fungal infections
- Erythema multiforme
- Pustular psoriasis

See also:

Bites and stings (p. 26)
Generalized rash (p. 118)
Localized rash (p. 185)
Common infectious diseases in children (p. 402)

Breast lumps

Breast lumps are relatively common but remain an understandable cause for anxiety both to the patient and to the doctor. Breast cancer must be confirmed or excluded in every woman who presents with a breast lump.

One in twenty women are at risk of developing breast cancer at some time in their lives. Approximately 85% of breast cancers are discovered in women presenting with a self-diagnosed breast lump.

Early detection appears to decrease morbidity, but the mortality as yet remains unchanged.

Fibroadenomata

Primary causes

Benign, firm, mobile, painless lumps

Occurs most commonly in the 20–30 year age group.

Fibroadenosis (mammary dysplasia)

Bilateral, tender, lumpy breasts, particularly premenstrually

Due to hormonal defect in breast tissue
Occurs most commonly in the 25–30 year age group
Indicates an increased risk of developing true breast cancer (4 times).

Carcinoma
Usually single, irregular, painless hard lump
May be attached to skin or underlying muscle
Associated supraclavicular or axillary lymphadenopathy
Rare in patients under 30 years of age
Pregnancy and breast feeding before the age of 35 years may be protective
Risk factors associated with carcinomas
- Family history
- Previous breast cancer
- Existing fibroadenosis
- Early menarche (≤16 years)
- Delayed menopause (>55 years)
- Delayed first pregnancy
- Combined contraceptive pill administered at a young age (possible association).

Other causes

Abscess – signs of infection
Mastitis of puberty – benign and hormone induced
Neonatal mastitis – benign and hormone induced
Fat necrosis – usually a history of trauma
Duct ectasia – usually bilateral around the time of menopause
Venous thrombophlebitis

History

Age
General health
Menstrual history
Associated symptoms
- weight loss
- skeletal pain
- skin changes

Contraceptive history
Obstetric history (including breast feeding)
Check for risk factors (see above)

Examination

Inspect both breasts with the patient sitting or standing with arms raised. Look for asymmetry, dimpling of the skin, elevation of the nipples or Paget's disease

Palpate both breasts and check for lymph nodes in the supraclavicular and axillary sites

Defining the lumps
- Size
- Site
- Surface outline
- Pain
- Mobility
- Skin involvement
- Nipple discharge

Clinical assessment

Probably benign
- Bilateral
- Multiple
- Smooth
- Mobile
- Tender
- No palpable lymph nodes

Possibly malignant
- Unilateral
- Single
- Irregular
- Attached to skin or muscle
- Painless
- Palpable supraclavicular or axillary nodes
- Recent change in the nipple

Investigation

- FBC
- ESR
- Alkaline phosphatase (boney secondaries)
- Cytology of fluid from cystic lumps

Options

Urgent referral if malignancy is suspected

Aspiration of a well defined cystic lump

Clinical review after next menstruation, followed by cautious reassurance if the lump is thought to be benign

Mammography for ill-defined lumps

Diuretics for fibroadenosis with premenstrual pain, e.g. bendrofluazide 5 mg daily during the second half of the cycle

Progestrogen for fibroadenosis, e.g. norethisterone 5 mg 8 hourly during the premenstrual week

Analgesia for breast pain, e.g. mefanamic acid 250–500 mg 8 hourly

Instruction and encouragement in self-examination.

Referral All cases of suspected breast cancer.

Screening for breast cancer

Self-examination

With the careful tuition and use of leaflets (e.g. *Breast Self Examination* published by the HEC) the patient can be encouraged to check regularly for breast lumps. Compliance is often poor and self-examination may raise patient anxiety.

Clinical examination

In order to be effective clinical examination should be carried out at regular intervals

Trained practice nurses can be co-opted to help with routine checks to avoid the inefficient use of skilled medical time.

Low-dose mammography

This is the most reliable screening method, but it is not considered to be cost effective. There is a theoretical risk of radiation induced carcinogenesis, thus routine mammography would be best limited to women over 50 years of age and those with major risk factors, e.g. a strong family history.

See also:

Health checks (p. 464)
Health education (p. 466)
Prevention (p. 489)

Bruising and purpura

Many patients complain that they bruise easily, particularly the elderly, but it is rare to discover an underlying bleeding disorder.

Patterns of presentation

Purpura

Purpura consists of numerous small haemorrhages into the skin. The lesions are flat, clearly defined and do not blanch on pressure. They are the result of increased capillary fragility and are usually associated with thrombocytopenia.

It may be seen in the elderly as part of the ageing process (senile purpura). Small lesions (< 2 mm) are sometimes known as petechiae.

Bruising

Bruises are larger areas of bleeding into the skin, usually subcutaneously. They may be associated with purpura in thrombocytopenia but if there is an underlying deficiency of clotting factors there is no purpura. They are also known as ecchymoses.

Bleeding

The usual complaint is of excessive nose bleeding, bleeding from the gums, prolonged bleeding after minor trauma or heavy periods.

Causes

Thrombocytopenia

Marrow infiltration

Leukaemia
Lymphoma
Myeloma
Secondary carcinoma

Marrow depression

Drugs
Irradiation
Renal failure
Severe systemic infection

Increased platelet destruction

Drugs
Hypersplenism

Platelet defects

Polycythaemia rubra vera
Chronic myeloid leukemia
Glanzmann's disease

Clotting defects

Idiopathic

Possibly follows viral infection

Inherited

Haemophilia (factor VIII)
Christmas disease (factor IX)
Von Willebrands (factor VIII deficiency and capillary fragility)

Acquired

Vitamin K deficiency (and vit. C deficiency)
Liver disease
Fibrin consumption coagulopathy
Post prostatectomy (? urokinase release)

History

Duration and severity of symptoms

nosebleeds
blood in urine
blood in stool
bleeding gums
heavy periods

associated trauma
unexplained joint swellings
Constitutional symptoms (fever, anorexia, weight loss)
Past history of bleeding tendency (operations, tooth extractions)
Family history of bleeding tendency
Medication
Dietary history

Examination

Extent of bruising or purpura and distribution
Assess for anaemia
Check
Nose
Gums
Joints
Retinal haemorrhages
Lymphadenopathy
Hepatomegaly
Splenomegaly

Investigation

FBC
ESR
Platelets
Prothrombin time
Kaolin – cephalin time
Hess test
Bleeding time

Options

Reassurance is all that is necessary if no underlying cause is found
Dietary supplements for vitamin and iron deficiency
Review drug therapy.

Referral

For further investigation and management if no obvious underlying cause is discovered
Urgent referral is indicated if the bleeding is excessive or uncontrolled
For management of haemarthrosis. This condition may lead to a fibrous ankylosis.

See also:

Heavy periods (p. 144)
Nose bleed (p. 219)
Chronic renal failure (p. 443)

Catarrh

Catarrh is the commonest presenting complaint of the various nasal disorders. Patients may also present with 'the common cold', 'runny nose', sneezing and snoring.

Nasal obstruction due to physical cause is considered on p. 214. Often more than one cause is present.

Causes for primary consideration

Infection viral – 50% due to Rhinovirus
bacterial – rarely

Allergy ingested – especially in children
inhaled – e.g. hay fever

Climatic, regional and topographical variations
Smoking, environmental irritants and pollutants
Nasal obstruction (see p. 214)
Excessive use of sprays and drops
Pregnancy
Mucosal atrophy
Psychological factors
Medication (some hypotensive agents, decongestant spray abuse)

Other causes

Migraine equivalent – with unilateral red eye and rhinitis
Syphilis – congenital or secondary
Staphylococcus carrier
Diphtheria

History

Allergic trait – inhaled or ingested allergens
Chronic sinusitis
URTI
Feeding difficulty – children
Foreign body
Nose bleed
Medication, e.g. use of hypotensives and nasal sprays
Seasonal onset
Smoking
Occupation and environment
Domestic chemicals or sprays
Psychological or social factors
LMP

Examination

Inspect nose, ears and throat
Check for
- Foreign body
- Septal deviation
- Nasal polypi
- Congestion of nasal mucosa
- Colour of mucosa
  - bluish in allergic rhinitis
  - red in vasomoter rhinitis
- Post-nasal drip
- Mouth breathing

Investigation

FBC and eosinophilia
Throat and nasal swabs
Skin prick testing or nasal provocation tests
X-ray paranasal sinuses

Options

Explanation of the underlying conditions
Self-help
- steam inhalations
- aspirin or paracetamol
- (avoid nasal sprays)

Avoidance
- of any known allergy
- advise on protective masks and cleaning of rooms

Antihistamine
- e.g. Phenergan 10–25 mg 8–12 hourly
- warn patient of sedative effect

Decongestants
- e.g. pseudoephedrine, 'Sudafed'

Antibiotics – only when indicated by fever and mucopurulent discharge.

Complications

Otitis media
Halitosis
Sinusitis
Headache

Referral

Removal of foreign body
Excision of nasal polyps
SMR for deviated nasal septum
Cautery for hypertrophied nasal mucosa
Full allergy testing and specific desensitization regimen.

See also: Migraine (p. 203)
Nasal obstruction (p. 214)
STD (p. 301)

Chest pain

In primary care the majority of patients presenting with chest pain probably have musculoskeletal pain. However, chest pain is the main feature in the presentation of several severe and life-threatening conditions. Patterns of presentation of these conditions are often recognizable but if the diagnosis is in doubt the more sinister causes must be excluded. In western society the significance of chest pain is well appreciated and the symptom is a potent source of anxiety for all concerned.

Patterns of presentation

Angina pectoris (p. 43)
Dissecting aneurysm (p. 45)
Myocardial infarction (p. 46)
Pericarditis (p. 49)
Pulmonary embolism (p. 50)

Oesophageal pain

Intrathoracic pain radiating to the T4–T6 dermatomes
'Burning', 'tight', deep discomfort or aching
Worse when supine
Associated with
- waterbrash
- reflux
- heartburn
- pain on swallowing.

Tracheo-bronchial pain

Upper sternum on both sides radiating to neck on the same side
Burning pain
Worse when coughing.

Diaphragmatic pain

Central diaphragm pain radiates to the shoulder tips
Lateral diaphragm pain radiates to the 5th and 6th ribs, epigastrium, lower abdomen or lumbar area
Pleuritic in character.

Chest wall pain

Localized pain and tenderness
Directly related to use of adjacent musculature

History of recent trauma or over-use or excessive coughing
Pain without use of the muscles may be a symptom of myositis.

Pleuritic pain

Localized pain without radiation
May be severe and is exacerbated by coughing, deep respiration and sudden movement
A pleural rub may be present
May be associated with pleural effusion.

Intercostal nerve pain

Whole dermatone involved
Usually is 'pleuritic' in character
A fractured rib results in a similar pain but is localized to site of periosteal disturbance. In Herpes zoster infection the pain is 'knife-like' or 'sharp' and persistent. This is associated with reduced sensation in the dermatone as well as the characteristic rash.

Aortic pain

Pain in upper aorta radiates to upper chest and shoulders
Pain in lower aorta radiates to the back, chest wall and epigastrium
Patients are very distressed and restless and may have signs of obliteration of peripheral circulation.

Functional pain

Usually situated in the left inframammary area
'Aching' pain at rest and a 'sharp' pain on exertion often in the later part of the day
Hyperventilation and other neurotic traits are often associated
If other members of the family have similar pain there may be an organic as well as a functional association.

History

Assessment of chest pain

- Site and radiation
- Mode of onset
- Character and severity
- Precipitating, exacerbating and relieving factors
- Associated symptoms

Cardiovascular, digestive and respiratory symptoms
Past history of

- angina
- diabetes

respiratory disease
physical or mental stress
Family history of cardiac disease
Smoking habits and medication

Examination

Observe the patient's hands during the description of the pain

Examine

cardiovascular and respiratory function
peripheral pulses
abdomen
fundi

Investigation

The selection of investigations will depend on the differential diagnosis, but consider the following

FBC
ESR
cardiac enzymes
ECG
CXR
barium swallow and meal

Options

Full explanation of clinical assessment
Education on preventive measures relating to diet, weight, exercise, stress and smoking
Advice on posture particularly with reflux oesophagitis
Analgesics for pain
Appropriate therapy for associated conditions.

Referral

Cardiological assessment including exercise ECG, 24 hour monitoring ECG, echocardiogram, cardiac catheterization
Respiratory assessment including CXR, tomograms, lung scans and bronchoscopy
Gastroenterological assessment including endoscopy and reflux studies.

Chest pain – angina pectoris

Angina pectoris is the commonest manifestation of Ischaemic Heart Disease (IHD). It is almost invariably related to exertion and is often present without any accompanying physical signs.

The history and recognition of the characteristic pain is therefore the most relevant part of the assessment of angina pectoris.

The chest pain

The site is usually central and retrosternal but may be referred to either arm or the jaw. Precipitation of the pain is by exertion – this is a cardinal feature in diagnosis.

The character of the pain may be described as
- pressure
- constriction
- tight band
- burning
- indigestion

It is rarely described as 'sharp'

The radiation of the pain is to the shoulders, arms or jaw in the C4–5 distribution. Associated symptoms include shortness of breath, syncope and anxiety

Cold or stress, particularly after food, can also result in pain. This pain will continue until relieved by rest, drugs or the removal of the precipitating factor.

History

Sex
Age
Weight
Diet and exercise
Smoking habits
Previous history of
- myocardial infarction
- diabetes
- hypertension
- hyperlipidaemia
- gout
- hypothyroidism
- anaemia

Family history of ischaemic heart disease

Examination

BP and pulse
Weight
CVS examination

Check for

Added heart sounds or murmurs
Signs of cardiac failure

Investigation

ECG

May appear quite normal at rest
Signs of previous infarction, ST or T-wave abnormalities or arrhythmias

CXR

To exclude alternative diagnosis
Heart size

Exclude

Diabetes
Thyroid disease
Anaemia
Hyperlipidaemia
Syphilis

Options

Minimize risk factors

Obesity (see p. 224)
Cholesterol levels – diet low in animal fats (see p. 472)
Smoking – stop
Hypertension (see p. 475)
Exercise – encourage, but advise to increase levels of exercise gradually.

Drugs

Nitrates
Glyceryl trinitrate sub-lingual 0.5 mg as required or in anticipation of exertion
buccal 1–2 mg 4 hourly (e.g. Suscard)
oral 2.6–6.4 mg 12 hourly (e.g. Sustac)
percutaneous 8 hourly (e.g. Transiderm)
Isosorbide dinitrate
sub-lingual 5–10 mg 2 hourly (e.g. Isordil)
oral 10–40 mg 12 hourly (e.g. Isordil)
Calcium antagonists
e.g. nifedipine oral 10–20 mg 8 hourly (e.g. Adalat)
Vasodilators (especially with associated hypertension)
e.g. prazosin (Hypovase) oral 0.5 mg 8 hourly initially
β-blockers
e.g. atenolol 100 mg daily (Tenormin)
metoprolol 100–200 mg daily (e.g. Betaloc)

Surgery
Coronary artery bypass grafts.

Follow-up

Review
- BP
- Pulse
- ECG (if pain continues)

Check for
- Effects of symptoms on life style and vice versa
- Change in smoking, exercise or dietary habits
- Family and patient's understanding

Differential diagnosis

Paroxysmal tachycardia
Associated LVF
Cardiomyopathy
Valve disease

Complications

Sudden cardiac death
Side effects of medication

Referral

All patients with unstable angina
Unacceptable levels of pain on standard therapy
All patients who are otherwise fit for consideration of coronary artery by-pass
For cardiologist's opinion when the diagnosis of IHD affects employment, e.g. PSV drivers, pilots.

Chest pain – dissecting aneurysm

This major medical and surgical emergency is seen only rarely by individual doctors in primary care. It is, however, important to recognize its pattern of acute presentation which may mimic acute myocardial infarction.

History

The pain is situated in the shoulder, interscapular area, chest wall or epigastrium depending on the level of dissection. The 'tearing' pain may be very severe and is usually of sudden onset, but symptoms may occasionally develop over several days. Cold extremities, shortness of breath, syncope and restless distress are often related in this condition.

Medical history
- hypertension
- coarctation
- atherosclerosis
- Marfan's syndrome

Examination

- BP
- Peripheral pulses
- Cardiac function

Check for
- Hemiplegia
- Cardiac failure
- Aortic diastolic murmurs

Emergency care

Refer all cases for hospital care

Chest pain – myocardial infarction

In western society cardiovascular disease is the commonest cause of death. Atherosclerosis is most commonly the underlying pathology. About one-third of patients die in the first few months of the episode; the majority of these within the first two hours.

The chest pain

The chest pain is usually of sudden onset, central in site but may radiate to one or both arms, the neck, jaw and/or back. The pain may be described as 'deep', 'gripping' or 'crushing', and is persistent and frightening. There may be associated nausea and vomiting, shortness of breath, anxiety and fear. The episode can be precipitated by physical exertion or psychological stress, but can also occur at rest. This type of chest pain cannot be relieved by rest or by coronary vasodilators (e.g. GTN).

Pain

Onset and precipitating factors site and radiation character and severity

History

Associated symptoms
- Shortness of breath
- Palpitations
- Sweating

Previous history of
- Angina
- Infarction
- Peripheral vascular disease
- Diabetes mellitus
- Stroke
- Hyperlipidaemia
- Hypertension
- Hypothyroidism

Family history of
- Cardiovascular disease
- Diabetes
- Hypertension

Medication
- Contraceptive pill

Social history
- Smoking habits
- Occupation

Examination

Pulse – rate and rhythm
BP
Signs of cardiac failure
Cyanosis or shock
Heart sounds – character and added sounds

Investigation

Cardiac enzymes
ECG to monitor resolution or extension of infarct
ECG changes (ST elevation) may take some time to develop and their absence in the early stages should not rule out the diagnosis

Management

Table 1.2. Home versus hospital management

Home	Hospital
Age >65 yrs	Age <65 yrs
Adequate pain relief	Cardiac arrest
No arrhythmia	Hypotension
No cardiogenic shock	Arrhythmia
Duration more than 8 hours	Collapse out of doors
Adequate family support	Poor family support
Unreasonable distance from hospital	Shock
Terminally ill with another clinical condition	Away from home

Options for home care

Pain relief
Oxygen therapy in the initial stages
Sedation if required
Treat associated cardiac failure (see p. 469)
Discontinue cardiac drugs during acute phase (e.g. digoxin, β-blockers)
Arrange nursing care.

Follow-up

Review daily initially
Assess level of pain
Check for signs of cardiac failure or dysrhythmia
Review medication
Advise on future life-style
- diet
- exercise
- weight loss
- sex
- smoking
- driving

β-blockade for at least a year after infarction may give protection against further infarction and sudden death

Mobilization

In uncomplicated cases bed rest for 48 hours followed by gradual mobilization over two weeks
Aim to achieve full mobilization within three months.

Complications

Continuing pain
Pericarditis
Dressler's syndrome – pericardial pain and friction rub with fever and leucocytosis
Dysrhythmia
Shock
Mitral or tricuspid valve damage due to ruptured papillary muscle
Cardiac failure – immediate or during mobilization
Ventricular aneurysm

Chest pain – pericarditis

Pericarditis may be mild and a complication of a more generalized disease, or it may be severe and disabling.

Pericardial effusion and constrictive pericarditis lie in the province of cardiology and are thus discussed only briefly.

The chest pain

The site is sub-sternal or para-sternal and sometimes occurs in the epigastrium
Radiation is to the left shoulder tip but not the left arm.
The pain is frightening, sharp and paroxysmal
Exacerbation is by inspiration and movement, or when supine. It is relieved by sitting forwards
Associated symptoms include dysphagia and other symptoms from adjacent organs.

Causes

Non-specific pericarditis
Post myocardial infarction
Infections – bacterial, viral or tuberculosis
Rheumatic fever
SLE
PAN
Giant cell arteritis
Uraemia
Hypothyroidism
Malignancy
Trauma
Medication – hydrallazine, anticoagulants
Radiotherapy

History

Check for history of, or symptoms suggestive of, any of the above causes of pericarditis

Examination

Record
- Temperature
- Pulsc
- BP
- Heart sounds

Check for
- Pericardial rub
- Atrial fibrillation
- Pulsus paradoxus
- Raised JVP
- Pericardial effusion
- Pleural effusion
- Pneumothorax

Investigation

ECG

Elevated ST segments concave upwards, maximal in lead II

CXR

To demonstrate large pericardial effusion or associated pulmonary malignancy or infection

Consider

- FBC
- ESR
- U & E
- Cardiac enzymes
- Thyroid function tests
- ANF

Referral

All cases for cardiological assessment.

Patterns of presentation

Pericardial effusion

Risk of cardiac tamponade

Symptoms as above, plus rapid development of shortness of breath and feeling faint except when supine

JVP raised, pericardial rub persists

Pulsus paradoxus, low voltage ECG.

Constrictive pericarditis

Insidious onset

Shortness of breath and weight loss

Ascites with ankle oedema

JVP raised, atrial fibrillation or pulsus paradoxus

Enlarged liver and spleen.

Chest pain – pulmonary embolism

Massive pulmonary embolism is a major medical emergency involving collapse, acute shortness of breath and cyanosis.

Smaller emboli may present with signs of pulmonary infarction and these can herald a more major event. The condition demands further investigation and treatment.

Recurrent emboli may result in pulmonary hypertension.

The chest pain

Sudden onset

Central constricting pain

With pulmonary infarction the pain is pleuritic in nature

History

Associated symptoms

Shortness of breath
Haemoptysis
Syncope
DVT

Predisposing factors

Immobility
Operations
Injury
Childbirth
Past history of DVT
Family history of DVT or pulmonary embolism
Medication – oestrogen preparations

Examination

Record

Colour
Pulse
Temperature
BP

Respiratory function

- respiratory rate increased
- PEF
- pink frothy sputum
- cyanosis
- pleural rub
- diminished breath sounds

Cardiac function

- oedema
- raised JVP
- ECG signs of RV strain
- palpable liver
- BP and pulse
- S wave in lead I and Q wave with inverted T wave in lead III ('$S_I Q_{III} T_{III}$ pattern')
- pulmonary murmurs, widely split second heart sound or gallop rhythm

Signs of DVT

Risk factors

Pill or pregnancy
Recent stress, surgery or injury
Immobility
Previous thrombosis

Emergency care

Lay the patient flat to assist respiration after massive embolism
Cardiopulmonary resuscitation
Oxygen therapy
Diamorphine 5 mg i.v. may relieve dyspnoea
Monitor pulse, BP and respiration
Arrange immediate transfer to hospital

Follow-up

Prophylactic elastic hosiery and exercises to prevent future thrombosis by minimizing stasis in leg veins.
Review existing medication – (stop administration of any oestrogen preparations)
Supervise anticoagulant therapy

Confusion and dementia

Confusion is a reversible state of impaired intellectual function that can occur at any age and for which a cause must always be sought.

Dementia is the irreversible and progressive state of impaired intellectual function that occurs in 1 in 10 people over the age of 65 years, and 1 in 5 over 80 years. Dementia develops insidiously with
- forgetfulness
- disorientation
- lability of mood
- loss of concentration
- sleep disturbance

The underlying pathology of dementia is not yet fully understood. Sympathetic support, by the family and the various agencies of primary care, is the most important aspect of management.

Causes of dementia

Multiple infarct
Post-traumatic
Tumours
Degenerative diseases, e.g.
- Alzheimer's syndrome
- Multiple sclerosis
- Alcohol-induced

Causes of confusion

Cranial

Cerebral ischaemia (TIA, stroke)
Hypoxia
Epilepsy
Head injury
Raised intracranial pressure (SDH, communicating hydrocephalus)
Tumour (primary or secondary)
Infection (meningitis, encephalitis, syphilis)
Cranial arteritis

Systemic

Infection (URTI, chest infection)
Anaemia (Folate and B_{12} deficiency)
Cardiac causes (arrhythmia, hypotension)
Hypothermia
Fever
Thyroid disorders
Hypoglycaemia
Electrolyte imbalance: (calcium, sodium, dehydration)
Kidney failure
Liver failure
Adrenal failure
Peripheral neurological disorders
Chronic pain
Constipation

Mental

Personality disorder
Change of environment
Bereavement
Sleep deprivation
Schizophrenia
Depression
Hypomania
Alcohol (intoxication or withdrawal)
Medication (e.g. hypnotics, sedatives, antidepressants, hypoglycaemia, antihistamines, digoxin, L-dopa, steroids)

History

From the patient, relative or friend
recent medical history
psychological psychotic symptoms
recent head injury
drugs
alcohol

sleeping, eating and bowel habits
bereavement or other 'life events'
previous personality, occupation and leisure
effect of dementia on the family and domestic affairs
patient and family health beliefs

Examination

General medical examination
- Vision
- Hearing
- BP
- Temperature
- Specific signs of systemic disease

Central nervous examination
- Focal signs
- Pupils
- Pyramidal signs

Mental assessment
- Emotional lability
- Orientation (time and place)
- Memory (long and short term)
- Concentration and attention span
- Current affairs
- Simple commands
- Arithmetic
- Abstract thought

Investigation

FBC
ESR
U & E, LFT, creatinine, calcium, glucose
B_{12} and folate
Thyroid function tests
MSU
CXR
ECG

Options

Inform and advise the family on
The changing expectations of the patient as the symptoms progress
The need for vigilance
The need to maintain involvement in activities and conversation ('reality reorientation')
The need to ensure a safe living area (floors, lighting, loud radio, etc.)
Night sedation – e.g. chlormethiazole 500 mg at night
Tranquillizers – e.g. thioridazine 100–200 mg daily or haloperidol 0.5–10 mg daily

Antidepressants – e.g. amitriptylline 10–25 mg 8 hourly
Anti-platelet drugs – e.g. aspirin 300 mg daily or dipyridamole 100 mg 8–12 hourly
Naftidrofuryl (Praxilene) in multi-infarct dementia
Anticoagulants in valvular heart disease
Vasodilation is of dubious benefit
Sheltered accommodation
Home help
Home care assistants
Meals on wheels.

Follow-up

Regular visits by Doctor, Health Visitor or District Nurse to relieve families of the sense of isolation
Regular standard questionnaire to assess change in mental function

Referral

Neurologist – to exclude intracranial lesion
Psychiatrist – for assessment and/or detoxification
Psychologist – for IQ assessment
Community psychiatric nurse
Social workers
Alcoholics Anonymous
Age Concern.

See also:

Constipation (p. 55)
Depression (p. 63)
Fever (p. 106)
Fits (p. 110)
Pallor/anaemia (p. 231)
Personality disorders (p. 242)
Problem drinking (p. 261)
Care of the elderly (p. 435)
Chronic renal failure (p. 443)
Multiple sclerosis (p. 483)
Stroke (p. 497)
Bereavement (p. 505)
Head injury (p. 523)
Hypoglycaemia (p. 525)
Hypothermia (p. 526)
Mental Health Act 1983 (p. 527)

Constipation

The definition of constipation is not precise. Epidemiological studies have shown that 99% of people open their bowels between three times every day and once every three days. Thus, constipation could be implied when defaecation takes place *less* than once every three days.

In practice constipation is taken as the infrequent passage of hard stools with difficult and straining defaecation.

The lay public often attribute other symptoms to constipation such as lassitude, depression, headache and 'bad breath'. They subsequently indulge, often inappropriately, in self-medication with laxatives.

The symptom presented may be part of a more complex problem and it is necessary to ascertain the real reason which prompts the consultation.

Causes

Inadequate bulk in the diet
Poor bowel habit
Immobility
Recent illness
Under-hydration
Pregnancy
Painful anal conditions
Irritable bowel syndrome
Diverticular disease
Colonic cancers
Neurological disease of the bowel
Depression and dementia
Hypothyroidism
Hypercalcaemia
Hypokalaemia
Medication
- anticholinergic drugs, e.g. tricyclic antidepressants
- some antacids
- opiates
- hypotensive agents
- diuretics

History

Usual bowel habit
Dietary history
Duration of symptoms
Weight loss
Frequency and consistency of stools
Rectal bleeding
Associated abdominal or anal pain
Symptoms of depression or hypothyroidism
Recent drug history

Examination

Weight
Abdominal distension, masses or tenderness

Rectal examination
Check for anal fissures and proctitis
Thyroid status
Mental state

Investigation

This is rarely required, but consider
- FBC
- ESR
- U & E
- Plasma calcium and phosphates
- Thyroid function tests
- Faecal occult blood
- Barium enema
- Sigmoidoscopy

Options

Diet
In bottle-fed infants the traditional remedy of extra sugar in the feed may help in the short term
Adequate fluid intake in hot weather is essential
Bulk forming agents and a fibre-rich diet help to reduce transit time
Drugs
Review and, if possible, withdraw exacerbating drugs
Faecal softener (e.g. liquid paraffin, dioctyl-sodium)
Stimulant (senna, bisacodyl)
Osmotic agents (lactulose)
Enemas
These may be necessary before barium studies, and for faecal impaction possibly combined with manual removal
Soothing creams
May ease the discomfort of an anal fissure
Treat appropriately
Depression (see p. 63)
Hypothyroidism (see p. 481)
Electrolyte disturbance.

Complications

Abdominal pain
'Overflow' incontinence (spurious diarrhoea)
Megacolon
Stercoral ulceration

Referral

Surgical assessment if neoplasm is suspected
Investigation and treatment of neurological disease and electrolyte disturbance.

See also:

Abdominal pain (p. 1)
Abdominal swellings (p. 4)
Anal bleeding (p. 8)
Anal irritation (p. 10)
Confusion and dementia (p. 52)
Depression (p. 63)
Headache (p. 133)
Piles (p. 249)
Symptoms in pregnancy (p. 352)
Hypothyroidism (p. 481)

Cough

Cough is one of the commonest symptoms presenting in primary care; it may be present in as many as one in eight consultations. It may be a voluntary or reflex response to irritation of the respiratory mucosa of the bronchi, trachea, larynx, pharynx and even the middle ear. The majority of causes are minor and self-limiting but a rational diagnostic approach is necessary in order not to miss the treatable and more serious causes.

Patterns of presentation

Sputum

A dry cough indicates congestion of the respiratory mucosa as in the early stages of infection, or after the inhalation of irritant dust or fumes.

A loose cough with clear sputum indicates free exudate in the respiratory passages.

A loose cough with purulent sputum (yellow or green) is usually indicative of infection, eosinophils. In allergic cases eosinophils may also colour the sputum.

Duration of symptoms

A transient cough is usually benign.

A chronic relapsing cough usually indicates a more serious underlying cause as in bronchitis, bronchiectasis, asthma, whooping cough, TB or cancer.

Nature of cough

A short sharp cough is usually present in upper respiratory infections or 'habit variety' or in the presence of painful pleurisy.

Paroxysmal coughing is more characteristic of chronic bronchitis or whooping cough.

Abrupt onset paroxysmal coughing may be due to an

inhaled foreign body especially in children. A severe paroxysm may be followed by vomiting or syncope.

A prolonged 'bovine' cough may indicate paralysis of the vocal cords as in tumours involving the recurrent laryngeal nerve.

Timing of cough

Morning cough on rising is often indicative of chronic bronchitis or bronchiectasis.

Nocturnal cough is common in bronchitis or with a 'post-nasal drip' of mucus, but cardiac causes and asthma should be considered.

Associated features

Fever and rhinitis would indicate an infective cause

Weight loss and haemoptysis may be noted with lung tumours or tuberculosis.

Environment

Smoking and occupational lung diseases

A change in temperature may precipitate coughing in bronchitics or asthmatics.

Examination

Inspect

- Cyanosis and finger clubbing
- Nares – blockage and discharge
- Pharynx – inflammation and post-nasal drip
- Trachea – check position
- Chest wall – deformity, intercostal recession with respiratory movements

Auscultate for localizing signs

Investigation

FBC eosinophil count
ESR
PEF (repeated after inhalation of bronchodilator)
Chest X-ray
Mantoux test
Sputum examination (apart from visual assessment) is rarely helpful in practice

Options

Reassurance is often all that is required

Advice against smoking and on taking adequate fluids. Suggest simple remedies such as steam inhalation, and improved sleeping posture. Warm, soothing drinks may give some symptomatic relief

Expectorants rarely help except with placebo effect or sedation by the antihistamine content

Cough suppressants such as codeine linctus may help the dry persistent cough associated with bronchial tumours

Antibiotics when appropriate for infections

Bronchodilators such as salbutamol for associated asthma (see p. 15)
Physiotherapy.

Failure to control
Inappropriate antibiotic
Obstructed bronchus (neoplasm or foreign body)
Tuberculosis
Pleural effusion
Lung abcess
Continued smoking

Referral
Suspected malignancy or tuberculosis
For reassurance of anxious patient or parent
Failure to control symptoms.

See also:
Asthma and wheezing (p. 15)
Haemoptysis (p. 129)
Influenza (p. 167)
Common infectious diseases in children (p. 402)
Chronic bronchitis (p. 440)
Pulmonary tuberculosis (p. 492)

Cyanosis

Cyanosis is the dusky blue coloration of the skin and mucosae seen in the presence of an excess of circulating reduced haemoglobin.

Peripheral cyanosis alone may simply be due to poor circulation in hands, feet and lips (see p. 254). Central cyanosis of the tongue and buccal mucosa always demands careful assessment.

Causes

Respiratory
- COAD
- Chronic bronchitis and emphysema
- Fibrosing alveolitis
- Pneumonia
- Severe asthma
- Pulmonary embolism

Cardiovascular
- Some cases of congenital heart disease
- Dehydration
- Cold exposure
- 'Pump failure' (usually peripheral cyanosis)
- Raynaud's phenomenon
- Mucus obstruction
- Peripheral circulatory disease

Haematological
Polycythaemia
Methaemalbuminaemia (very rare)
Haemoglobinopathy (very rare)

History

Mode of onset – acute or insidious
Associated symptoms
Cough
Sputum
Haemoptysis
Shortness of breath
Chest pains
Palpitations
Ankle swelling
Relationship to exercise in congenital heart disease
Past history of heart or lung disease
Medication

Examination

Check hands, lips and tongue for skin colour (and clubbing)
Full assessment of cardiovascular and respiratory systems

Investigation

FBC
Sputum culture (if appropriate)
Chest X-ray
ECG

Options

Oxygen therapy
May be life saving in acute onset central cyanosis while arranging urgent hospital admission
It may also improve the quality of life when given in the domiciliary situation for a housebound 'respiratory invalid'
Physiotherapy
Antibiotics – for chest infection; choice depends on sputum culture, if available
Bronchodilators – for asthma (see p. 15)
Digoxin and diuretics or alternatives in cardiac failure
Venesection – in polycythaemia.

Referral

Acute onset central cyanosis
Congenital heart disease for assessment
Respiratory assessment.

See also:

Asthma and wheezing (p. 15)
Chest pain – pulmonary embolism (p. 50)
Poor circulation (p. 254)
Chronic bronchitis (p. 440)

Deep vein thrombosis

The painful purple swollen calf due to deep vein thrombosis (DVT) is not a commonly presenting sign in general practice, but because of its association with pulmonary embolism it is an important condition to exclude.

As many as 50% of patients with serious DVT have no clinical signs or symptoms.

Risk factors

Age
Immobility
Oral contraception
Pregnancy
Trauma
Heart failure
Obesity
Major surgery
Cancer

History

Onset and nature of pain or swelling
Associated symptoms
- breathlessness
- chest pain
- haemoptysis
- syncope

Past history of thrombophlebitis
Contraceptive pill
Recent pregnancy
Major surgery
Assess previous mobility

Examination

Measure calf sizes
Check for
- discoloration
- calf muscle tenderness
- venous distention

Rectal/vaginal examination if indicated from the history
Temperature (may be marginally raised in larger VTs)
Auscultation of the chest for signs of pulmonary infarction

Investigation

Hospital based venography and ultrasound studies

Management

Once the diagnosis is suspected the patient should be urgently referred to hospital for investigation and initial treatment if the diagnosis is confirmed. After discharge the control of anticoagulation is often the responsibility of the family doctor

Follow-up

Oral anticoagulant control: warfarin or phenindione

The dose should be adjusted to maintain a blood prothrombin time at about twice normal. The particular test varies between laboratories

The frequency of blood tests may be twice weekly initially, reducing to monthly when stable

Check for any bruising or epistaxis and test for haematuria

Duration of treatment may vary between 6 weeks and 6 months (sometimes longer)

It is probably wiser to 'taper off' dosage at the end of therapy rather than to attempt abrupt withdrawal

Drugs interacting with oral anticoagulants

(All current drug therapy must be carefully reviewed)

- aspirin and related drugs
- antibiotics – particularly tetracycline and sulphonamides
- alcohol
- barbiturates and phenothiazines
- hypoglycaemic drug – tolbutamide

Documentation

Anticoagulant advice cards for patients

Possibly recommend an emergency alert bracelet/medallion for patients on long term treatment

See also:

Chest pain – pulmonary embolism (p. 50)
Ulcers (p. 317)

Depression

Most people will suffer from some sort of depression at some time in their lives. It is a normal companion to grief, disappointment, and many illnesses. As such it is a transient and subjective experience which only becomes abnormal when there are persistent and objective changes in vitality, mood or function.

Depression is presented in primary care more frequently by women than by men (ratio of 2:1); this may reflect its common occurrence during the premenstrual phase of the female reproductive cycle.

It is more common in patients
of low socio-economic grouping
living in the city
without a confidante
with loss of parent at an early age
with sibling rivalry
who are unemployed

Patterns of presentation differ according to the personality and experience of the sufferer. Certain recognized characteristics of depression may help in assessment – for example, of the cyclothymic (i.e. manic-depressive), the psychotic (i.e. unrealistic), the retarded or the agitated depressive.

The conventional distinction between reactive and endogenous depression in which symptoms are understandable or inexplicable respectively, has only limited value in the primary assessment and management. The **relative severity** of the depression is the most important aspect to assess.

Patterns of presentation

Retardation

Inefficiency at job or housework
Lack of interest
Lack of energy
Inflexible demeanour
Heavy gait
Dull monotonous speech
No sense of time
Retarded body functions (see below)

Agitation

Restless
Fidgety
Garrulous
Repetitive
Agitated body function (see below)

Mood

Suicidal (see p. 307)
Sad
Guilty
Low self-esteem
Paranoid
Compulsive phenomena
Depersonalized
Irrationally pessimistic
Anxious
Irritable

Attacks of panic
Diurnal variations in mood

Body functions

No appetite
Weight loss
Loss of libido
Sleep disturbance
Poor concentration
Pain in face, chest or abdomen

Retarded functions

Constipation
Indigestion
Dry mouth
Amenorrhoea
Palpitations
Tremor
Sweating
Urgency of micturition
Tight chest

Differential diagnosis

Anaemia
Diabetes
Dementia
Cancer with secondaries
Hypothyroidism
Hypoparathyroidism (very rare)
Porphyria (very rare)
Food allergy

Assessment

Attitude towards
- Enjoyment
- Interests
- Attitude to the future
- Decision making
- Moodiness
- Level of energy
- Sleep
- Appetite
- Sex
- Pain
- Weight loss
- Retardation
- Severity – subjective
  objective (e.g. Hamilton rating scale)
- Suicide risk (see p. 307)

Onset and duration of symptoms
Psychiatric history

Previous personality
Medication
Menstrual history
Family history
Social or psychological factors
Exclude the differential diagnosis
Discussion with friend or relative

Prevention

Restricted prescribing habits
Recognition
Availability
Sympathetic response to presenting problems
Counselling through life-events
Lithium carbonate (in consultation with a psychiatrist)

Options

Full physical examination and investigation for reassurance

Counselling or psychotherapy after exclusion of
- No interest
- No concentration
- Inflexible demeanour
- Diurnal variation of mood
- Retardation
- No appetite
- Weight loss
- Guilt

Tricyclic (or bicyclic or tetracyclic) **antidepressants**
- *Sedative*, e.g. amitriptyline initially 75–150 mg at night or divided dose
- *Neutral*, e.g. imipramine initially 75 mg at night or divided dose
- *Stimulant*, e.g. protriptyline initially 5–10 mg 6 hourly during the day
- Continue therapy 3–6 months longer
- Withdraw therapy cautiously
- Use the safer tetracyclines, e.g. mianserin if there is a potential risk of suicide
- The clinical response to amitriptyline and imipramine has not yet been superseded by more recent introductions

MAOI (Mono-amine-oxidase inhibitors) are used rarely as an alternative to tricyclics, e.g. phenelzine 15 mg 6–8 hourly. Avoid all foods containing tyramine and sympathomimetics

If possible give the patient a list of those substances
Delay therapy for 14 days after the withdrawal of tricyclics.

Referral

Continuing suicidal risk
Psychiatric assessment of ECT and lithium
Psychotic behaviour
Medical management when appropriate
Failure to control
Further support and counselling with alternative agency.

Follow-up

Planned consultations – on a frequent basis until mood improves
Review medication – compliance
– side effects
Assess severity of depression – subjective
– objective (e.g. rating scales)

The elderly depressive

Prevalence rises over 50 years of age
Recurrent depression becomes more common
Suicide rates rise with age
Physical symptoms become the commonest form of presentation
Drug dosage must be modified
Drug interaction is more likely
Social support must be rallied

Failure to control

Review
Drug side-effects
Patient compliance
Drug dosage

Exclude
Differential diagnosis
Other psychiatric disorders
Pre-menstrual syndrome
Menopause
Suppressed emotion, e.g. grief
Change in life style as cause or effect of depression

Consider stopping
Steroids
Contraceptive pill
Sedatives
Alcohol
Narcotic drugs

See also: Food allergy (p. 113)
Menopause (p. 199)
Pre-menstrual syndrome (p. 257)
Suicide (p. 307)
Post-natal depression (p. 383)
Care of the elderly (p. 435)

Diarrhoea

This is a commonly presented complaint in primary care. It is particularly important to establish the nature of the complaint as what is accepted as normal by one patient may be abnormal to another. The condition usually implies a change in bowel habit with increased frequency of stools which may be soft or watery.

The vast majority of cases are a result of self-limiting gastrointestinal infection or dietary indiscretion. Much less commonly bacterial infections may be the cause.

In children under 5 years up to 50% have rotaviruses isolated in the stools.

If the symptom persists for more than two weeks it is unlikely to be due to a simple infection.

Causes

Acute

Infections

Viral
Rotavirus
Echovirus
Coxsackie virus

Bacterial
Shigella
Salmonella
Clostridium
Cholera
Yersinia enterocolitica
Staphylococcus enterotoxin
Campylobacter

Protozoan
Giardia lamblia
Entamoeba histolytica

Dietary indiscretion

Medication
Antibiotics
Laxative abuse

General infections in children

Appendicitis
'Imported diarrhoea' after travel abroad

Chronic or recurrent

Gastrointestinal
- Irritable bowel syndrome
- Ulcerative colitis
- Crohn's disease
- Constipation with overflow incontinence
- Diverticulitis
- Tumours of the large bowel
- Post-gastrectomy
- Malabsorption syndrome
- Ischaemic colitis

General
- Psychogenic
- Chronic pancreatitis
- Diabetes
- Thyrotoxicosis
- Addison's disease
- Food allergy

Medication
- Aspirin
- Indomethacin
- Magnesium salts
- Digoxin
- β-blockers
- Antibiotics

History

Nature of stools
- colour
- consistency
- presence of blood or mucus

Frequency of stools
Alternating bowel habit
Infective contact
Travel abroad
Weight loss
Abdominal pain
Recent appetite and diet
Occupation (e.g. food handler)
Recent history of medication
Past history of gastrointestinal operations

Examination

Temperature
Hydration
Tongue

Jaundice
Abdominal examination – tenderness and masses
Rectal examination – digital and proctoscopy

Investigation

Unnecessary for minor, self-limiting conditions. If the symptoms persist for more than five days consider
- FBC
- ESR
- U & E
- LFT
- Serum iron and TIBC
- Serum B_{12} and folate
- Thyroid function tests
- Serum proteins
- Plasma calcium
- Amylase
- MSU
- Stool examination and culture
- Faecal fats and occult blood
- Barium enema
- Sigmoidoscopy

Options

Diet

Fluids and starving settles most acute cases in 48 hours
Bulk-forming agents or fibre-rich diets may be helpful in irritable bowel syndrome, inflammatory bowel disease or diverticulosis
Exclusion diets for food allergy (see p. 113)
Gluten-free diet in coeliac disease
Iron, folate and vitamin D supplements should be given when indicated.

Drugs

Symptomatic treatment with
- kaolin and morphine mixture 10 ml 4 hourly
- codeine phosphate 30 mg 4 hourly
- diphenoxylate HCl } may be suitable alternatives
- loperamide HCl }

Antispasmodics may relieve cramping pain
- mebeverine 135 mg 8 hourly
- dicyclomine 10–20 mg 8 hourly
- hyoscine 20 mg 6 hourly

Salazopyrine 1 gm 12 hourly. Steroid tablets or enemas may be helpful in inflammatory bowel disease
Metronidazole 400 mg 12 hourly for ten days is indicated in *Giardia lamblia* infections
Antibiotics are rarely helpful and may in fact be harmful in

cases of salmonella infections (by promoting a carrier state). However, erythromycin is indicated in campylobacter infections

Reconsider any existing drug therapy.

Recommend additional contraceptive measures in female patients using oral contraception.

Referral

To a surgical unit for assessment in cases of appendicitis, suspected bowel cancer or longstanding ulcerative colitis

To an infectious diseases unit in more severe cases of infective diarrhoea

To a gastroenterologist for investigation of persistent diarrhoea.

See also:

Abdominal pain (p. 1)
Constipation (p. 55)
Food allergy (p. 113)
Imported disease (p. 157)
Malnutrition and malabsorption (p. 195)
Diabetes (p. 457)

Difficulty in swallowing

Many factors cause difficulties in swallowing. However, if a patient complains of recent and persistent difficulties with solid food carcinoma of the pharynx or oesophagus must be excluded. Carcinoma of the pharynx is commoner in women, carcinoma of the oesophagus is commoner in men. Young women are not exempt from carcinoma of the pharynx whereas men usually only suffer from oesophageal carcinomas when over the age of fifty.

Epiglotitis in children may lead to respiratory distress and even death and requires urgent referral.

The symptom of a 'lump in the throat' makes the swallowing of saliva uncomfortable, but solid food is usually taken without difficulty.

Causes

Malignant and benign tumours

Pharynx
Post cricoid
Oesophageal
Brachial
Gastric

Premalignant condition
- Plummer–Vinson syndrome or Paterson–Kelly syndrome

Inflammatory conditions
- Tonsillitis
- Pharyngitis
- Dental sepsis
- Smoking
- Sclerodema
- Sjögren's syndrome
- Chagas' disease

Structural causes
- Foreign body
- Oesophageal pouch
- Oesophageal compression by thyroid or thymus
- Tracheo-oesophageal fistula (neonatal)
- Oesophageal stricture
- Aberrant subclavian artery
- Pericardial effusion
- Achalasia
- Post-radiotherapy stricture

Psychological
- A 'lump in the throat' (globus hystericus)
- Oesophageal spasm

Paralysis
- Pseudobulbar palsy
- Motor neurone disease
- Myasthenia gravis
- Bulbar polio
- Diphtheria neuritis

History

Onset, duration and nature of swallowing (solids and liquids)

Associated symptoms
- Altered appetite
- Earache
- Reflux
- Fever
- Weight loss
- Hoarseness
- Substernal pain

Thyroid status

Smoking habits

Social and psychological factors

Examination

Inspect
  Throat and teeth
  Lymph glands
  Signs of anaemia
Record weight
Chest and abdominal examination
Signs of scleroderma (in hands, eyes and mouth)

Investigation

FBC
ESR
Serum iron and TIBC
Thyroid function tests
Throat swab
Faecal occult blood
Barium swallow and meal

Options

Advice on diet
  mouth breathing
Stop smoking
Treat nasal polypi – e.g. Beconase inhaler
Antibiotics – e.g. penicillin V 250 mg 6 hourly
Iton supplements – e.g. ferrous gluconate 300 mg 12 hourly.

Referral

Two weeks persistent symptoms, to exclude carcinoma
Total obstruction, with dehydration
Impacted foreign body
Suspected Plummer–Vinson syndrome
Suspected achalasia.

See also:

Ptosis (p. 270)

Dizziness

Dizziness, or giddiness, has no universal definition but it is understood to relate to an imbalanced sense of movement of oneself and the surroundings due to a loss of equilibrium.

The term 'vertigo' has a similar usage but actually describes the specific sensation of rotation within oneself or the surroundings.

A reasonably reliable diagnosis can often be made from constructing a detailed history, but referral may be indicated for more detailed investigation.

Causes

Physiological
- Roundabouts, etc.

Labyrinth and VIIIth nerve
- Benign postural vertigo
- Labyrinthitis
- Vestibular neuronitis
- Menière's disease
- Acoustic neuroma
- Ototoxic drugs

Brainstem and cerebrum
- Multiple sclerosis
- Tumours (primary and secondary)
- Hydrocephalus
- Cerebral ischaemia
- TIA
- Stroke
- Migraine

Cardiovascular
- Fluid loss
- Low-output states
- Dysrhythmia
- Transient vertebrobasilar ischaemia (cervical spondylosis)

Psychosomatic

History

Accurate description of dizziness including
- onset
- duration
- frequency
- precipitating factors

Associated ENT symptoms
- otalgia
- hearing loss
- ear discharge
- tinnitus

Associated neurological symptoms
- headache
- visual disturbance
- loss of consciousness
- speech disturbance
- fits
- ataxia

Associated cardiovascular symptoms
- palpitations
- breathlessness
- angina

Family history
Drugs/alcohol
Social and psychological factors
Health beliefs

Examination

Inspection of ears, throat and neck
Tuning fork tests for hearing
Cardiovascular examination
Neurological examination
- cranial nerves (especially V, VII and VIII)
- fundi
- brainstem/cerebellar signs – ataxia, dysarthria, diplopia

Investigation

FBC
ESR
U & E
Blood glucose
Syphilis serology
X-ray
- internal auditory meatus
- cervical spine
- chest

ECG

Options

Discuss the condition and likely prognosis
Consider life style, stress and potentially dangerous situations
Cervical collar
Medication
- antihistamines e.g. promethazine 25 mg 8 hourly
- phenothiazine e.g. prochlorperazine 5 mg 8 hourly
- betahistine 8–16 mg 8 hourly.

Referral

Persistent or progressive symptoms and signs
Failure of simple therapy
Suspected diagnosis of
- acoustic neuroma
- suppurative labyrinthitis
- cholesteatoma.

See also:

Menopause (p. 199)
Migraine (p. 203)
Multiple sclerosis (p. 483)

Tinnitus (p. 314)
Stroke (p. 497)

Dysuria and frequency

These are extremely common symptoms. Studies have shown that up to 50% of women have suffered these symptoms at some time in their lives. Only about half of the patients presenting have associated bacteruria although clinically the two groups are indistinguishable.

History

Severity and duration of symptoms (including coincidence with sexual activity)

Associated symptoms

- Abdominal pain
- Loin pain
- Fever
- Vaginal discharge/or irritation
- Urethral discharge
- Uterovesical prolapse
- Haematuria

Past history

- UTI
- Renal disease
- STD
- Food allergy

Examination

(Not usually helpful but consider)
In women: urethra and vaginal examination
In men: foreskin, urethra and prostate examination
Palpate for renal enlargement or tenderness

Investigation

MSU
Vaginal, cervical and urethral swabs
IVP indicated in the following

- Females
  - under 5 years of age
  - recurrent bacteruria
  - persistent haematuria and pyuria
- Males
  - all male patients

Options

Advice

- High fluid intake (>3 litres/day)
- Regular and complete emptying of bladder particularly

after intercourse if the symptoms are related
Careful perineal toilet.

Antibiotics

Await bacteriological examination of the urine if possible, but consider a broad spectrum antibiotic earlier if the symptoms are severe
Single dose or 2–3 day courses of antibiotics are usually successful in the uncomplicated case
In recurrent cases of bacteruria a full 7–10 day course may be more appropriate
A single dose antibiotic after intercourse may help to prevent associated bacteruria
Long term night time dose of antibiotic may prevent frequently recurring bacteruria.

Potassium citrate mixture

Can be used to 'alkalinate' the urine and relieve symptoms while awaiting results of bacteriological examination of the urine.

Topical oestrogen

Senile vaginitis is sometimes associated with dysuria and frequency in the presence of sterile urine
Dienoestrol cream is occasionally helpful in some cases.

Referral Any case not responding to the above management.

See also:

Abdominal pain (p. 1)
Fever (p. 106)
Haematuria (p. 127)
Polyuria (p. 251)
Pelvic pain (p. 240)
Vaginal discharge (p. 320)
Symptoms in pregnancy (p. 352)

Earache

Earache is common, especially in children. It may be produced by local trauma or inflammation, or may be referred from other sites in the head. The commonest cause is bacterial otitis media which can affect up to 1 in 4 of all children under 10 years. Up to 40% of cases will recur and hearing loss is a significant complication. The following account applies to the management of the common causes of earache.

Common causes

Otitis media
- bacterial
  - *Streptococcus pneumoniae* 40%
  - *Haemophilus influenzae* 20%
- viral (25%)

'Glue ear' with or without adenoid hypertrophy

Otitis externa (see p. 80)

Other causes

Local pain
- Trauma to pinna
- Perichondritis of pinna
- Herpes zoster
- Mumps
- Myringitis bullosa
- Impacted wax
- Foreign body
- Trauma to drum
  - instrumentation
  - blast injury
  - pressure changes
- Tumour

Referred pain
- Cervical lymphadenopathy
- Tonsillitis
- Sinusitis
- Tooth decay
- Impacted wisdom tooth
- Tempero-mandibular joint arthritis
- Cervical spondylosis
- Carcinoma of tongue or pharynx
- Bell's palsy

History

Onset, progress and nature of pain

Associated symptoms
- running nose
- mouth breathing
- discharge from ear
- snoring
- exacerbation of pain when supine

Previous history of URTI, ear problems, ENT operations

Hearing loss – achievement at school or work
– social development

Examination

Auriscopic examination of the drum

Otitis media: Increased vascularity, reddening,

bulging cobblestone pattern of the drum and possible performation.

'Glue ear': Variable colour, some increased vascularity, fluid level and retraction of the drum.

Tuning fork tests
Temperature
Throat and voice
Cervical lymph glands

Investigation

Ear swab if discharging
X-ray post-nasal space
Audiogram

Options

Explain aetiology and natural history of ear infections
Analgesics, e.g. paracetamol or aspirin
Nasal decongestant drops for one week, e.g. xylometazoline
Systemic decongestant in extended cases (2–3 months) for 'glue ear', e.g. pseudoephedrine
Antibiotics (if indicated)
- Amoxycillin in children under 5 yrs (in whom *Haemophilus influenzae* is more common)
- Penicillin
- Septrin

Avoid atmospheric pressure changes if possible, e.g. flying, diving
Advice on nose blowing (it is probably more physiological to 'sniff').

Follow-up

Check again after 2 weeks in otitis media or 1–2 months in 'glue ear'
Inspect drums
Assess hearing

Prevention of recurrent otitis media

Systemic and topical decongestants used prophylactically with uppper respiratory infections in susceptible individuals
Antibiotics – low dose, long term over 2–3 months or prophylactically with each upper respiratory infection
Myringotomy for 'glue ear' with or without the insertion of grommets
Adenoidectomy.

Referral

Removal of foreign body or impacted wax
Full hearing assessment

Surgery, e.g. adenoidectomy or myringotomy
Suspected carcinoma.

Complications of otitis media

Hearing loss and attendant social disadvantage
Recurrence
Perforation
Cholesteotoma
Mastoiditis
Facial nerve palsy
Lateral sinus thrombosis, brain abscess

See also:

Blisters (p. 29)
Ear discharge (p. 80)
Facial palsy (p. 96)
Hearing loss (p. 137)
Sinusitis (p. 287)
Common infectious diseases in children (p. 402)

Ear discharge

The ear may discharge a variety of substances including wax, pus, blood, serum or epithelial debris. Bacterial otitis externa is the commonest cause of a pusy discharge and may be recurrent in patients who are staphylococcus carriers.

A head injury leading to a fractured petrous temporal bone may lead to a discharge of CSF from the ear.

Local skin conditions e.g. eczema may become secondarily infected with *Candida* or fungus.

Causes

- Otitis externa
  - Infective
    - *Pseudomonas aeruginosa*
    - *Staphylococcus pyogenes*
    - *Klebsiella*
    - *Proteus*
    - *E. coli*
    - *Candida*
    - *Aspergillus*
  - Allergic
  - Eczematous
  - Psoriatic
- Suppurative otitis media with a performation of the drum
- Boils in the external auditory canal

Foreign body
Trauma
Head injury
Cholesteatoma
Tumour
Wax

History

Onset, duration and nature of discharge
Associated pain
Associated hearing loss
History of ear problems
Foreign body or trauma
History of general illness or skin disorder
Occupation

Examination

Inspection of ears
Tuning fork tests
Associated skin disorders

Investigation

Ear swab
Nose swab
Urinalysis

Options

Advice
- avoid scratching
- avoid wetting, e.g. swimming
- avoid chemical irritants
- discuss preventive measures with hearing aid wearers or swimmers

Local therapy
- aural toilet
- syringe wax (unless there is an underlying perforation of the drum)
- antiseptic, e.g. aqueous gentian violet
- antibiotic for limited course, e.g. gentamycin drops
- antifungal, e.g. miconazole cream
- steroids, e.g. prednisolone drops
- steroid/antibiotic/antiseptic combinations, e.g. Otosporin or Locorten-Vioform

Systemic therapy
- antibiotics for ottis media (see p. 79)
- for otitis externa, if cellulitis is associated, consider amoxycillin or flucloxacillin.

Complications

Recurrent infections
Meatal stenosis
Trauma to the drum

Reactions to medication
Bacterial resistance to antibiotics
Perichondritis

Referral

Removal of foreign body
Aural toilet in complicated cases
Perichondritis
Suspected mastoiditis
Cholesteatoma.

See also:

Earache (p. 77)
Hearing loss (p. 137)
Localized rash (p. 185)
Head injury (p. 523)

The elbow

The elbow may be the site of local joint pathology, or be the site of pain referred from the neck or shoulder. Most types of arthritis can affect the elbow joint.

The ulnar nerve lies in a groove behind the medial epicondyle and is prone to involvement in trauma. It may be affected in a variety of elbow conditions.

'Tennis elbow' is one of the most common elbow conditions seen in primary care. It is due to an epicondylitis at the muscle insertion on the lateral side.

History

Onset and timing of pain, stiffness or locking
Exacerbating and relieving factors
Associated symptoms of
  deformity
  sensory changes (especially in the ulnar distribution)
History of trauma
History of other joint disease

Examination

Inspect
  Asymmetry or deformity
  Swelling or effusion
  Wounds, scars and subcutaneous nodules

Palpate
  Site of maximum pain
  Displacement of bony prominences
  Active and passive movements
  Range of movement compared with normal side
    flexion/extension 0–150°
    pronation 0–90°

supination 0–90°
lateral stability and valgus/varus movement

Check

Peripheral pulses at elbows and wrists
Peripheral nerve involvement (especially the ulnar nerve)

Investigation

FBC
ESR
Uric acid
Culture of aspirated effusions
X-ray
Consider
calcium and phosphate
rheumatoid factor
clotting studies
ANF

Patterns of presentation

Arthritis

See pp. 485, 493.

Trauma

Fracture or dislocation of the elbow often affects the nerves and vessels to the forearm.

Check both radial pulses, signs of pallor or cyanosis and change in power or sensation in the wrist and hand.

Immobilize joint in the position of least pain and transfer to accident unit.

Pulled elbow

This occurs in children of about 2–4 years of age. There is a history of being pulled by the arm which may produce subluxation of the radial head. Forced supination during examination may reduce the subluxation with an audible 'click'.

Osteochondritis desiccans

The capitulum of the elbow is the second most common site involved after the knee.

It may follow trauma and can result in loose body formation.

This can predispose to subsequent osteoarthritis.

The symptoms include pain, effusion and limitation of movement, later the joint may lock in the presence of a loose body.

An X-ray confirms the diagnosis.

Referral for orthopaedic assessment is recommended.

Loose bodies

These are usually the result of osteochondritis desiccans, previous fracture or following arthritis. They may give rise to pain, swelling and locking of the joint. This is often followed by a spontaneous recovery after a few days but repeated attacks are common.

If they cause significant and repeated symptoms surgical removal is recommended.

Haemophiliac arthritis

After the knee, the elbow is the second most commonly affected joint. Repeated intra-articular haemorrhages lead to joint damage. Treatment is by immobilization in a plaster splint, and rest. Referral to hospital is usually necessary for Factor VIII therapy. Orthopaedic care is advised to limit degeneration of the joint.

Olecranon bursitis

The bursa between the olecranon and the skin may become enlarged as a result of pressure or friction. Treatment is by aspiration and firm bandaging. Occasionally surgical excision is necessary in chronic conditions. If the fluids become infected incision and drainage with antibiotic cover may be more appropriate.

Nodules

The elbow may be the site of rheumatoid nodules which should be distinguished from gouty tophi. They rarely cause symptoms but if they do then surgical excision may be necessary.

Epicondylitis

This may occur on the lateral (tennis elbow) or medial (golfer's elbow) epicondyles. There is pain on pressure over the epicondyle. The pain is often referred into the forearm particularly on stressing the extensor and flexor movements of the wrist respectively.

In the early stages, many cases will improve with a course of non-steroidal anti-inflammatory drugs, but standard treatment is by rest or local injection of a steroid/local anaesthetic mixture. The latter should be avoided with golfer's elbow because of the proximity of the ulnar nerve.

Refractory cases should be referred for orthopaedic assessment.

Ulnar nerve neuritis

The ulnar nerve passes behind the medial epicondyle and is exposed to trauma, by direct injury or compression from elbow joint deformity with OA or cubitus valgus deformity. There is usually pain at the medial epicondyle with numbness and tingling in the little and ring fingers as well as along the ulnar border of the hand. There may be wasting of the associated interossei muscles.

The condition may be transient, and will settle with rest. If it persists or is associated with muscle wasting, surgical transposition of the ulnar nerve will be necessary.

See also:

Shoulder (p. 284)
Wrist and hands (p. 341)
Osteoarthritis (p. 485)
Rheumatoid arthritis (p. 493)

Enlarged liver

In adult patients the liver may just be palpable under the right costal margin. It should be regarded with suspicion if it is palpable lower than this. The upper border is best discerned by percussion since a liver may appear enlarged in association with a hyper-inflated chest.

Causes

Congestion due to heart failure
Metastatic disease
Viral hepatitis
Cirrhosis

Other causes

Anatomical variation (Riedel's lobe)
Biliary obstruction
Hepatic vein thrombosis*
Polycystic liver diease
Infectious mononucleosis*
Malaria*
Weil's disease*
Hydatid disease*
Liver abscess
Pernicious anaemia
Sickle cell disease*
Reticulosis*
Myeloproliferative disorder*
Amyloidosis
Haemochromatosis
Inherited storage disease

*May be associated with an enlarged spleen

History

General health
Symptoms of cardiac failure
Systems enquiry to exclude malignancy
Past history of hepatitis or liver disease
Past history of blood transfusion
Travel abroad
Occupation
Contact with animals
Alcohol ingestion
Drug abuse

Examination

General
- Temperature
- Weight change
- Enlarged lymph nodes

Skin
- Jaundice
- Bruising and purpura
- Spider naevae
- Liver palms

Abdomen
- Size
- Shape and consistency of the liver
- Associated enlargement of the spleen
- Ascites
- Palpate for other masses (including rectal examination)

CVS
- Raised JVP
- Peripheral oedema
- Heart rate, rhythm and murmurs

CNS
- Signs of peripheral neuropathy

Investigation

FBC
MCV
ESR
U & E
LFT
Alcohol level (if appropriate)
Hepatitis B antigen
Chest X-ray
Plain abdominal X-ray
Liver scan

Options

Heart failure should be treated in the usual way (see p. 469)
Infective hepatitis (A and B) patients should be advised on hygiene and the appropriate precautions to avoid transmitting the disease
Drug therapy should be reviewed
Alcohol should be avoided or taken in moderation. Refer to Alcoholics Anonymous or detoxification unit if appropriate (see p. 261)

Follow-up

Regular review for patients suffering from cirrhosis. Check liver function tests and assess alcohol consumption

Referral

Further investigations to establish diagnosis
Treatment for
- suspected or proven malignancy
- evidence of liver failure with ascites, flapping tremor or confusion
- haematemesis and melaena from ruptured oesophageal varices.

See also:

Enlarged spleen (p. 91)
Glandular fever (p. 122)
Imported disease (p. 157)
Pallor/anaemia (p. 231)
Problem drinking (p. 261)
Heart failure (p. 469)

Enlarged lymph nodes

'Swollen glands' are a very common finding in primary care. Most commonly they are due to an infective process, especially in children.

Some less common but more sinister causes are important to detect and treat early and these must be considered.

Causes

Infections
Focal enlargement
- tonsillitis

boils
skin lesions
General enlargement
glandular fever
cytomegalovirus
toxoplasmosis
rubella
Chronic inflammatory skin disease
Vaccination and immunization response

Rare but sinister causes

Lymphatic spread of malignant tumour
Lymphoma
Leukaemia (particularly chronic lymphatic leukaemia)
Tuberculosis

Other causes

Brucellosis
Secondary syphilis (see p. 301)
Toxocara
Tropical diseases (see p. 157)
Sarcoidosis
Collagen disease
Myeloma
Histiocytosis
Anticonvulsant drugs
AIDS

History

General health including
appetite
weight loss
fever
rash
bruising
nose bleeds
Symptoms of focal infection
History of contact with infectious disease
History of recent vaccination
Systems enquiry particularly when malignancy is considered

Examination

Nodes
Site
Size
Consistency
Mobility
Attachment
Tenderness

Associated lymphangitis and infection in the area of drainage

General

Temperature
Tonsils and pharynx
Bruising and purpura
Breast lumps
Spleen and liver enlargement
Systems examination as indicated by the history

Investigation

FBC
Blood film and differential white count
ESR
Glandular fever screening tests
Other virus antibody screens when indicated
Toxoplasma dye test
Swab local infected lesions, e.g. tonsils
Mantoux or Heaf test for tuberculosis
Chest X-ray
Barium studies if occult malignancy is suspected

Options

Reassurance and general advice if a self-limiting infection is the cause – including glandular fever (see p. 122)
Topical antiseptics or antibiotics with or without systemic antibiotics for local bacterial infections
Antihistamines, e.g. chlorpheniramine 4 mg 6–8 hourly for vaccination reaction.

Follow-up

Most local causes will settle in 1–2 weeks and require no follow-up
Generalized viral infections may take longer to settle and should be reviewed as required
Neoplastic causes will require regular and careful follow-up both in hospital and primary care

Referral

For lymph node biopsy if no cause is found and lymph node enlargement persists after 3–4 weeks
For investigation and treatment if an underlying lymphoma, leukaemia or malignancy is suspected or proven.

See also:

Glandular fever (p. 122)
Imported disease (p. 157)
STD (p. 301)
Common infectious diseases in children (p. 402)
Pulmonary tuberculosis (p. 492)

Enlarged prostate

Benign enlargement of the prostate is a common problem in men. The incidence increases with age and it is estimated that 75% of 80 year olds show benign hypertrophy of the gland at post-mortem.

Prostatic cancer is the fourth most common cancer in men. Histologically 20% of men over the age of 50 show microscopic depositis of cancer in the prostate. In many cases the cancer lies dormant for years and is discovered on routine examination or post-mortem. Most cases of cancer that present with symptoms are inoperable unless there is coincident benign hypertrophy leading to earlier discovery.

History

Onset and duration of symptoms
- urgency
- frequency
- nocturia
- hesitancy
- poor stream
- haematuria
- bone pain

Exclude
- urinary tract infection
- prolapsed intervertebral disc
- urinary retention due to drugs (anticholinergics, antidepressives)

Examination

Anaemia
Weight loss
Abdominal masses
Hydronephrosis
Distended bladder
Enlarged liver
BP
Per rectum
- smoothly enlarged prostate with an obvious median sulcus suggests benign hypertrophy
- indurated nodules with obliteration of the sulcus is a more serious presentation

Investigation

FBC urea and creatinine
Acid phosphatase
MSU
IVP
Chest X-ray

X-ray spine and pelvis if indicated, to exclude bony secondaries

Options

Review drug therapy
Avoid large fluid intake
Advise emptying the bladder frequently to avoid over-distention
Oestrogen therapy might be considered for carcinoma of prostate after consultation with a urologist
Analgesia, e.g. aspirin or steroids for bony pain with spinal secondaries.

Referral

Acute retention
Chronic retention with overflow incontinence
Suspected carcinoma.

Follow-up

Check for infections
Catheter care
Review renal function periodically
Monitor oestrogen therapy

Complications

Urinary obstruction
Infection
Hydronephrosis with or without renal failure
Metastatic tumour deposits with bone pain
Urinary obstruction is exacerbated by certain drugs (e.g. antidepressives, anticholinergics, potent diuretics)

See also:

Haematuria (p. 127)
Oliguria and anuria (p. 229)

Enlarged spleen

This is uncommonly presented in primary care. The spleen is only palpable when enlarged but it may easily be missed unless specifically checked. Traditionally it can be distinguished from other masses in the left hypochondrium by:

a distinct medial border with palpable 'notch'
a dullness to percussion over the anterior surface
the upper border is only discernible by percussion, not palpation.

Causes

Infections
glandular fever

brucellosis
septicaemia (SBE)
infectious hepatitis
tuberculosis

Vascular
cirrhosis
hepatic vein thrombosis

Haematological
leukaemia
haemolytic anaemia
myelofibrosis
reticulosis
polycythaemia vera
idiopathic thrombocytopenic purpura

Other rarer causes

Tropical disease, e.g. malaria, kala-azar, trypanosomiasis
Sarcoidosis
Syphilis
Hydatid disease
Collagen disease
Felty's syndrome
Amyloidosis
Storage disease (lipoidoses)

History

General health and recent trauma
Associated symptoms of fevers, appetite, weight loss
Nosebleeds, bruising readily
Contact with infectious disease
International travel
Drugs and alcohol, use and abuse
Past history of liver, haematological or rheumatic heart disease

Examination

Size, site, shape and consistency of the spleen
Associated signs
ascites
liver enlargement
bruising
purpura
pallor
striae
liver palms
leukonychia
clubbing
splinter haemorrhages

enlarged lymph nodes (local and generalized)
heart murmurs

Investigation

FBC
Blood film with differential white count
ESR
Liver function tests
Serology for glandular fever and brucella
Chest X-ray
Mantoux test for tuberculosis

Options

Reassurance if the spleen is only minimally enlarged and due to self-limiting infective illness
Hygienic procedures should be explained to limit the spread of infection in acute infective hepatitis
Antibiotics as indicated for infective causes
Regular follow-up for the alcoholic with enlarged liver and spleen (this carries a poor prognosis).

Referral

Further investigation and treatment of the haematological and chronic infective causes
Liver biopsy if cirrhosis is suspected.

See also:

Enlarged liver (p. 85)
Glandular fever (p. 122)
Imported disease (p. 157)
Pallor/anaemia (p. 231)
STD (p. 301)
Pulmonary tuberculosis (p. 492)

Enlarged thyroid

Patients may complain of difficulty in swallowing, shortness of breath, swelling, or fullness in the neck. A goitre may also be detected by routine examination or via other symptoms or signs of thyroid disease. Thyroid cancers can present with enlargement of the thyroid, but are rare. However, the diagnosis must be excluded in every case.

The prevalence of goitre varies from country to country according to local availability of iodine. Iodine deficiency is unusual in the UK.

Causes

Hyperthyroid

Diffuse toxic goitre (Graves' disease)

- Nodular toxic goitre (Plummer's disease)
- Toxic adenoma

Euthyroid

- Physiological changes
  - puberty
  - pregnancy
  - menopause
- Carcinoma
  - follicular
  - anaplastic
  - medullary

Hypothyroid

- Autoimmune disease (Hashimoto's disease)
- Iodine deficiency
- Enzyme deficiency
- Antithyroid drugs, e.g. carbimazole

History

Rate of growth swelling
Country of origin and family history
Symptoms of thyroid malfunction (see p. 479)
Symptoms of compression in the neck
History of irradiation
Medication

Examination

Size, position, consistency and mobility of the goitre
Thyroid status (see p. 480)
Lymph gland involvement or skin lesion

Investigation

T_3 (hyperthyroid suspected)
T_4 and TSH (hypothyroid suspected)
CXR with thoracic inlet
Thyroid antibodies
TRH studies (in consultation with the laboratory)

Referral

Hospital investigations and the exclusion of a carcinoma in most cases
Radio-iodine therapy
Surgery
Goitre due to Graves' disease, Hashimoto's disease, iodine deficiency, drugs or physiological changes can be diagnosed and managed in primary care without referral.

Options

No action – if benign
Iodine supplement in diet – especially in children

Drugs
hypothyroidism (p. 481)
hyperthyroidism (p. 479)
Surgery
Radio-iodine

Follow-up

Supervision of medication
Neck circumference, pulse rate, weight
Clinical assessment of thyroid status (regularly over a long term with thyroid functions tests at intervals)

Complications

Haemorrhage
Obstruction of thoracic inlet (resulting in voice change, stridor, shortness of breath, dysphagia)
Radiation disease
Metastatic disease
Medullary carcinoma may occur in other members of the patient's family

See also:

Difficulty in swallowing (p. 71)
Hyperthyroidism (p. 479)
Hypothyroidism (p. 481)

Epidemic myalgic encephalomyelitis

This obscure and incapacitating epidemic condition is often diagnosed as merely a viral illness. The cause is probably viral but none has been isolated. The incubation period is 1 week. Women are affected more than men.

Patterns of presentation

Muscle pain, generalized weakness, exhaustion with depression and emotional irritability are constant features in an often confusing presentation. Other symptoms include
headache
lightheadedness
lassitude
exhaustion
sore throat
fever
enlarged glands
There are no associated clinical signs
The condition, though without serious complications, can run a protracted course.

Options

Symptomatic management

Exclude other cause of PUO (see p. 106)
(Cautious use of this diagnosis).

See also: Fever (p. 106)

Facial pain

In children, facial pain is normally directly related to an inflammatory or dental condition. In the elderly the diagnostic range is wider and occult carcinoma or cranial arteritis, trigeminal neuralgia and migrainous neuralgia should be excluded.

In the younger adults, who are often successful but obsessive, the syndrome of 'atypical facial pain' may seriously disrupt their lives. Their families may collude with their problem: they are always affected, and often adversely. The description of the pain is inappropriate for the physical signs and an organic cause is seldom found.

There is a wide range of causes.

Causes

Dental
- Malocclusion
- Dental caries
- Apical abscess
- Impacted teeth
- Pericoronitis

Vascular
- Migraine
- Migrainous neuralgia
- Cranial arteritis

Inflammatory
- Sinusitis
- Otitis externa
- Tonsillitis
- Iritis
- Glaucoma
- Herpes zoster

Arthritis
- Temporo-mandibular joint dysfunction
- Rheumatoid arthritis
- Osteoarthritis
- Cervical spondylosis

Neurological
- Trigeminal neuralgia
- Post-herpetic neuralgia
- Referred pain
- Angina
- Myocardial infarction

Psychogenic
'Atypical facial pain'

Other causes

Vincent's angina
Quinsy
Salivary gland infection
Mental nerve compression
Head injury
Carotid aneurysm
Acoustic neuroma
Meningioma
Intracranial tumour
Carcinoma of maxillary antrum or nasopharynx

History

Facial pain
- onset
- duration
- periodicity
- site
- precipitating and relieving factors

Associated symptoms
- loss of sensation
- loss of vision
- red eye
- congestion
- trismus

Psychological/social factors
- occupation
- leisure pursuits
- age
- alcohol intake
- depression
- cancer phobia
- obsessional traits
- neurotic traits
- family support
- 'life events'
- health beliefs

Examination

ENT
- nose
- mouth
- teeth
- LAP
- indirect laryngoscopy

Joints
- temporo-mandibular
- cervical spine

Eyes
- general examination and visual acuity

Cranial nerves
loss of sensation may indicate a carcinoma
Peripheral nerves
exclude stroke

Investigation

FBC
ESR
X-ray teeth, paranasal simuses, temporo-mandibular joint
Temporal artery biopsy

Options

Dental care initially confined to definite dental pathology or remoulding dentures
Simple analgesics, e.g. paracetamol 500 mg 3–6 hourly
Tranquillizers, e.g. diazepam 2–5 mg 6–8 hourly
Antidepressants, e.g. tricyclics or MAOI in migrainous neuralgia
Local anaesthesia
Carbamazepine (200 mg daily initially) in trigeminal neuralgia and post-herpetic pain
Ergot preparations at night – for migrainous neuralgia
Steroids, e.g. prednisolone 60 mg daily initially – for cranial arteritis
Psychotherapy according to patient's needs.

Referral

Dentist
Neurologist – to exclude carcinoma or neurological cause
Psychiatrist – (the patient may characteristically resent the implied psychological basis of the facial pain)
Pain relief unit
Neurosurgeon – as a last resort since surgery may complicate the complaint.

Complications

Post-operative recurrence
Substitution of alternative symptoms if and when facial pain is relieved
Blindness in cranial arteritis
Multiple sclerosis may present with trigeminal neuralgia

See also:

Blisters (p. 29)
Chest pain – angina pectoris (p. 43)
myocardial infarction (p. 46)
Ear discharge (p. 80)
Migraine (p. 203)
Red eye (p. 271)
Sinusitis (p. 287)
Osteoarthritis (p. 485)
Rheumatoid arthritis (p. 493)
Head injury (p. 523)

Facial palsy

Lower motor neurone facial palsy, or 'Bell's palsy', is a benign condition with complete recovery in 90% of cases. Symptoms develop over four days, recovery starts within a week, and is usually complete within six weeks. It occurs equally in both sexes and at any age, but maximally between the ages of 20 and 50 years.

The exact cause is unknown but is probably due to swelling of the nerve in the facial canal.

The facial palsy is lower motor neurone in type, i.e. smooth brow on the affected side and inability to close the eye. The weakness is occasionally associated with pain in the mastoid area. There are also other much rarer causes of facial palsy that are usually more persistent.

Associated conditions

Diabetes
Hypertension
Pregnancy – third trimester
Dental anaesthesia

Causes

Idiopathic – 'Bell's palsy'
Hypertension in children
Herpes zoster
Glandular fever
Cholesteatoma
Suppurative otitis media
Carcinoma of the parotid
Polio
Multiple sclerosis
Head injury
Guillain–Barré syndrome

History

Rate of onset
Associated symptoms
- preceding pain
- ENT symptoms
- change in taste
- change in speech
- difficulty eating
- dribbling
- watery eye
- dry eye
- vertigo
- diplopia
- loss of co-ordination

Check for contraindications to steroid therapy

Examination

Confirm lower motor neurone lesion
Taste in anterior 2/3 of tongue
Eye – ability to close lid, eye movements, lacrimation, corneal relex
Ears – cholesteatoma, tuning fork tests
BP (in children)

Options

Reassurance
- **not** a stroke
- **not** a cause of blindness
- full recovery to be expected

Facial massage – may help morale more than the facial nerve
Oral hygiene
Artificial tears, e.g. hypromellose
Analgesics, e.g. paracetamol 500 mg 3–6 hourly
Steroids, e.g. prednisolone 20 mg 6 hourly reducing over 10 days. Must be started within the first week. (The effectiveness of steroid therapy is still debated.)

Complications

Conjunctival or corneal damage
Loss of self-confidence
Adverse effects of steroid therapy
Incomplete recovery (assess after 3 months)
Axonal degeneration in 10–20% cases
Synkinesis due to misdirection in axonal regeneration

Differential diagnosis

Upper motor neurone weakness
Horner's syndrome
Facial hemispasm

Referral

Neurologist
- gradual onset
- upper motor neurone lesion
- brainstem symptoms or signs
- incomplete recovery after 3 months.

See also:

Blisters (p. 29)
Earache (p. 77)
Facial pain (p. 96)
Glandular fever (p. 122)
Symptoms in pregnancy (p. 352)
Diabetes (p. 457)
Hypertension (p. 475)

- Multiple sclerosis (p. 483)
- Head injury (p. 523)

Faints (syncope)

Fainting, or syncope, is a sudden but transient loss of consciousness that may result from a variety of causes. A detailed history is paramount in reaching a diagnosis.

Causes

Cerebral
- Epilepsy
- Hydrocephalic attacks
- (Cerebrovascular disease does not generally result in syncope)

Cardiovascular
- Vertebrobasilar attacks
- Cardiac dysrhythmias
- Postural hypotension from
  - fluid loss
  - drugs
  - autonomic neuropathy
- Low output state from myocardial infarction or valve disease

Vasovagal
- Cough syncope
- Micturition syncope
- Reflex syncope (carotid sinus)

Metabolic
- Alcohol excess
- Hypoglycaemia

Psychogenic
- Hyperventilation
- Breath-holding in children

History

- From the patient and eye witness if possible
- Frequency and duration of attacks
- Precipitating factors
  - psychological stress
  - febrile illness
  - hunger
  - lack of sleep
  - relationship to change in posture, cough, micturition and exertion

Eye witness report
- warning signs
- rate and mode of onset
- meaning
- movements
- colour
- incontinence
- injury

After fainting
- automatic behaviour
- confusion
- headache
- sleep

Neurological symptoms
- Speech and vision
- Confusion and sleepiness
- Weakness of limbs
- Headache

Cardiovascular symptoms
- Palpitations
- Breathlessness
- Chest pain

Past medical history
- Epilepsy
- Cardiovascular disease
- Head injury
- Meningitis

Family history of epilepsy

Medication
- Hypoglycaemic agents
- Antihypertensives
- Diuretics

Examination

Pulse – rate and rhythm
BP lying and standing
Cardiac murmurs or bruits in carotid arteries
Signs of internal bleeding
Neurological examination
Range of neck movement
Mental state

Investigation

FBC
U & E
Blood sugar
ECG

Chest X-ray
X-ray cervical spine

Options

Management plan for epilepsy (see p. 110)
Reassurance – simple faints are benign provided serious pathology can be excluded. Be sure that patient does not fear a sinister cause
Patients with postural hypotension should be advised against standing up quickly or taking strenuous exercise after rests
Cervical collar – may prevent vertebrobasilar attacks by restricting neck movements
Elastic hosiery – useful in postural hypotension. This can be supplemented with indomethacin 25--50 mg 8 hourly
Psychiatric opinion for hysterical faints in adults or breath-holding attacks in children
Glucagon 0.5–1.0 mg i.m. to reverse hypoglycaemic attacks
i.v. glucose 20 ml of 50% solution into a large vein (as an alternative to glucagon).

Referral

Urgent referral for acute internal haemorrhage
For investigation of unexplained cases
For investigation and control of epilepsy
For correction of cardiac dysrhythmias, valve defects or carotid stenosis.

See also:

Cough (p. 58)
Fits (p. 110)
Problem drinking (p. 261)
Fits and funny turns (p. 423)
Convulsion (p. 518)
Hypoglycaemia (p. 525)

Female subfertility

10–14% of all couples are unable to conceive without intervention. A much larger proportion present for advice on relative delay in conception.

Subfertility in the male is discussed separately (see p. 192) although the couple should be seen and assessed together.

Causes

Psychosexual problems (see p. 266)

Ovulation disorders
- pituitary/hypothalamic lesions
- chronic illness

Tubal occlusion
- congenital
- post-infective
- adhesions

Uterine abnormality
- congenital
- poor endometrium
- uterine adhesions
- sub-mucous fibroids
- (retroversion)

Cervical disorders
- 'hostile' cervical mucus
- cervicitis

Genetic disorders
- intersex states

History

Sexual history and contraception

Menstrual history

Parity

Gynaecological history (including previous venereal disease)

History of abdominal surgery

Medication

Examination

General
- distribution of body hair
- secondary sexual development
- lower abdominal scars

Introitus
- hymen
- congenital abnormality

Vagina
- septate vagina
- vaginal discharge
- vaginismus

Cervix
- cervicitis

Uterus
- shape, size and position
- fibroids

Fornices
- ovarian masses
- tenderness over fallopian tubes

Investigation

Menstrual charts
Cycles less than 21 or more than 42 days are usually anovulatory
Temperature charts
To assess ovulation
Cervical mucus
Ovulatory mucus is clear, copious and can be stretched 10–15 cms (spinnbarkheit). On drying it forms a ferning pattern
Post-coital test
Aspirate the cervical mucus within 2 hours of coitus. View under a low power microscope to demonstrate motile sperm
Hormone assays
Luteinizing hormone (early cycle) – if increased exclude polycystic ovaries
Prolactin (early cycle) – if increased exclude pituitary adenoma
Progesterone (20th to 22nd day of cycle) if reduced indicates defective ovulation
Tubal patency – refer to specialist for assessment

Options

Discussion
Range of normal time for conception
Sex technique and timing in relation to ovulation
Hormone treatment
This is best left to the specialist who may consider
Clomiphene 50–100 mg on the first five days of menstrual cycle to induce ovulation
Ethinyloestrodiol 10 mg daily for 3 days preceding expected ovulation to improve cervical mucus.

Referral

Investigation after 18 months for apparently healthy young couples, or earlier if the patient is over 35 years
Surgery for correction of abormalitities or tubal occlusion if appropriate
In vitro fertilization for assessment and selection
Artificial insemination for consideration and assessment
Adoption as a realistic alternative.

See also:

Male subfertility (p. 192)
Psychosexual problems (p. 266)
STD (p. 301)

Fever

The body temperature fluctuates in circadian rhythm usually between 36.5° and 37.5° centigrade. A control system for these daily changes is situated in the thermoregulatory centre of the hypothalamus.

Fever is the elevation of body temperature above the patient's normal range.

'Pyrexia of unknown origin' (PUO) is a term to be used with some caution. In 1961 three classical criteria were proposed to define PUO.

1. A fever of more than 38.3°.
2. A fever lasting more than 3 weeks.
3. A situation in which no diagnosis has been reached after 1 week in hospital.

In the 1980s PUO is generally used to describe a persistent fever that remains undiagnosed after initial assessment.

Table 1.3. Causes of fever

Infection–systemic	
Septicaemia	Meningococcus
Glandular fever	Cytomegalovirus
Chickenpox	Leptospirosis
Measles	Brucellosis
Mumps	Toxoplasmosis
Rubella	Toxocara
Other viral illness	Worms
Whooping cough	Imported disease
Tuberculosis	
Infection–local	
Encephalitis	Subacute bacterial
Meningitis	bronchiolitis
Otitis media	endocarditis
Sinusitis	STD
Dental sepsis	Herpes zoster
Tonsillitis	Septic arthritis
Bronchitis	Cholangitis
Pneumonia	Abscess
Cholecystitis	peri-tonsillar
Enteritis	sub-phrenic
Appendicitis	para colic
UTI	renal
Pelvic inflammatory disease	

Connective tissue disorders

Rheumatoid arthritis
Polymyalgia rheumatica
Temporal arteritis
Systemic lupus erythematosus
Still's disease
Polyartertis nodosa
Other autoimmune diseases

Cancers

Hodgkin's disease
Lymphoma
Leukaemia
Carcinomatosis
Hypernephroma
Hepatoma
Pancreatic tumour
Atrial myxoma
Sarcoma

Miscellaneous

Post-myocardial infarction
Post-pulmonary infarction
Post-traumatic
Post-anaesthetic
DVT
Dehydration
Sun stroke
Thyrotoxicosis
Sarcoidosis
Familial mediterranean fever
Malignant hyperpyrexia
Anaphylaxis
Drug reaction, e.g. sulphonamides
Faked fever
Whipple's disease
Phaeochromocytoma
CVA affecting hypothalamus

History

Associated symptoms

Non-specific
- malaise
- lethargy
- anorexia
- general headache
- moderate abdominal pain
- muscle aching

Specific
- earache
- toothache
- breathlessness
- diarrhoea
- rash
- thyrotoxic symptoms
- dysuria
- dyspareuria
- sore throat
- facial pain

chest pain
vomiting
arthritis

Past medical history
Diabetes
Leukaemia
Immunosuppression

Medication

Social factors
Contacts
Travel
Trauma
Anaesthetics
Pets
Social and dietary neglect

Examination

Record
Temperature – oral, rectal or axillary site
Temperature chart
Pulse
BP

Check for
Ear disease
Mouth signs
LAP
Erythema nodosum
Skin changes
Jaundice
Finger clubbing
Splinter haemorrhage
Added heart sounds
Recent heart murmurs
Lung 'crackles' or rub
Swollen tender red joints
Abdominal masses or tenderness
Rectal lesions
Localizing neurological signs
Retinopathy
Pelvic masses and tenderness

Investigation

FBC film
ESR
Glandular fever screening test
U & E
LFT

Serology – as indicated
Viral titres in paired samples ten days apart
Culture of
- blood
- urine
- faeces
- sputum

Urinalysis
Throat swab
Nasal swab
Chest X-ray

Options

Cool the patient
- remove clothing
- open windows
- fan
- cool baths
- tepid sponging

Encourage fluid intake (regular drinks of clear fluids, ice-lollies, etc.)
Aspirin or paracetamol
Treat underlying pathology
Avoid antibiotics unless there is clear indication of a bacterial infection.
Notify the community physician (Environmental Health) when appropriate.

Referral

All cases with PUO (by the definition in current usage)
On suspicion of imported disease
To confirm or exclude the diagnosis or rare or serious disease, e.g. atrial myxoma or temporal arteritis
For hospital care when there is associated debilitation, extreme age, complications or intercurrent illness
For specialist or surgical treatment, e.g. ischiorectal abscess or STD.

See also:

Blisters (p. 29)
Glandular fever (p. 122)
Imported disease (p. 157)
Infection and parasites from pets (p. 165)
Influenza (p. 167)
Pelvic pain (p. 240)
Sinusitis (p. 287)
STD (p. 301)
Worms (p. 339)

Common infectious diseases in children (p. 402)
The feverish child (p. 420)
Chronic bronchitis (p. 440)
Pulmonary tuberculosis (p. 492)
Rheumatoid arthritis (p. 493)
Anaphylactic shock (p. 513)

Fits

These are episodic disturbances of cerebral function of abrupt onset and short duration (seconds or minutes). These fits or seizures are the hallmark of epilepsy. They may be local or generalized and in the latter, consciousness is almost always affected.

Patterns of presentation

Generalized

Absence – brief loss of awareness
Myoclonic – single or multiple jerking movements
Atonic – loss of postural tone (drop attacks)
Tonic-clonic – sustained muscular contraction followed by generalized rhythmical jerking

Focal

Motor
Sensory
Cognitive
Psychosensory

The incidence is 3 per 1000. The aetiology is not well understood but primary seizures may have some association with genetic factors.

Secondary seizures may result from

Head injury
Birth trauma
Cerebral tumour
Cerebrovascular disease
Cerebral infection
Metabolic disorder
Drug or alcohol withdrawal

The detailed history is most crucial to the diagnosis. The report of a witness is essential.

History

Complete history of the seizure
precipitating factors

loss of consciousness
injury
abnormal movements
duration
incontinence
behaviour after the event
patient's memory of the event

Past medical history of meningitis, head injury or birth trauma

Family history of epilepsy

Drugs and alcohol intake

Examination

This is rarely positively helpful after the event

Teeth marks on the tongue and incontinence are suggestive signs

Focal neurological signs persisting for more than 2–3 hours may indicate underlying cerebral disease

Investigation

These are usually carried out by the hospital specialist
EEG
CT scan
Chest X-ray

Other investigations would be necessary if an underlying cause such as a metabolic disorder or cerebral infection is suspected

Options

Drug treatment

Start drug treatment if it is certain that the patient has had two or more fits

Use a single drug if possible (see Table 1.3)

Aim for a twice daily dosage for better compliance

Increase dosage gradually to achieve seizure control, otherwise side-effects supervene

Consider measuring plasma concentration of the drug if control or compliance appear inadequate

Measure regularly during pregnancy

Treatment must be continuous

Continue for at least three years after the last seizure before considering gradual withdrawal of treatment.

Advice

Driving

The patient has a legal obligation to notify the licensing authority that he is undergoing medical treatment for episodic fits

If the fits occur only during sleep he may continue to drive

Table 1.4

Drug	Recommended adult daily dosage (mg/kg)	Appropriate for
Sodium valpropate	20–30	Most types
Phenytoin	5	Tonic-clonic Focal
Phenobarbitone	2	Tonic-clonic Focal
Carbamazepine	20	Tonic-clonic Focal
Clonazepam	0.2	Absences Myoclonic Atonic
Ethosuximide	15	Absences

If no fits have occurred during waking hours for two consecutive years then the licence may be reapplied for

Sport

Should be encouraged

Each case must be considered individually

Swimming is not precluded if it is under careful supervision

Genetic counselling

If one parent has generalized epilepsy the child has a 1:10 chance of being affected. If both parents are affected the risk is about 1:4

By the time that the child is 10 years old and seizure-free the risk is reduced to 1:50

Referral

Prescriptive exemption can be applied for

Initial full assessment

Inadequate control

Status epilepticus.

Complications

Status epilepticus – repeated seizures with short intervals. It is a medical emergency since hypoxia and brain damage can occur

Options

diazepam 5–10 mg i.v., i.m. or rectally

or phenobarbitone 200 mg i.m.

or paraldehyde 5–10 ml i.m.

Injury – the patient may be injured in a fall or during the clonic phase of a tonic-clonic seizure

Drug side-effects – several of the drugs have harmful

effects in the long term. It is important to assess for these particularly with phenytoin

Differential diagnosis

Simple faints
Stoke–Adams attacks
Vertebrobasilar attacks
Transient ischaemic attacks
Narcolepsy
Hysterical fits

Follow-up

see opposite

See also:

Faints (p. 101)
Fits and funny turns (p. 423)
Convulsion (p. 518)
Head injury (p. 523)

Food allergy

Patients may ascribe a variety of different symptoms to food allergy. If suspected, excellent results may be achieved by practising simple avoidance. To identify food allergies doctors must have a high index of suspicion, especially where there is a personal history or family history of other allergies. However, time consuming investigations will often be unrewarding.

Food allergy must be distinguished from food intolerance which may be due to enzyme deficiency.

Presenting symptoms

Wheezing
Sneezing
Urticaria
Abdominal pains
Diarrhoea
Vomiting
Eczema
Mouth ulcers
Painful joints
Swollen legs
Frequency
Bed wetting
Palpitations
Anxiety
Tiredness
Depression
Loss of concentration

Disturbed sleep
Failure to thrive
Overactive children
Migraine
Angioneurotic oedema

Investigation

Diary of exact diet and symptoms
Elimination of suspected food from the diet and then reintroduction after 2–3 weeks (see table 1.4)
Monitor symptoms objectively, e.g. pulse rate or PEF rate

Options in management

Avoid any proven allergens
Avoid commonest allergens
Resort to low allergy diet (see table 1.5)
Referral to allergy clinic
Referral to dietician
Advice on breast feeding
Medication with antihistamines and/or sodium cromoglycate.

Table 1.5. Common food allergens

Coffee	Tea	Alcohol
Cows' milk	Eggs	Chocolate
Wheat	Rice	Soya
Cane sugar	Yeasts	Nuts
Pork	Shellfish	Other fish
Tomatoes	Oranges	Other pipped fruits
Colouring	Preservatives	Strawberries

Low allergy diet

Lamb	Tea
Sago	Soda water
Green leaf vegetable	Sugar
Celery	Salt
Lettuce	Fresh rhubarb
Carrots	

Failure to control

Resort to 5 day fast – water only – with 5 day interval between reintroduction of each group of foodstuffs
Consider all components of ingested matter (including colouring and preservatives in drinks and drugs, etc.)

Complications

Anaphylactic collapse
Anaemia – iron loss
Oedema – protein loss
Complications of the above symptoms if severe

The foot and ankle

The foot is the site of much disability. There are several congenital problems and as with most synovial joints it is affected by the common forms of arthritis. However, much of the disability is self-induced through injury, over use, excessive stress from obesity, ill-fitting footwear or poor care of the feet. Problems with the feet are also significant complications of diabetes and vascular disease which are not considered here (see pp. 457, 254).

History

Onset duration and severity of symptoms
History of trauma
Exacerbating and relieving factors
Site of radiation
Associated symptoms
- swelling
- discoloration
- effect on ADL and mobility

Examination

Inspect for symmetry, swelling, skin changes or deformity
Palpate for site of maximal pain
Assess active and passive range of movement
Check
- weight
- Achilles tendon
- neurological signs
- footwear

Patterns of presentation

Arthritis

The painful swollen first metatasophalangeal joint is the classic presentation of gout (see p. 462).

Metatarsalgia

This is a painful condition of the metatarsal heads. It usually occurs in the degenerate feet of middle age onwards. It is also associated with degrees of flat foot, hallux valgus or claw-toe. However, it may result from
- tight footwear
- disease – RA and osteochondritis
- injury – arch fracture
- intercristal neuroma of Morton.

On examination there is usually a callosity under a tender metatarsal head, most often the 2nd or 3rd. In the case of the neuroma the pain is between the metatarsal heads. If the pain occurs after a particularly long walk or excessive exercise an X-ray should be arranged to exclude a fracture.

Acute symptoms can be relieved by changing to a more comfortably fitting shoe or using an insole with support under the metatarsal shafts to relieve pressure on the heads. In the case of a neuroma or more serious underlying disease referral is necessary for operative treatment.

Plantar fasciitis

There is pain under the heel at the insertion of the plantar fascia into the calcaneum. X-ray examination may show a bony spur at the site of maximum tenderness.

Treatment is usually simple with an injection of local anaesthetic mixed with cortisone into the site of maximum tenderness. If this fails consider NSAIDs, small heel raise and ultrasound (if available). Ultimately referral for surgical correction may be required.

Cramps

Muscle cramp in the foot is a common condition particularly in the elderly. It frequently causes sleep disturbance. Treatment is unsatisfactory but quinine sulphate may be helpful (300 mg at night).

Peripheral vascular disease

This condition is discussed separately (see p. 254) it may be the cause of rest pain in the feet particularly at night.

Sprains

This is an extremely common presentation. The majority are due to inversion injuries with strain on the lateral ligament. If a fracture is suspected particularly with inversion injuries then X-ray examination is necessary. Otherwise a firm support or stirrup strapping with elasticated adhesive bandage should be applied for a week followed by graded exercises until normal function is recovered. This is usually achieved within 3 weeks.

If there is marked swelling over the lateral ligament and the patient is completely unable to bear weight then it is often advisable to immobilize the joint in plaster for 3–4 weeks. This injury may result in a lax lateral ligament with chronic instability.

The Achilles tendon

Tendon strains are quite common in sportsmen. The patient complains of pain in the tendon after exercise. On examination there may be tender thickening. Treatment is best with immobilization and gradual return to normal activities. Steroid injections may provide early relief but the condition may become chronic as a result of repeated trauma to the damaged tendon.

Complete rupture of the tendon is possible, particularly as the tendon degenerates with ageing. The onset is very acute usually during strenous exercise and the patient often feels he has been hit at the back of the heel. On examination the tendon is swollen and painful. When the patient kneels on a chair squeezing the gastrocnemius will cause plantar flexion of the foot. This fails to happen if the tendon is ruptured.

Treatment is by operative resuturing followed by immobilization for six weeks.

Club foot

This is a congential abnormality comprising plantar flexion, adduction and inversion of the foot. In the absence of proper treatment a persisting deformity develops which is often bilateral.

The foot cannot be passively stretched through its usual range of movement. Even with treatment the outcome is uncertain and early referral is essential. It is more common in boys.

Flat feet

This is a common condition which is usually congenital

In the past undue emphasis has been placed on this as a cause of subsequent disability. The condition is frequently asymptomatic and reassurance is all that is needed. If it causes foot strain the treatment is by arranging for special footwear with a medial wedge in the heel of the shoe to be fitted. Physiotherapy may also assist the discomfort.

Hallux valgus

This is predominantly a condition found in women in whom there is often a strong family history. The big toe deviates laterally. A bursa may be evident over the first metatarsal head. If this becomes inflamed it is termed a bunion. Gout, rheumatoid arthritis and ill-fitting shoes may predispose to this deformity. If the condition causes pain referral is necessary for operative treatment. In the younger patient surgery might be considered for cosmetic reasons.

Hallux rigidus

There is pain and stiffness of the first metatarsophalangeal joint as a result of trauma and secondary OA. The symptoms may be controlled by wearing a shoe with a firm sole – possibly with a metatarsal bar. NSAID analgesics may be helpful. If this fails surgery is recommended.

Claw-toes The smaller toes are flexed at both IP joints. This may occur as a result of rheumatoid arthritis, neuromuscular disease or ill-fitting shoes. It may lead to pain or pressure symptoms and is best treated by surgery with arthrodesis and advice regarding appropriate foot wear.

Hammer-toes In this condition the proximal IP joint is flexed and the distal IP joint extended. It particularly occurs in young adults. It may cause pressure symptoms and requires arthrodesis.

See also:

Hip (p. 146)
Knee (p. 179)
Nail problems (p. 212)
Poor circulation (p. 254)
Diabetes (p. 457)
Gout (p. 462)
Osteoarthritis (p. 485)

Generalized rash

Probably the most common causes of a generalized rash seen in primary care are the acute exanthemata seen in children. (See pp. 402–407).

There are other, non-infective causes. The recognition of their patterns of presentation depends upon a careful history and assessment of the distribution of the rash and of the associated features.

Drug eruption

History

Many drugs can cause a rash in sensitive individuals
May occur as first or subsequent exposure to the drug
Usually sudden onset
Some drugs share a cross-sensitivity, e.g. ampicillin and cephalosporins

Skin lesion

Maculopapular erythematous rash
Widespread distribution
May become more confluent

Associated features Itching

Urticaria
Angioneurotic oedema
Constitutional upset with fever, malaise, and joint pains

Options

Remove offending drug
Oral antihistamines (e.g. chlorpheniramine 4 mg 6 hourly)
Topical calamine lotion
Systemic steroids in more severe cases.

Urticaria

This is due to localized vasodilation and increased vascular permeability due to a release of histamine and other chemical mediators in the skin.

Causes

Allergy to drugs or foodstuffs
Temperature sensitivity
Sunlight
Trauma
Anxiety

History

Contact with allergen
Usually sudden onset and short duration (<24 hrs)
May be recurrent or chronic
Intensely itchy

Skin lesion

Erythematous patch with raised, white centre
Variable outline and size
Usually widespread

Associated features

Dematographism
Angioneurotic oedema
Joint pains and swelling
Wheezing
Anaphylactic shock

Options

Avoidance of any identified precipitating factors
Antihistamines (e.g. chlorpheniramine 4 mg 6 hourly)
Systemic steroids and adrenaline in more serious cases.

Pityriasis rosea

This rash has a characteristic appearance but undefined aetiology. It may follow a presumed viral illness with mild sore throat and malaise. There is little constitutional upset or irritation. It mainly affects young adults, females more than males. It is more common in the spring and autumn.

Skin lesion Annular scaly, red-brown patches
Preceded by a single patch, with scaly margins, usually on the trunk ('Herald patch')
Oval shaped patches with long axis in lines of cleavage of the skin; gives a 'christmas tree' distribution on the back

Differential diagnosis Eczema
Guttate psoriasis
Fungal infection
Drug eruption
Secondary syphilis
Rubella
Glandular fever

Associated features Frequently symptomless but can cause itching
Clears spontaneously in 8 weeks
Rarely recurrent

Options Reassurance and explanation is usually all that is necessary
Topical steroids may produce partial suppression.

Tinea versicolor This is caused by a fungus, *Malassezia furfur*. The rash is also known as Pityriasis versicolor. Common in the tropics but also seen in temperate climates this condition often presents after the patient has been on holiday. It may appear to change colour – fawn-coloured in fair-skinned patients, or pale in tanned patients (because the lesions fail to pigment).

Skin lesion Pale fawn-coloured macules which may coalesce
Vary in shape and size
Become finely scaly on scraping
Distribution on upper trunk, neck and upper arms

Associated features No irritation or constitutional disturbance

Options Whitfield's ointment (half-strength) applied daily for 3 or 4 weeks
Selenium sulphide shampoo applied topically and left overnight before washing off. It may be applied weekly until clear.

Purpura

Purpura is due to leakage of red cells through the capillary vessel wall.

Causes

Vascular fragility or damage
- ageing
- infections
- systemic disease
- vitamin C deficiency
- allergic vasculitis
- emboli (SBE)
- hereditary fragility

Platelet deficiency
- idiopathic
- secondary to drugs, infections, leukaemias

Disorders of coagulation

Skin lesions

Red-brown or purple patches (from a few millimetres to a few centimetres in size)
The patches do not blanch on pressure
Particularly affects the lower limbs

Options

Full medical and haematological assessment because of the seriousness of some of the causes
Management depends on the precise cause.

Erythema multiforme

This is probably an immunological disorder affecting cutaneous blood vessels. It is usually idiopathic but can be associated with viral or bacterial infection, or drug sensitivity. It may be recurrent.

History

Recent infection
Drug history
Symptoms of mouth ulcers

Skin lesion

Variable morphology – erythematous macules, urticarial lesions blistering or pupuric
Classically erythematous macule with central clearing (target lesion)
Usually affects the distal upper limb
Occasionally more generalized

Associated features

Mouth ulcers
Uveitis
Genital ulcers
Usually asymptomatic but can be associated with a

severe illness which may be fatal (Stevens–Johnson syndrome)

Options

Reassurance in mild cases which clear in 2 or 3 weeks
Avoidance of precipitating factors (drugs)
Oral antihistamines for itching irritation (e.g. chlorpheniramine 4 mg 6 hourly)
Systemic steroids in Stevens–Johnson syndrome.

See also:

Food allergy (p. 113)
Itch (p. 174)
Localized rash (p. 185)
Stress and anxiety (p. 303)
Common infectious diseases in children (p. 402)
Anaphylactic shock (p. 511)

Glandular fever

Glandular fever is a clinical diagnosis. It is recognized as the familiar pattern of presenting symptoms occuring predominantly in the 'teens and twenties in males and females equally. There is low infectivity, it is more common in winter and recurrences do occur. It is characterized by the appearance of atypical lymphocytes and mononuclear cells.

Causes of glandular fever-like illness

EB virus – gives a positive Paul–Bunnell test and is the commonest cause
Cytomegalovirus – may follow blood transfusions
Toxoplasma gondii – from cysts in raw or undercooked meat, e.g. pet food
Rubella
Infectious hepatitis
Adenovirus

Differential diagnosis

Infection
- leptospirosis
- streptococcal pharyngitis
- diphtheria

Vincent's angina
Leukaemia
Lymphoma
Agranulocytosis
Aplastic anaemia
Drug reactions

Patterns of presentation of glandular fever

Pharyngitis with or without exudate
Palatal petechiae
Prolonged 'flu-like' illness
Malaise
Lymphadenopathy
Fever or PUO
Enlarged spleen
Rashes (including the ampicillin rash)
Swollen eyes
Jaundice

History

Onset and duration of symptoms
Previous similar symptoms
Family history of symptoms
LMP
Recent contacts, uncooked meats, blood transfusions
Exclude (or confirm) pregnancy

Examination

Temperature
Lymph node enlargement
Liver or spleen enlargement
Throat
Skin

Investigation

Blood film
ESR
Monospot or Paul–Bunnell test
Serology (including Rubella titre)
LFT
Throat swab
MSU
CXR

Options

Information about the condition
Symptomatic relief – bed rest, gargles, etc.
Steroids may be appropriate with
- severe pharyngitis
- excessive fever and malaise
- rash

abnormal liver function tests
e.g. prednisolone 30–60 mg daily for 5 days
Antibiotics, e.g. phenoxymethylpenicillin 250 mg 6 hourly when T/S indicates streptococcus, e.g. Septrin 2 tablets, 12 hourly for 3 months
Avoid contact sports if spleen is enlarged
Avoid alcohol for 6 months if liver function is disturbed.

Follow-up Return to normal activities should be dictated by subjective well-being and not by blood analysis.

Complications
Death in the immunosuppressed patient
Depression
Cranial nerve palsies
Meningo-encephalitis
Haemolysis
Thrombocytopenia
Pneumonitis
Arthritis
Ampicillin rash

Pregnancy
EB virus – no risk
CMV
Toxoplasma gondii
Rubella
Infectious hepatitis
} Consult with virologist and obstetrician (CMV, *Toxoplasma gondii*, Rubella, Infectious hepatitis)

Referral
For immunofluorescence studies
Fetal infection
Lymph node biopsy.

See also:
Fever (p. 106)
Imported disease (p. 157)
Influenza (p. 167)
Flu-like illness (p. 169)

Gynaecomastia

In any culture breast development in a man is an embarrassing if not humiliating experience. When the low levels of circulating oestrogens are unopposed by androgens gynaecomastia will develop. This can occur at any age but the neonatal period, puberty and old age are most common.

The size can range from the five pence sized 'blue-disc-of-puberty' – so called because of its apparent translucency – to full breast development.

The causes are many and most are extremely rare.

Causes

Neonatal gynaecomastia
Puberty
Old age
Obesity
Tumours
- pituitary
- testes
- adrenals
- breast

Drugs
- steroids
- digoxin
- tricyclics
- cannabis
- spironolactone
- methyldopa
- oestrogens
- griseofulvin
- phenothiazines
- amphetamines
- cyproterone acetate
- cytotoxic alkylating agents

Hyperthyroidism
Liver disease
Renal disease

Other causes

Hermaphroditism
Klinefelter's syndrome
Addison's disease
Hypopituitarism
Orchitis
Testicular feminization
Kallman's syndrome
Acromegaly
Cushing's syndrome
HCG secreting bronchial carcinoma

History

Age of onset and progress of breast development
Age of onset and progress of puberty
Associated symptoms
- pain
- lethargy
- thyrotoxic symptoms
- urinary symptoms
- anosmia
- visual changes

Previous history (if considering testosterone therapy)
- liver disease
- epilepsy
- migraine
- prostatic carcinoma
- nephrosis

Family history of sexual development
History of medication
Social and psychological effects

Examination

Weight and height and general demeanour
Breast size, shape, consistency and mobility
Genitalia
Secondary sexual characteristics
Check for visual field defects
Check for signs of
- acromegaly
- Addison's disease
- Cushing's syndrome
- hyperthyroidism
- hypopituitarism

Investigation

U & E
LFT
T_3
LH
FSH
Digoxin level
MSU
CXR
Skull X-ray

Options

Dietary advice
Revise drug regimen
Allow spontaneous resolution usually within 18 months
Testosterone replacement, e.g. 100 mg implant 6 monthly

Other medication
- danazol 100 mg 12 hourly (initially)
- tamoxifen 10 mg 12 hourly
- clomiphene 50 mg 12 hourly

Mastectomy.

Referral

Endocrine assessment
Chromosome assessment
Surgical intervention
Failure of resolution of gynaecomastia
Suspicion of carcinoma (1% occur in males).

See also:

Obesity (p. 224)
Chronic renal failure (p. 443)
Hyperthyroidism (p. 479)

Haematuria

Blood in the urine is an important sign that demands further investigation to elucidate a cause. Microscopic haematuria is only noticed if looked for and may occasionally be found on routine testing.

The phenomenon of haematuria can occur at any age.

Causes

Infections
- Urethritis
- Prostatitis
- Cystitis
- Acute pyelonephritis

Trauma
- Urethra – postal-coital, catheterization, self-inflicted
- Bladder – pelvic injuries
- Kidney – crush injuries

Urinary calculi
- Bladder
- Ureteric

Renal disease
- Glomerulonephritis
- Bacterial endocarditis with embolization

Tumours
- Prostate
- Bladder
- Kidney

Bleeding disorders – spontaneous or drug-induced
Contamination from menstrual bleeding

Other causes of red coloured urine

Porphyria – urine may change to pink or red on standing in daylight

Foods – beetroot and blackberries may give pink coloured urine

History

Onset, frequency and timing of the bleeding
- blood passed before micturition is more likely to be urethral or prostatic
- blood evenly mixed in urine is more likely to be from the kidney or bladder
- a small amount of blood may give a smoky appearance in urine

Associated symptoms
- dysuria
- frequency
- nocturia
- loin pain
- vaginal discharge

Recent history of
- trauma (urethral, pelvic and abdominal)
- sore throat
- fever

Menstrual and sexual history
Family history of renal disease or bleeding disorder
Drugs including anticoagulants

Examination

Pallor, bruising or purpura
BP
Signs of fluid retention
Abdominal tenderness
Renal enlargement
P.R. or P.V. examination to assess prostatic enlargement or pelvic tumours

Investigation

FBC
ESR
MSU – microscopy
Culture
Cytology for malignant cells
Urea, electrolytes and creatinine
High vaginal swab if indicated
Cervical smear
IVP

Options

Infection – high fluid intake and appropriate antibiotic therapy

Ureteric calculi – high fluid intake and adequate analgesia, e.g. Pethidine 50–100 mg 6 hourly by injections or orally.

Referral

For further investigation if it is not possible to confidently diagnose a benign cause

Failure to control pain of ureteric colic or if the stone has not been passed after 48 hours of conservative treatment

To trace contacts in sexually transmitted urethritis.

See also:

Dysuria and frequency (p. 76)
Enlarged prostate (p. 90)

Haemoptysis

Coughing up blood is a relatively uncommon complaint in primary care. The ratio of serious to non-serious causes is estimated at 1:7 but this symptom always warrants careful assessment.

Causes

Acute respiratory infection
Chronic bronchitis and bronchiectasis
Epistaxis
Neoplasm in lungs or upper respiratory tract
Tuberculosis
Pulmonary embolism
LVF and mitral stenosis
Trauma
Aortic aneurysm

History

Onset, duration and periodicity of haemoptysis

Volume and nature of haemoptysis – bleeding from the respiratory tract is usually pink and frothy whereas in gastrointestinal haemorrhage the blood is dark and altered

Associated symptoms
- cough, with or without sputum
- weight loss
- ankle oedema
- chest pain
- shortness of breath

History of TB contact or inhalation of foreign body

Past history of heart or lung disease

Drugs – especially anticoagulants
Smoking

Examination

Record
Weight
Pulse
Temperature
BP

Check for
Clubbing
Bruising and purpura
Bleeding site in nose, mouth or throat
Respiratory signs on auscultation
Mitral stenosis

Investigation

FBC
ESR
Mantoux text
Chest X-ray (P.A. and lateral) – a normal CXR does not exclude an early carcinoma

Options

When serious pathology can confidently be excluded consider
reassurance
advise against smoking
antibiotics for infection
physiotherapy when appropriate for bronchtis or bronchiectasis.

Follow-up

Review in one to three months and repeat tests if indicated

Failure to control

Review diagnosis and consider rarer causes
Blood clotting disorder
Gastrointestinal bleeding
Inhaled foreign body

Referral

To control massive haemoptysis
To confirm or exclude serious causes:
tuberculosis
neoplasm
pulmonary embolism
bleeding disorder
trauma.

See also:

Chest pain – pulmonary embolism (p. 50)
Nose bleed (p. 219)
Chronic bronchitis (p. 440)
Pulmonary tuberculosis (p. 492)

Hair loss

Excessive loss of scalp hair is a socially embarassing condition, particularly for women.

The adult scalp contains around 100,000 hairs of which 20 to 100 are lost daily. Growth is dependent on hormonal influence. In women, oestrogens have a stimulant effect on scalp hair growth while androgens have an opposite effect. Axillary and pubic hair are dependent on adrenocortical androgen production in women, in men testosterone will contribute to growth in these areas. Testosterone has an inhibitory effect on the growth of male scalp hair; eunuchs rarely develop typical male baldness.

Patterns of hair loss

Diffuse loss

Male balding

This is extremely common and perhaps should not be considered abnormal. It occurs in the fronto-temporal regions and also at the vertex. It often begins in the late teenage years and is progressive.

Female balding

Diffuse hair loss occurs mainly from the vertex. It particularly affects middle-aged and elderly women. The cause is usually unknown but it can occur as a result of a constitutional disturbance such as hypothyroidism, iron deficiency or Addison's disease. Over-processing with perming lotions, bleach and heat may damage hair.

Telogen effluvium

Large numbers of hairs pass into the resting phase and are prematurely shed. It can occur after a pregnancy, a period of stress or febrile illness. Regrowth occurs in a few months.

Drugs

Cytotoxics
Excess vitamin A
Heparin.

Inflammatory dermatoses

Hair loss can occur in exceptional cases of seborrhoeic eczema or psoriasis. The trauma of scratching may be a contributing factor.

Patchy loss

Alopecia areata

This is a relatively common condition. It is of sudden onset and leads to round or oval patches of loss. The remaining hair stubbles have the appearance of exclamation marks. These are easily removed with the follicular bulb attached. The underlying skin may be pink but is not scaly. The patches may be multiple and include the eyebrows and beard area. Very occasionally all the body hair is affected (alopecia universalis). The larger the affected area the worse the prognosis.

Trichotillomania

Rubbing the scalp or pulling the hair can lead to bald patches particularly in children.

Congenital

There is complete absence of the hair follicle.

Secondary

A severe inflammatory response leads to scar formation and destruction of the hair follicle. This may be due to
burns
infections
irradiation
lichen planus
scleroderma
discoid lupus erythematosus.

History

Onset, duration and distribution of hair loss
Recent febrile illness, pregnancy or stress
Over-processing with hairdressing
Habit of hair pulling
Symptoms of constitutional disease (endocrine or iron deficiency)
Past history of skin or scalp disease
Family history of hair loss
Medication

Examination

Distribution of scalp hair loss
Associated body hair state
Check the condition of the scalp for disease or previous scarring
Signs of constitutional disease

Investigation

Rarely necessary but consider
Lost hair count after brushing on 4 consecutive days (>100 per day is abnormal)
Scalp scrapings and affected hairs for mycology
Thyroid function tests
Serum iron and TIBC
ANF and LE cells

Options

Reassurance – in telogen effluvium and minor forms of alopecia areata many will regrow in a few months
Steroids – topical steroids are helpful in seborrhoeic eczema and scalp psoriasis

Intradermal injection of steroids into the lesions of alopecia areata have been recommended but are rarely successful for long-term or more severe cases

Antifungal agents, e.g. griseofulvin 125 mg 6 hourly for one month for tinea capitis

Other specific therapy – as indicated for underlying disease (thyroxine, iron, etc).

Referral

Plastic surgery – can be helpful in patchy type of scarring alopecia if the area involved is small and the condition non-recurring

Psychiatric opinion – may be useful for patients with persistent trichotillomania

Wigs – may be all that can be offered for severe hair loss.

See also:

Hypothyroidism (p. 481)

Headache

The assessment of headache depends primarily on a careful and comprehensive history.

Tension headaches and migraine are the most common presentation in primary care. Serious intracerebral causes such as tumours are fortunately rare but must always be considered. Headaches are not a symptom of mild to moderate hypertension.

Serious causes

Sub-arachnoid haemorrhage (SAH)

Very sudden onset of severe pain. – 'like a kick in the head'. Photophobia and sometimes neck stiffness are associated features.

Meningitis or encephalitis

The onset is usually more gradual than SAH. There is usually associated fever, neck stiffness and possibly meningococcal rash. Drowsiness or focal signs carry a more grave prognosis.

Raised intracranial pressure

Usually secondary to sub-dural haematoma, cerebral tumour, abscess or hydrocephalus. Initially an aching pain, especially in the mornings and exacerbated by coughing or stooping. It may be associated with vomiting, dizziness, diplopia, visual disturbance or other focal symptoms. Gradual deterioration in time with the development of focal symptoms and signs including failing intellect, change in mood, convulsions, peripheral signs and drowsiness and finally coma.

Cranial arteritis

Non-specific constant or throbbing pain sometimes with local tenderness over the arteries. Tends to occur in patients over 60 years of age. There is an association with polymyalgia rheumatica. There is a risk of blindness from retinal artery thrombosis.

Other causes

Tension headaches

These are fronto-occipital or bitemporal and are described as a 'tight band', 'pressure' or 'fullness'. There is usually no pain on waking, but it tends to worsen towards the end of the day. It is not usually relieved by simple analgesics, but may be with alcohol. There is usually an association with stress or anxiety however it can also be a symptom of depression.

Tension headache should be a diagnosis of exclusion.

Migraine (see p. 203)
Facial pain (see p. 96)
Glaucoma (see p. 325)
Iritis (see p. 271)
Retrobulbar neuritis
Stroke (see p. 4[illegible])
Thyroid disorder (see p. 93)
Herpes zoster
Paget's disease of skull
Malignant hypertension
Fever
Dehydration
Hypoglycaemia
Syphilis
Post-epidural or lumbar puncture
Post-traumatic
Pre-menstrual
Alcohol
Tobacco
Caffeine

History

The headache

Onset
Periodicity
Site
Character

Duration
Precipitating factors
Relieving factors

Associated symptoms

Visual disturbance
Eye pain
Facial pain
Dental pain
Ear pain
Nasal congestion
Neurological symptoms
Depression
Weight loss
Myalgia
Waking at night
Head injury

Diet

Including alcohol, caffeine

Social and psychological factors

Smoking
Working conditions
Financial, family or marital stress
Health beliefs and fears of patient and family

Examination

Temperature
Hydration
Lymphadenopathy
Rash
BP
Cranial arteries
CNS examination
- consciousness level
- pupil response
- neck stiffness
- Kernig's sign
- fundi
- photophobia
- localizing signs
- visual activity

Investigation

FBC
ESR
U & E
LFT
Blood glucose

Thyroid function tests
Syphilis serology
X-ray – skull and nasal sinuses

Options

Simple analgesics, e.g. aspirin and paracetamol
Psychotherapy
Relaxation techniques
tranquillizers, e.g. diazepam 2–5 mg 6–8 hourly for a limited period
Antibiotics and decongestants in sinusitis
Idoxuridine may be helpful if started early in Herpes zoster infections
Steroids in temporal arteritis
Anti-migraine treatment (see p. 203).

Referral

Suspicion of more serious causes requires urgent hospital referral for
raised intracranial pressure
subarachnoid haemorrhage
meningitis
A history suggestive of temporal arteritis may need referral for urgent biopsy before starting steroids (certainly within 24 h of starting treatment)
A significant head injury with loss of consciousness or amnesia may need observation for 24 hours
If glaucoma is suspected referral is necessary for tonometry
If a tumour is suspected a neurological opinion may be necessary
Children with headaches of uncertain origin should be referred.

See also:

Blisters (p. 29)
Facial pain (p. 96)
Fever (p. 106)
Food allergy (p. 113)
Influenza (p. 167)
Migraine (p. 203)
Pre-menstrual syndrome (p. 257)
Red eye (p. 271)
STD (p. 301)
Stress and anxiety (p. 303)
Visual loss (p. 325)
Hypertension (p. 475)
Stroke (p. 497)
Head injury (p. 523)
Hypoglycaemia (p. 525)

Hearing loss

Deafness implies any degree of hearing loss. 1–2 in every 1000 liveborn babies are deaf, 10,000 children are in special schools for the deaf in this country and between 60 and 160 in every 1000 adults will become deaf at some point in their lives.

In conductive deafness there is a disruption of transmission of the sound waves between the inner and outer ear.

In sensorineural deafness the defect is proximal to the oval window involving the cochlea, the VIIIth cranial nerve or the central pathways.

There is an opportunity for case finding and prevention of deafness during routine development checks in the first years of life and by careful checking of all ear infections during the first 10 years.

Causes

Conductive

Obstruction in the external canal
- wax
- otitis externa
- foreign body
- cholesteatoma
- tumour
- atresia

Damage to the ear drum
- infection
- trauma
- pressure changes

Discontinuity in the ossicular chain
- otitis media
- trauma

Immobility in the ossicular chain
- otosclerosis
- tympanosclerosis

Obstruction in the eustachian tube
- secretory otitis media
- 'glue ear'
- adenoidal hypertrophy in children
- carcinoma of the nasopharynx in adults

Sensorineural

Bilateral
- Ageing – presbycusis
- Noise – acoustic trauma

Ototoxic drugs
- i.v. diuretics
- salicylates – reversible
- aminoglycosides – neomycin/streptomycin/gentamycin

Infective
- measles
- mumps

Congenital
- teratogenic drugs
- rubella
- birth trauma
- anoxia
- kernicterus

Unilateral
- Menière's disease
- Acoustic neuroma
- Syphilis

History

Onset and duration of symptoms
- hearing loss
- tinnitus
- dizziness
- pain trauma
- foreign body discharge

Maternal suspicion of hearing loss

Age

Occupation

Leisure pursuits

Medication

Risk factors
- family history of deafness
- complicated pregnancy
- complicated perinatal period
- cerebral palsy
- speech defects

Family attitude to deafness

Examination

Examination of drums, external canal, nose and pharynx

Routine screening at 8 months, 3 years and 5 years

'Startle test' watch for response to sudden loud noise

'Distraction test' 3 tones (e.g. cup and spoon, paper and voice) are sounded 3 metres behind and to one side of the child, who must first be distracted by a third party. He will then turn to the side from which the sound is coming

Tuning fork tests (tuning fork of 512 Hz)

Rinne's test

Compares intensity of sound through external canal AC (air conduction) and mastoid process BC (bone conduction)

negative = BC > AC = conduction defect

positive = AC > BC = conduction normal

Weber's test

Tuning fork placed over the midline of the skull

sound lateralizes to the ear with a conductive loss

sound lateralizes away from the ear with a sensorineural loss.

Investigation

FBC

ESR

Viral studies

Serology for syphilis

X-ray internal auditory meatus

Pure tone audiometry (125–8000 Hz) hearing loss of 40 db in any frequency is significant (see Fig. 1.2)

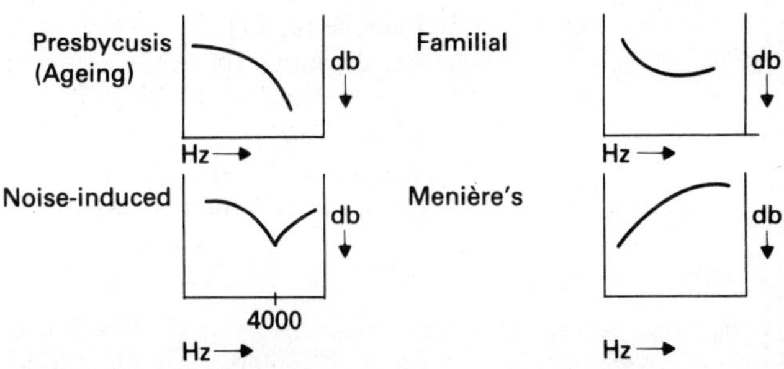

Fig. 1.2. Characteristic patterns in pure tone audiometry

Options

Syringe wax

Antibiotics for otitis media

Decongestants (see p. 288) for eustachian tube obstruction

Ear drops

If infections are acute or grommets *in situ* avoid swimming

Treat underlying disease for otitis externa

Advise families on lip-reading, adjustments to TV, telephones, etc.

Avoid ototoxic drugs.

Referral

Suspicion of hearing loss – for audiometry and assessment for hearing-aid
Conductive deafness – for surgical assessment and management
Sudden onset of unilateral sensorineural deafness – to exclude
acoustic neuroma
syphilis
perilymph fistula
If educational difficulties are involved – seek the advice of Special Schools for the Deaf
For general advice and support – seek the advice of the Royal National Institute for the Deaf.

Complications

Associated tinnitus
Speech defects
Social and emotional isolation
Depression

See also:

Catarrh (p. 38)
Depression (p. 63)
Dizziness (p. 73)
Earache (p. 77)
Ear discharge (p. 80)
Speech disorder (p. 291)
STD (p. 301)
Tinnitus (p. 314)
Common infectious disease in children (p. 402)

Heart murmurs

Extra heart sounds and murmurs may be suspected by deduction from the pattern of presenting symptoms and signs. More often they are detected incidentally or at routine screening examination. Once detected all murmurs should be carefully and systematically assessed.

Primary causes

Congenital malformation
Atheroma
Rheumatic fever
Endocarditis
Syphilis
'Floppy valve'

Other causes

Marfan's syndrome
Carcinoid syndrome
Dissecting aneurysm
Ankylosing spondylitis

History

Cardiovascular symptoms
- shortness of breath
- chest pain
- palpitations
- ankle oedema
- orthopnoea

Pyrexia
Previous suspicion of murmurs by other doctors
Previous history of
- rheumatic fever
- neonatal cyanosis
- growth retardation

Gestational diabetes during mother's pregnancy
Social and psychological implications of any symptoms – e.g. 'hole in the heart'

Examination

Inspect
- Visible pulsation on the chest
- JVP
- Ankle oedema
- Cyanosis or anaemia
- Splinter haemorrhages

Palpate
- Apex beat for site and pressure
- Thrills
- Enlarged liver

Auscultate

Heart sounds (Table 1.7)
Murmurs – timing, site, loudness (Table 1.7)
Added sounds
- opening snap
- friction rub
- prosthetic valves

Positions of patient
- reclining position (45° to horizontal)
- left lateral after exercise (mitral stenosis)
- leaning forward in expiration (aortic incompetence – murmur will be accentuated after exercise)

Table 1.6. Heart sounds

Sound	Best site	Origin
I	Apex	Closure of mitral and tricuspid valves
'Ejection' click	Upper sternum	Opening of aortic and pulmonary valves
II	2 LICS	Closure of aortic and pulmonary valves
'Opening snap'	Apex to 4 LICS	Opening of mitral and tricuspid valves
III	Apex	Left ventricular filling
IV	Apex	Atrial contraction

Leaning forward in expiration (aortic incompetence – murmur will be accentuated after exercise)

Heart murmurs

Grades of loudness (see Table 1.7)

- I barely audible
- II soft
- III moderately loud
- IV loud
- V very loud
- VI no stethoscope needed

Less common murmurs

Systolic

- Tricuspid incompetence
- Coarctation

Diastolic

- Tricuspid stenosis
- Pulmonary incompetence
- Increased atrio-ventricular flow in ventricular septal defect
- Persistent ductus arteriosus
- Atrial septal defect

Continuous

- Venous hum (in children)
- Aorto-pulmonary septal defect
- Combined AS and AI
  - MI and AI

Table 1.7. Heart murmurs

Timing	Site and radiation	Thrill	Origin	Associated features
Mid-systolic	2RICS and apex neck	2 RICS 3 LICS 4 LICS	Aortic stenosis	A loud murmur. Reduces with inspiration. LVH and AI often associated
	2 LICS	Left parasternal heave	Pulmonary stenosis	Reduced pulmonary 2nd sound. Increases with inspiration. Check for Fallot's tetralogy
	2 LICS		Atrial septal defect	Common in neonates Fixed splitting of second sound
Pan-systolic	Apex to axilla	Apex	Mitral incompetence	Check for 3rd sound. Reduces in inspiration. LVH and MS often associated
	3 LICS 4 LICS	3 LICS 4 LICS	Ventricular Septal defect	Loud 'rough' murmur
Diastolic	2 LICS 3 RICS to apex		Aortic incompetence	'Blowing' murmur
	Apex	Apex	Mitral stenosis	'Rumbling', opening snap presystolic accentuation. Loud first sound. Reduces in inspiration
Continuous	2 LICS 3 LICS in M.C.L	Left sternal edge	Persistent ductus arteriosus	'Machinery murmur' Maximal in late systole

'The innocent murmur'

This is a common occurence in childhood particularly in febrile children. It may also occur in pregnancy, anaemia or hyperthyroidism
- maximal in pulmonary area
- not loud – grades I or II – no thrill
- no pan-systolic
- no cardiac enlargement
- no abnormal heart sounds
- no associated symptoms or signs
- variable with changes in posture

Referral

Refer all cases, except the most obviously 'innocent murmurs', for cardiological opinion.

See also:

Heart mumurs in children (p. 425)

Heavy periods

Menorrhagia is excessive vaginal blood loss, either heavy or prolonged. It is usually a feature of the early menopause, although it can also occur in younger age groups. When menstruation is irregular both in timing and volume, uterine pathology must be considered.

Causes

Dysfunctional uterine bleeding
Fibroids
IUCD
Early pregnancy
Chronic pelvic infection
Cervical polyp
Cervical erosion
Endometriosis
Carcinoma of uterus
Carcinoma of cervix
Thyroid disorder (hypothyroidism)
Hypothalamic disorder

History

Menstrual history
Assessment of blood loss
Patient's tolerance of the blood loss
Gynaecological and obstetric history
Social and psychological factors
Other endocrine symptoms
Details of any hormone therapy

Examination

BP
Anaemia
Pelvic examination

Investigation

FBC + platelets
ESR + platelets
LFT
Thyroid function tests
Cervical smear

Emergency care

Assess shock
Assess blood loss
Establish i.v. line
Transfer to gynaecological unit

Options

Prostaglandin synthetase inhibitors – e.g. mefaminic acid 250 mg 8 hourly
Antifibronolytis – e.g. amino caproic acid 3 g 6 hourly
Progestogens – e.g. norethisterone 5 mg 8 hourly
The Pill (after exclusion of organic disease or pregnancy)
Antigonadotrophins – e.g. danazol 200–800 mg 6 or 12 hourly
Iron preparations – e.g. ferrous gluconate 300 mg 12 hourly.

Follow-up

Menstrual charts
FBC + clotting factors
Review social and psychological factors

Failure to control

Check for
Liver disease
Pituitary disorder
Clotting defect
Psychiatric disorder

Referral

Symptoms affecting life style
Suspected carcinoma of uterus
Investigation of clotting defect.

See also:

Menopause (p. 199)
Hypothyroidism (p. 481)
Vaginal bleeding in pregnancy (p. 544)

The hip

The hip joint is the site of disease and occasionally major disability both for adults and children. Pain and stiffness are the predominant symptoms. Hip pain may radiate to the groin, the thigh and the knees; similarly pain from other structures may radiate to the region of the hip making accurate diagnosis difficult. In children hip pathology commonly presents as knee pain.

Cause of hip pain

Children
- Congenital dislocation of the hip (CDH)
- Irritable hip
- Perthes' disease
- Slipped epiphysis
- Septic arthritis

Adults
- Osteoarthritis
- Rheumatoid arthritis
- Septic arthritis
- Bursitis
- Polymyalgia rheumatica
- Fracture and dislocation
- Osteomalcia and osteoporosis
- Paget's disease
- Avascular necrosis
- Ankylosing spondylitis
- Reiter's syndrome
- Psoriasis
- Tumours

Referred pain
- Lumbar spine disc disorders
- Sacro-iliac disease
- Pelvic inflammation
- Aorto-iliac vascular disease

History

Onset duration and severity of pain

Exacerbating and relieving factors especially rest and exercise

Site and radiation of pain
- groin
- buttock
- thigh
- knee

Associated symptoms
- delayed development in children

limb stiffness
disturbed sleep
effect on ADL and mobility

History of trauma

Examination

Inspect
Gait
Scars and skin changes
Pelvic and spinal symmetry
Trendelenburg test

Measure
Leg lengths

Palpate
Bony prominences, including pubic rami, abdomen, and femoral canals
Test for dislocation in infants
Active and passive movements

Check
Multiple injuries or fractures after trauma

Patterns of presentation

Congenital dislocation of the hip (CDH)

This is found in 1–2 per 1000 newborn babies, but there are racial and cultural variations which relate to the mode of carrying new-born babies. It is more common in females (6:1) and can be familial. All newborn babies should be screened for instability of the hip joint using Ortolani's test and the 'telescoping' test.

The sooner the condition is discovered the easier the treatment and better the outcome. Irreversible changes occur if the hip remains dislocated.

In the older child there is more obvious limitation of abduction in flexion, limb shortening and altered skin creases. The child usually exhibits delay in walking, or later, a 'waddling' gait. Bilateral CDH can easily be missed as there is no apparent asymmetry.

Treatment is left to the orthopaedic specialist; in the younger child a splint will often suffice. In the older child traction or operative intervention may be necessary.

Irritable hip

This occurs in children, most often in boys, and sometimes following an injury although there is frequently a history of URT viral illness. The child complains of pain in the hip, thigh or knee and often limps. There is limitation in the range of movement, particularly abduction in flexion. Investigations are all normal; treatment is with bed-rest for a few days. Referral is usually necessary to exclude other important diagnoses including septic arthritis.

Perthe's disease

This is an avascular necrosis of the upper femoral epiphysis thought to be due to vascular occlusion, probably as the result of repeated trauma.

It occurs predominantly in boys aged 5–10 years. The patient limps and complains of hip pain. There is a limited range of movement particularly of abduction in flexion. The diagnosis is made on X-ray changes.

Treatment is by rest, splintage and occasionally by operation, depending on severity of progress. The disease process lasts 2–3 years, and if left untreated it can lead to joint deformity and severe degenerative changes. The prognosis is variable but tends to be more severe in older children.

Slipped femoral epiphysis

In this condition the upper femoral epiphysis slips down on the femoral neck in the line of the growth plate. It may become bilateral in 30% of cases.

It occurs towards the end of puberty and again is more common in boys, who are often overweight during this period of development. It can occur in association with hypothyroidism and vitamins D and C deficiency.

The patient complains of pain and limps. In more acute cases it may present like a fracture.

Damage to the blood supply to the femoral head may lead to avascular necrosis. Treatment is by operation and requires urgent referral with advice to avoid weight-bearing on the affected leg.

Trauma

In the elderly, metabolic bone disease may predispose to the fracture of the hip; a common result of falling. Pain is not always severe and a full assessment is essential after any fall.

The signs are leg shortening with external rotation pain, crepitus on movement, and bruising and swelling in the thigh. Check for associated fractures in the pelvis, ribs and arms, and crush fractures of the vertebrae. Also check for the effects of blood loss.

The same signs are evident in younger patients especially after a road traffic accident when multiple fractures, internal injuries and head injuries must also be considered.

All suspected cases should be immobilized and transferred to an accident unit with due attention to analgesia and shock

Avascular necrosis

Avascular necrosis of the head of the femur can follow
- trauma
- liver disease or pancreatitis
- alcoholism
- pregnancy
- steroid therapy
- haemoglobinopathies.

In many cases no cause is found. Patients present with incapacitating pain and limitation of movement. Diagnosis is confirmed by X-ray although radiological signs may not be obvious in the early stages.

In the young, conservative measures include rest and non weight-bearing; in the older patient total hip replacement is indicated.

See also:

Knee (p. 179)
Localized rash (p. 185)
Children that limp (p. 399)
Osteoarthritis (p. 485)
Rheumatoid arthritis (p. 493)

Hirsutism

In our culture hairiness is a symbol of masculinity and as a corollary western society imposes unreasonable and inhibiting stress on the hairy woman.

The doctor must be alert to the pathological features and associations of hirsutism but there is rarely a treatable medical cause for the condition. Sympathetic advice on the cosmetic solutions is often the most that can be offered.

'Idiopathic hirsutism'

Common features
- starts at the menarche
- normal secondary sexual characteristics
- regular periods
- facial hair predominates
- family history
- racial variation – especially Mediterranean women

Associated conditions

Pregnancy
Menopause
Obesity
Anorexia nervosa
Acne
Cushing's disease
Acromegaly
Ovarian tumours
Intersex status
Drugs
- Phenytoin
- Androgens
- Streptomycin
- Steroids

History

Menarche
Menstrual history
Family history
Social, psychological and cultural factors
Medication

Examination

Distribution of hair
Weight
BP
Distribution of fat
Skeletal and muscular form
Skin lesions
Pelvic examination

Options

Education on the condition
Advice on depilatories
- electrolysis
- wax
- creams
- shaving
- plucking
- abrasives

Advice on bleaching darker hair
Steroid/oestrogen/progestogen preparations (after discussion with endocrinologist).

Referral

Associated amenorrhoea
Associated virilism
- enlarged larynx
- enlarged clitoris
- muscular 'male' form

excessive hair on the trunk
Pre-pubertal hirsutism
Hirsutism starting in early middle-age
Idiopathic hirsutism for reassurance (as indicated by patient's anxiety).

See also:

Anorexia (p. 12)
Menopause (p. 199)
Obesity (p. 224)
Spots (p. 294)

Hoarseness

Hoarseness usually indicates disease of the larynx and may vary from a mild disturbance of phonation to an almost total loss of voice.

The acute condition is usually self-limiting, but chronic laryngitis, lasting more than four weeks, should be referred to exclude a laryngeal carcinoma.

In children laryngitis presents as croup (see p. 537).

Causes

Inflammatory
- primary viral infection
- secondary bacterial infection
- trauma, e.g. shouting excessively
- abuse of alcohol and tobacco

Neoplastic
- squamous cell carcinoma (more common in men than women)

Neurological
- vagus nerve palsy
- recurrent laryngeal nerve palsy

'Hysterical aphonia'

Other causes

Inflammatory
- Mouth breathing
- Allergies
- Toxic fumes
- Polyp
- Singer's nodule
- Hypertrophy of false cords
- Hyperkeratosis of true cords
- Tertiary (gummatous) syphilis
- TB

Benign tumours
- Papilloma
- Chondroma
- Haemangioma
- Cylindroma

Arthritis of laryngeal joints

History

Onset and duration of symptoms
Associated symptoms
- fever
- malaise
- dysphagia
- cough
- pain in ear

History of ENT or chest disease or surgery to the neck
Alcohol or tobacco
Occupation and leisure pursuits, e.g. singing, football

Examination

Temperature and cervical lymphadenopathy
Nasal obstruction
Post-nasal discharge
Mouth-breathing
Thyroid status
Indirect laryngoscopy

Investigation

FBC
ESR
Thyroid function tests
Nasal and throat swabs
X-ray chest and paranasal sinuses
Barium swallow

Options

Self help
- rest the larynx – stop talking!
- humidify atmosphere
- steam inhalations

Avoid alcohol and tobacco
Antibiotics – rarely indicated
Treat associated
- sinusitis
- nasal polypi
- carious teeth
- chronic bronchitis
- TB.

Referral

All cases with persistent hoarseness after 6 weeks for assessment and speech therapy.

Follow-up

Regular follow-up for patients with tracheostomy to help rehabilitation after laryngectomy

See also:

Sore throat (p. 289)
Respiratory distress – croup (p. 537)

Hypochondriasis

Hypochondriasis is a persistent, anxious pre-occupation with health or illness. The patient may actually have a physical disorder but the concern is out of proportion to the implications of the underlying condition. It may dominate the life style of the patients and their families. It commonly occurs in association with anxiety or depression. When the tendencies are life-long it may be regarded as a specific personality disorder.

It is more common among men, the elderly and the lower social classes.

Assessment of hypochondriacal symptoms

Pain
- Head
- Lower lumbar region
- RIF

Gastrointestinal symptoms
- Nausea
- Dysphagia
- Regurgitation of acid
- Bad taste in the mouth
- Flatulence
- Abdominal pain

Cardiovascular symptoms
- Palpitations
- Left-sided chest pain
- Shortness of breath
- Worries about blood pressure

Other
- Sweating
- Body shape or appearance

Examination

As appropriate for reassurance

Options

Treat underlying depression or anxiety

Support

Sympathetic understanding of the patient's suffering, but try to deflect attention away from symptoms to discuss the possible underlying problems which might be causing the symptoms. Occasionally the symptoms are a defence against overwhelming feelings of personal inadequacy. To expose this may lead to a serious depressive illness.

Caution: hypochondriacs can develop real physical illness.

See also: Depression (p. 63)
Stress and anxiety (p. 303)

Hypothermia

Hypothermia is a body temperature of less than 35°C recorded by a low reading thermometer inserted rectally for 5 minutes. Hypothermia can occur in an adequately heated environment and will only be detected if the doctor is alert to the possibility. The elderly are most commonly affected but hypothermia is a significant complication in the newborn, in victims of road traffic accidents and, of course, in exposure.

The mortality is 50% with body temperatures below 32°C; hypothermia must be considered a medical emergency.

Causes

Environmental
Exposure to cold with inadequate clothing or insulation

Inadequate thermoregulation
- Immature mechanism in neonates
- Head injury
- Coma
- Stroke
- Parkinsonism
- Dementia

Impaired metabolism
- Hypothyroid
- Pituitary failure
- Addison's disease

Medication
- Phenothiazines
- Barbiturates
- Antidepressants
- Benzodiazepines
- Alcohol

Illness
- Immobility – arthritis, neurological disease

- Weight loss
- Anaemia
- Pneumonia
- Myocardial infarction
- CCF

Psychological

- Loneliness
- Depression

Social

- Housing
- Isolation
- Neglect
- Poverty

History

From both patient and family (or attendants)
Symptoms of associated conditions
Social circumstances
Psychological factors
Drugs – consider abuse

Examination

Rectal temperature
- low reading thermometer for 5 minutes
- record ambient temperature

Skin temperature
- abdominal skin feels cold 'like marble'

Level of consciousness
Cardiovascular signs
- arrhythmia
- bradycardia
- hypotension

Respiratory rate – slow
Signs of hypothyroidism
CNS signs
- extensor plantar response
- increased muscle tone
- slurred speech
- tremor
- sluggish pupil response

Investigation

FBC
ESR
Thyroid function tests
Electrolytes
CXR
ECG

Options

Emergency care (see p. 526)

Home care is appropriate if rectal temperature is more than 32°C, if room temperature is 25–28°C, and if there is adequate supervision available.
Slow rewarm with blankets and hot drinks (0.5°C per hour)
Monitor rectal temperature, pulse and BP
Antibiotics
Steroids, e.g. 100 mg hydrocortisone i.v. 4 times daily
No alcohol or vasodilators which can increase mortality
Treat hypothyroidism
Advice on prevention
- clothing
- insulation
- heating and fuels
- visitors and family
- financial help.

Referral

To hospital
- temperature less than 32°C
- coma
- arrhythmia
- cardiac failure
- overdose of drugs
- stroke
- respiratory difficulty
- head injury

To social worker for advice and supervision.

Follow-up

Review social circumstances
Plan routine visiting especially during cold weather – recurrence is common

Complications

Recurrence – especially during cold weather
Hypothermic cardiac arrest is reversible
Death
Hypotension during rewarming – stop the rewarming till BP is stable
Arrhythmia during rewarming – stop the rewarming till pulse is stable
Coma
Inhalation of vomit

Imported disease

Imported disease in this context implies infectious diseases carried into the UK by travellers; it does not include the health hazards of canned disease (e.g. botulism) nor deep-frozen disease (e.g. in meat).

Traveller diseases such as jet lag and motion sickness are not discussed.

History

Onset and duration of symptoms

Fever
Weight loss
Abdominal pain
Muscle pain
Skin lesions
Lymphoedema
Diarrhoea
Worms
Rectal bleeding
Haematuria
Asthma
Red eye

Travel details

Itinerary
Duration of travel
Mode of travel
Sanitation
Water supplies
Food and drink
Contact with disease
Immunization status
Medication – especially malaria prophylaxis
Self care
Contacts in UK

Examination

Record

Temperature
Weight
BP
Fundi appearance
Hydration state

Check for

Skin changes
Spleen enlargement
Neurological signs

Jaundice
Anaemia

Investigation

FBC
ESR
Blood film for eosinophilia
Thick film for malarial parasites
U & E
LFT
Hepatitis B antigen
Fresh stool culture and microscopy ('Sellotape slide')
CXR
IVP
Skin biopsy if leprosy is suspected

Referral

To infectious disease unit for immediate isolation or for further investigation.

Prevention

The World Health Organization emphasizes the importance of prevention in the primary medical care of diseases such as schistosomiasis. This implies a need for political and social change in developing countries to improve water supplies and maintain eradication programmes before medical measures in primary care can be effective.

In the UK prevention will only succeed with careful surveillance of travellers to and from affected countries, and with effective measures for immunization and prophylaxis.

Immunization practice is constantly changing with the changing recommendations for different countries. Advice on immunization should be based on current information.

Prophylaxis is essential for travellers to endemic malarial zones and details of drugs and dosage will depend on destination and duration of stay. All travellers from non-endemic areas should take prophylaxis (including recent immigrants returning to their country of origin).

Filariasis

Wuchereria bancrofti
Brugia malayi
Brugia tumori
Found in Africa, Indonesia, Australia, Central and South America.
3 months incubation (minimal).
Characteristic 'elephantiasis' of legs and genitalia, eye involvement, pulmonary eosinophilia, fever, itching, sub-cutaneous swellings.

Treatment with diethylcarbamazine in specialist care (risk of anaphylaxis.

Onchocerca volvulus with its ocular lesions is a disease of major international importance.

Schistosomiasis

Schistosoma japonicum
Schistosoma haematobium
Schistosoma mansoni

Found in N. Africa, S. America, Asia and Middle East.

4–6 weeks incubation.

Transmitted in water, it starts with an itchy rash, and is followed by fever with enlargement of the liver and spleen. Portal hypertension follows and then CNS involvement.

Diagnosed by microscopy of blood (eosinophilia), stool and urine, cystoscopy and sigmoidoscopy

Treatment with Niridazole or antimony compounds.

Trypanosomiasis

Tsetse fly in Central, East and W. Africa – 'Sleeping Sickness'.

'Triatomids in S. America – 'Chagas' disease'.

2 weeks to 3 months incubation.

Non-immune presentation is of malaria-like illness not responding to chloroquine with associated chancre, and spleen and liver enlargement.

Immune presentation is asymptomatic in the first stage then headache, fever, LAP, lethargy, tremor and dizziness supervene.

Diagnosis by serology and thick film microscopy

Treatment with arsenic compounds, Suramin or Pentamidine.

Leishmaniasis

Mediterranean, Central and South Africa, Central and South America and Indonesia – 'Kala-Azar'.

2–4 months incubation.

Fever is intermittent and associated with sweating, marked liver and spleen enlargement, weight loss, anaemia, leucopenia, skin pigmentation and ulceration.

Treatment is with antimony compounds.

There is 70% mortality in untreated cases.

Leprosy

Mycobacterium leprae

Worldwide distribution of major importance.

Incubation period of months or years.

Onset is insidious with nerve or skin lesions, especially depigmentation. The spectrum of presentations lies between tuberculoid (nerve involvement greater than

skin involvement) and lepromatous (skin involvement greater than nerve involvement). A combination of these features carries the worst prognosis.
Assessment and treatment requires specialist units.

Malaria

Worldwide except Europe, USSR, USA and Australasia.
10–14 days incubation.
Presenting symptoms include cyclical fevers and chills, sweating and tachycardia. Signs include jaundice and spleen and liver enlargement.
Infection by *Plasmodium falciparum* can result in haemolysis, renal failure, LVF and coma. It is potentially fatal.
Treatment with chloroquine, quinine and other drugs.
Prophylaxis for *all* travellers visiting endemic areas.

Polio

Worldwide distribution.
3–21 days incubation.
Mild polio is a flu-like illness
Paralytic polio presents with meningitis, personality changes, flaccid paralysis, asymmetrical signs but no sensory involvement.
Diagnosis by stool and CSF culture.
Prevention by immunization.

Yellow fever

Group B Arbovirus
Africa and Central and South America.
3–6 days incubation.
Mild form – flu-like illness with fever and headache
Severe form – sudden onset of fever headache and petechial haemorrhages, followed in 3–4 days by abdominal pain, vomiting, jaundice and generalized bleeding
50% mortality – with renal failure, heart failure, hypothermia and septicaemia.
Supportive care and bed rest.
Immunization for all travellers to endemic areas.

Rabies

Rhabdovirus
UK, Scandinavia, Australasia, Japan and Antarctica are rabies-free areas.
A flu-like illness progressing to hydrophobia, fits, excitability and coma or paralysis.
Rabies encephalomyelitis is fatal.

Full surgical toilet of animal bite wounds, heavy sedation and intensive nursing is required.

Post-exposure vaccination in infectious disease units is now advised in all suspicious cases.

Hepatitis A

Worldwide distribution especially where area has poor sanitation.

2–6 weeks incubation.

Malaise, anorexia, weight loss and fever are followed after 4–5 days by obstructive jaundice, itching and liver enlargement.

Manage with rest and careful hygeine. Avoid alcohol and drugs metabolized by the liver for 2 months after clinical recovery.

Prevention by treatment with human immunoglobulin before exposure.

Anthrax

Bacillus anthracis

Found in Africa and India.

2–5 days incubation.

Presentation with isolated oedematous necrotic but painless ulcers, complicated by haemorrhagic bullous lesions, gross oedema and renal failure

Treatment with i.m. penicillins or streptomycin.

Prevention by vaccination.

Legionnaires disease

Legionella pneumophilia

The symptoms of fever, sweating, anorexia, and weight loss progress to a productive cough and mental confusion. This is complicated by respiratory failure, arrhythmia and renal failure.

Treatment with erythromycin early in the illness.

Typhus

Worldwide wherever there are lice.

1–2 weeks incubation.

Initial flu-like illness with haemorrhagic maculo-papular rash progresses to confusion, weakness, hypotension and spleen enlargement.

If recovery occurs there are no sequelae.

Cholera

Vibrio cholerae

Found in the tropics and subtropics.

1–6 days incubation.

Painless profuse diarrhoea, vomiting and muscle cramps.
Immunization gives 60–80% immunity for 6 months.
Treatment by fluid and electrolyte replacement.

Plague

Yersinia pestis
Found in Indonesia.
2–5 days incubation.
Sudden onset of oedematous LAP – the 'bubo' – with headache, anorexia, vomiting and delirium.
Treatment with tetracyclines or chloramphenicol and streptomycin. Supportive care is of importance.
Pneumonic plague presents with viral illness, haemoptysis and rapid deterioration.

Flukes

Fasciola hepatica
Worldwide distribution.
Fever, abdominal pain and liver enlargement are associated with eosinophilia.
Diagnosis is by stool culture.
Treatment is with bithionol.

Amoebiasis

Entamoeba histolytica
Found in the tropics and subtropics, in areas with poor water supplies.
21 day incubation period.
Intestinal amoebiasis gives mild abdominal symptoms or severe symptoms with colonic ulceration, amoebomata and rectal bleeding.
Hepatic amoebiasis is insidious in onset with malaise, liver enlargement and pulmonary and cerebral involvement.
Diagnosis by stool culture, serology, barium enema and liver scan.

Hydatid disease

Echinococcus granulosus
Found in the tropics and subtropics.
1 week to 1 year incubation period.
Allergic manifestations and cyst formation in gut, liver and lungs and the CNS.
Treatment in specialist units.

See also: Infections and parasites from pets (p. 165)
Worms (p. 339)

Indigestion

The patient complaining of indigestion may be suffering from a variety of symptoms. The combination may vary from patient to patient. Usual complaints include

- right hypochondrial, epigastric or restrosternal discomfort
- bloatedness
- wind
- anorexia
- nausea and vomiting
- flatulence

It is very difficult to evalute the pathology involved but it is usually attributed to increased gastric tone, hyperacidity, aerophagy and oesophageal reflux.

The cause may be a functional problem and so psychological factors must be considered. However this diagnosis is usually made by exclusion of other possible underlying causes.

Causes

- Peptic ulceration
- Cholelithiasis
- Reflux oesophagitis
- Ischaemic heart disease
- Pancreatitis
- Irritable bowel syndrome
- Intra-abdominal malignancy (oesophageal, gastric, pancreatic or large bowel)
- Mesenteric ischaemia
- Drinking problems
- Smoking

History

- Duration and severity of symptoms
- Pain and radiation
- Associated symptoms
  - weight loss
  - stress
  - wind
  - change in bowel habit
- Precipitating and relieving factors

Relationship with
- food
- coffee or tea
- alcohol
- smoking
- posture
- current life events

Family history and health beliefs
Medication

Examination

Check for
- Anaemia
- Jaundice
- Lymphadenopathy (Virchow's node)

Palpate abdomen for
- Tenderness
- Enlarged liver
- Enlarged kidney
- Enlarged spleen

Assess mental state

Investigation

Consider
- FBC
- ESR
- LFT
- barium meal or endoscopy
- cholecystogram
- chest X-ray
- ECG
- ultrasound of pancreas and gall bladder
- barium enema

Options

Simple advice about diet, regular meals and restriction of alcohol, tobacco and irritant drugs (e.g. aspirin). For reflux oesophagitis recommend upright posture, avoiding stooping, and sleeping propped up

Antacids: are often used as a therapeutic trial and may relieve some of the symptoms, e.g. magnesium trisilicate mixture B.P. 10 ml 6–8 hourly

Antiflatulants may relieve distressing wind, e.g. Peppermint water

Antispasmodics may relieve some of the pain particularly in irritable bowel syndrome, e.g. mebeverine (Colofac) 135 mg 8 hourly, hyoscine (Buscopan) 20 mg 6 hourly

Increased roughage (the popular panacea!), e.g. bran, Normacol, advice on intake of dietary fibre

H_2 antagonists, e.g. ranitidine 150 mg 12 hourly after objective evidence of peptic ulceration

Psychological assessment and support – many patients, presenting with these symptoms have an underlying anxiety state, dependent personality or alcohol problem. These difficulties must be tactfully explored and dealt with appropriately. Often the placebo effect of antacids coupled with a sympathetic explanation of the symptoms is all that is required.

Referral

Further investigation such as endoscopy
Specialist treatment of more serious causes
Detoxification of the alcoholic patient.

See also:

Anorexia (p. 12)
Chest pain – angina pectoris (p. 43)

Infections and parasites from pets

Several animals both in the UK and abroad share their parasites with man. Air travel enables rapid importation of some of these parasites but the following table includes parasites endemic to the UK.

Tetanus

Clostridium tetani

Worldwide distribution.

Early malaise and fever with dysphagia and 'lock jaw', progresses to rigidity and the classic syndrome.

Treatment by prophylactic penicillin and intensive care.

Prevention by immunization with anti-tetanus toxoid and thorough cleaning of all wounds.

Brucellosis

Brucella abortus

Found in the UK and Australia (other strains found in N. America and the Mediterranean).

Incubation period 7–12 days.

Acute forms of the disease last 2–3 weeks with fever and fatigue, headaches, sweats and joint pains.

Chronic forms of the disease include periods of fever and fatigue, headaches, backache and depression.

Treatment by tetracyclines.

Table 1.8. Hosts and parasites

	Dogs	Cats	Birds	Fish	Horses	Cows	Sheep	Goats	Pigs	Rats and mice
Fleas	x	x								
Leptospirosis	x					x			x	x
Toxocara	x	x								
Microsporum canis V	x	x								
Rabies	x									
Cat scratch fever		x								
Ornithosis (including psittacosis)			x							
Salmonella				x						
Tape worm				x		x			x	
Tetanus					x	x	x			
Brucellosis						x	x	x	x	
Anthrax						x	x			
Flukes						x	x			
Trychophyton						x				
Verrucosum (ringworm)						x				
Hyatid disease							x			
Orf							x	x		

Orf

Worldwide distribution affecting sheep handlers.
Self-limiting vesicular lesions on the hands which become crusted over within 2 weeks. There is associated fever and LAP.

Ornithosis

Chlamydia
Worldwide distribution.
Initial flu-like illness with pneumonia can be complicated by myocarditis and cardiac failure.
Treatment by tetracycline early in the illness.

Leptospirosis

Leptospira interrogans
Worldwide distribution.
The initial flu-like illness of 4–7 days is associated with headache, vomiting, photophobia, muscle aches, fever and meningism. It may be complicated by jaundice, haemorrhage, renal failure and visual failure.
Treatment with i.m. penicillins.

Toxocara

Toxocara canis
Affects children
Flu-like illness which may be complicated by involvement of the liver, spleen, heart, lungs, muscles, eyes and brain.
Diagnosis is by blood film (eosinophilia) and tissue biopsy.
Treatment is with thiabendazole.

See also:

Imported disease (p. 157)

Influenza

The viral illness caused by the myxoviruses, influenza A, B and C, occurs in epidemics usually 2–3 years apart and more rarely as a devastating pandemic. The changing antigen characteristics of the viruses make eradication programmes impracticable and even the anticipatory programmes of immunization are of unproven value.

The pattern of presentation is consistent and the diagnosis can be made, particularly during an epidemic, on clinical grounds alone. During an epidemic many cases might never present to a doctor but despite this and the sudden increase in work load, vigilance must be maintained for the rare but serious complications of the disease.

Patterns of presentation

Fever
Headache and aching eyes
Backache and aching muscles (myositis)
Cough – dry, becoming productive (bronchitis and pneumonitis)
Sore throat (pharyngitis)
Chest pains (tracheitis)
Meningism
Conjunctivitis
Nosebleeds
Loss of interest, loss of energy
Duration 4–14 days
All ages (teenagers present most often)

History

Details of presenting symptoms
Onset and duration of symptoms
Contacts
Self-care

Examination

Temperature
Chest signs
ENT
CNS including signs of meningism

Investigation

Throat swabs
'Paired sera' for serology with blood samples taken 10 days apart

Prevention

Immunization is available but of unproven benefit; it might be indicated in
- the elderly
- institutions
- patients with chronic infections
- patients with heart disease
- health workers

Options

Advice and information
Rest
Increase fluid intake
Inhalants, e.g. Karvol
Linctus, e.g. Simple linctus BP
Antipyretic analgesics, e.g. aspirin
Antibiotics for secondary bacterial infection, e.g. broad spectrum – amoxycillin 250 mg 8 hourly

anti-staphylococcal – flucloxacillin 250 mg 6 hourly.

Complications

Death
Chest infections
- bronchitis
- pneumonitis
- lobar pneumonia
- empyema

Depression

See also:

Cough (p. 58)
Fever (p. 106)
Glandular fever (p. 122)
Headache (p. 133)
Flu-like illness (p. 169)

Influenza-like illness

'Flu-like-illness' or 'viral illness' are descriptive terms used freely by patients and doctors alike. Such a term is appropriate only when the symptoms of localized inflammation with associated malaise and fever remain self-limiting and benign.

The prodromal phase of several recognizable viral illnesses may initially be described as 'flu-like-illness'. The term 'influenza' should be reserved for the characteristic epidemic illness. (See p. 167)

Causes

URTI
Pharyngitis and tonsillitis
Sinusitis and otitis
Tracheitis and croup
Bronchitis and bronchiolitis
Prodromal phase of
- glandular fever
- mumps
- measles
- rubella
- Herpes zoster
- polio
- rabies
- leptospirosis
- brucellosis
- psittacosis

malaria
Guillain–Barré disease
encephalitis
meningitis
pneumonia, e.g. *Mycoplasma, Chlamydia*
epidemic myalgic encephalomyelitis

Complications

Secondary bacterial infections with
Streptoccocus pyogenes
Pneumococcus
Haemophilus influenza

Management

Advice and information on self-care
Analgesics, e.g. aspirin
Antibiotics for secondary bacterial infection

See also:

Blisters (p. 29)
Epidemic myalgic encephalomyelitis (p. 95)
Fever (p. 106)
Glandular fever-like illness (p. 122)
Headache (p. 133)
Imported disease (p. 157)
Infection and parasites from pets (p. 165)
Influenza (p. 169)
Sinusitis (p. 287)
Common infectious diseases in children (p. 402)
Chronic bronchitis (p. 440)
Respiratory distress – croup (p. 537)

Insomnia

This common symptom occurs in up to one-third of the population and is more frequent in women. It is often associated with other symptoms and then its significance must be assessed in the context of those other symptoms. The definition of a disturbed sleep pattern or insomnia, is subjective as it reflects the patient's feeling that the quantity or quality of sleep is less than adequate.

A disturbed sleep pattern is especially significant as a cardinal symptom of depression.

Causes

Pain
Illness
Disturbing environment – noise, uncomfortable bed, excessive light, etc.

Depression
Anxiety
Bereavement
Other 'life events'
Dieting
Stress
Nightmares
Night terrors
'Idiopathic insomnia'
'Shift-work'

History

Sleep pattern – falling asleep and early waking
Actual and expected amount of sleep – any recent change
Total amount of time in house – nights, days and weekends
Quality of sleep – light or deep sleep, refreshed or tired in the morning
Associated symptoms
 pain
 shortness of breath
 nocturnal cough and cramps
 symptoms of depression or anxiety
 effect on family, work, and leisure time
 psychosexual problems
Medical history
Psychiatric history
Social history

Options

Self help
Attention to exercise and relaxation
Hot milky drinks, hot baths, preparation of the bed, bedroom temperature, noise and darkness
Attention to life style (e.g. shift workers) and to environment (e.g. double glazing for insulation and noise)
Avoid stimulants (e.g. coffee, tea, alcohol)
Advice on relaxation techniques
Special advice to patients with asthma, left ventricular failure or hiatus hernia
Advice to parents about the wide range of 'normal' sleep patterns in children and also about nightmares, night terrors (which are transient) and sleep-walking (which may warrant investigation and sedation).

Medical help
Adequate control of medical conditions (e.g. thyroid disease, shortness of breath, pain, skin complaints, cramps)
Treatment and supervision for depression or anxiety

Counselling for bereavement or marital crisis, etc.
Short term use of hypnotics
- Benzodiazepines, e.g. Temazepam 10 mg at night
- Chloral derivatives, e.g. chloral hydrate 0.5–2 g at night
- Antihistamines, e.g. promethazine 25–75 mg at night
- Antidepressants, e.g. amitriptyline 50–100 mg at night.

Failure to control

Excessive sedation in paediatric and geriatric age groups and in patients with respiratory disease
Inadequate sedation in terminal illness
Emergence of withdrawal symptoms after long term use of night sedation
Alternative or less common diagnoses
- drug abuse
- marital and/or sexual problems
- enuresis
- food allergy
- sleep apnoea (may be exacerbated by night sedation)

Referral

General physician or rheumatologist for intractable pain or other symptoms
Psychiatrist for assessment and therapy in complicated cases of insomnia
Clinical psychologist for behavioural therapy and relaxation techniques
Guidance counsellors for marital and other stressful life crises (e.g. bereavement).

See also:

Depression (p. 63)
Food allergy (p. 113)
Psychosexual problems (p. 266)
Stress and anxiety (p. 303)
Bereavement (p. 505)

Irregular periods

Irregular bleeding may be due either to normal periods of irregular timing or to regular periods with unexpected bleeding in between – 'intermenstrual bleeding'. This latter category may be directly related to sexual intercourse, (post-coital bleeding), and warrants full investigation.

Causes

Hypothalamic
- Trauma

Stress (physical or emotional)
Change in life style
Ovarian
The slight blood loss at ovulation
'Break through bleeding' with use of the Pill
IUCD
Chorionic carcinoma
Endometrial polyp
Endometrial carcinoma
Cervical polyp
Cervical erosion
Cervical carcinoma
Vaginitis
Clotting disorder
Pre-pubertal bleeding
trauma
pituitary or ovarian tumours
precocious puberty
accidental ingestion of oral contraceptive pill

History

Menstrual history
Obstetric history
Gynaecological history
Contraceptive history
Associated symptoms

Examination

Anaemia
BP
Abdominal examination
Pelvic examination
Weight

Investigation

HVS
Urethral swab
MSU
FBS
Platelets
Syphilis serology
Cervical smear

Options

Exclude urethral or rectal bleeding
Discuss patient's concept of 'normality'
Review contraception
Exclude contraindications to hormone therapy
Progestogens, e.g. norethisterone 5 mg 8 hourly
Discuss sex technique.

Follow-up

Menstrual chart
Check for side effects of hormone therapy
Investigate any other source of bleeding, e.g. haematuria

Complications

Indefinite dating of pregnancy
Disruption of contraception

Referral

Fertility investigations
Cryotherapy of cervical erosions
Investigation of suspected cervical carcinoma
D & C in all cases of unexplained intermenstrual bleeding.

See also:

Stress and anxiety (p. 303)
Cervical cancer screening (p. 438)
Contraception (p. 446)

Itch

Itching is a tiresome symptom that can usually be effectively assessed and relieved in primary care. In some cases referral to hospital is advisable especially when an itchy rash is the result of a systemic disorder.

Causes

Itching rashes

- Eczema
- Urticaria
- Parasites, e.g. scabies, filariasis (see p. 158)
- Insect bites
- Fungal infections of skin
- Viral infections, e.g. chickenpox
- Miliaria rubra
- Pityriasis rosea
- Lichen planus
- Lichen simplex
- Dry skin – ichthyosis
- Neurodermatitis

Systemic causes without rashes

- Obstructive jaundice
- Pregnancy (see p. 355)
- Drugs
    - The Pill
    - Chlorpromazine
    - Chloroquine
    - Narcotic drugs

Diabetes (see p. 457)
Thyroid disorders (see pp. 479, 481)
Uraemia (see p. 443)
Iron deficiency

Systemic causes with rashes

Drugs, e.g. antibiotics
Occult carcinoma
Leukaemia
Lymphoma
Polycythaemia
Dermatitis herpetiformis
Thalamic tumour
Syphilis
Pruritus ani (see p. 10)
Pruritus vulvae (see p. 321)

History

Onset and duration of the itch
Timing and distribution of the itch
Associated symptoms
Recent medical history
Medication
Contacts
Job
Travel
Pets
LMP

Examination

Inspection of skin
- colour
- hydration
- mucous membranes
- distribution of rash
- character of rash
- urticaria
- bites and burrows
- visible parasites

Thyroid status
Signs of liver disease
Signs of kidney disease
Anaemia

Investigation

FBC & ESR
Iron & TIBC
U & E
LFT

T_3 & TSH
Syphilis serology
Urinalysis
Stool
- occult blood
- ova and parasites

CXR
Skin scrapings for microscopy

Options

Topical preparations
- Calamine as lotion, oily lotion, ointment or cream
- Crotamiton (i.e. Eurax) 10% lotion or ointment
- Simple ointment (e.g. emulsifying ointment BNF)
- Simple creams (e.g. Boots E45)
- Simple soap
- 'Oilatum Emollient' added to bath water
- Topical steroid creams – only in selected cases
- Coal tar, dithranol and salicylic acid preparations – for psoriasis
- Gamma benzene hexachloride 1% cream – for scabies
- Occlusive bandages – for neurodermatitis

Systemic preparations
- Systemic anthistamines, e.g.
  - Chlorpheniramine 4 mg 8 hourly
  - Promethazine 10–25 mg 8–12 hourly
- Sedatives, e.g. hydroxyzine 10–25 mg 8 hourly
- Systemic steroids *only* in selected cases
- Iron supplements as indicated.

General advice

Cut nails
Cool room
Cool bath
Cool clothes
Avoid skin irritants, e.g. drugs, chemicals, woolly clothes
Avoid topical local anaesthetic or antihistamine creams because of risk of sensitization.

See also:

Anal irritation (p. 10)
Bites and stings (p. 26)
Generalized rash (p. 118)
Localized rash (p. 185)
STD (p. 301)
Symptoms in pregnancy (p. 352)
Common infectious diseases in children (p. 402)
Diabetes (p. 457)

Hyperthyroidism (p. 479)
Hypothyroidism (p. 481)

Jaundice

Jaundice is yellow discoloration of the skin mucosae and sclera which is noticeable when the serum bilirubin level is greater than 35 mmol/l.

It must be distinguished from the yellow pigmentation of carotinaemia and brown pigmentation of Addison's disease or chronic liver disease.

Common causes

Infective hepatitis (hepatitis A)
Gall stones
Drugs
Malignant disease

Rarer causes

Hepatocellular jaundice
Serum hepatitis (hepatitis B)
Alcoholic liver disease
Poisons
Chronic aggressive hepatitis
Portal cirrhosis

Obstructive jaundice
Primary biliary cirrhosis
Carcinoma of the pancreas
Carcinoma of the ampulla of Varter
Lymphadenopathy at the porta hepatis

Haemolytic jaundice
Spherocytosis
Haemoglobinopathy
Malaria
SLE

History

Mode of onset and duration
General health
Associated abdominal pain, fever, anorexia or lethargy
Colour of faeces and urine
Past history of jaundice or liver disease
Recent blood transfusion or contact with a jaundiced person
Alcohol intake and drugs
Occupation and visits abroad

Examination

General – appearance mental state and lymphadenopathy
Eyes – assess conjunctivae in natural light
Skin – 'Spider naevae', liver palms, bruising, purpura and venepunctive marks
Hands – finger clubbing, leukonychia and flapping tremor
Abdomen – liver size, shape and consistency
palpable gall bladder
splenomegaly and ascites
caput medusae

Investigation

All cases

FBC
MCV
ESR
PTT
Urine (for bilirubin)
Bilirubin conjugated
Bilirubin unconjugated
Alkaline phosphatase
Aspartate transaminase
γ Glutamyl transferase
Hepatitis B antigen

Selected cases

5′ nucleotidase
Protein electrophoresis
Antinuclear factor
Mitochondrial antibodies
Syphilis serology
Glandular fever screening test
Random serum alcohol level
Plain abdominal X-ray
Barium meal
Cholecystogram
Liver scan
Blood film for malaria

Management

Review drug therapy and reduce to essential medication
Ban alcohol for at least 3 months
Quarantine arrangements should be discussed for patients with infective hepatitis B
Special diets are probably unnecessary except in liver failure
Cholestyramine may be helpful for itching associated with jaundice

Reasons for referral

Urgent relief of obstructive jaundice
Further investigation of persistent jaundice lasting longer than one month
Management of liver failure with ascites, confusion and flapping tremor
Management of malaena and haematemesis from ruptured oesophageal varices.

See also:

Imported disease (p. 157)

The knee

The knee is the site of many orthopaedic conditions. It is very prone to injury and most kinds of arthritis. Pain may also be referred from other sites,notably the hip.

Its stability is maintained by the collateral and cruciate ligaments and the powerful quadriceps muscle. The latter rapidly wastes in joint disease; this is a good sign of underlying abnormality. Curiously a strong quadriceps muscle can support an otherwise lax knee joint.

History

Onset duration and severity of symptoms
Detailed history of previous trauma
Exacerbating and relieving factors
Site and radiation
Associated symptoms
- swelling
- instability
- locking
- crepitus
- effusion
- weakness

Social and psychological effects
ADL and earning capacity

Examination

Inspect for deformity, swelling and muscle wasting
Palpate for effusion and site of maximal tenderness
Assess
- active and passive range of movement
- ligamentous stability – including cruciates
- McMurray's test – for torn meniscus

Check for signs of
- hip disease
- peripheral neurological signs (e.g. drop foot)

X-ray
Synovial fluid for
microscopy
culture

Patterns of presentation

Arthritis

(See pp. 485, 493)

Trauma

Strains can often be associated with delayed onset of an effusion, which will usually settle with rest, support, analgesics and subsequent physiotherapy if necessary.

Haemarthrosis is painful and the blood damaging to the joint. Aspiration is therefore desirable.

Sprains or ligamentous tears, without instability can be managed as a strained knee. However a complete rupture of the ligaments with clinical instability is a case for referral.

Locked knees may result from loose bodies or meniscal tears. They should not be forcefully manipulated but analgesics and muscle relaxants, e.g. diazepam 5–10 mg should help in a gentle manipulation of the joint into extension again.

Any suspected fracture should be referred to an accident unit.

The ligaments

The collateral and cruciate ligaments are partly responsible for stability of the knee. They may be stretched or ruptured in injuries. Usually, more than one ligament is involved and sometimes the menisci also, causing pain and swelling. If the injury leads to instability an orthopaedic opinion is essential. Minor injuries may be compensated for by strengthening the quadriceps muscle.

The cartilages

The menisci or cartilages are moon-shaped fibro-cartilage pads forming part of the internal architecture of the joint. They are prone to injury and because they do not have a blood supply they cannot heal.

The medial mensicus is most often affected. It may be torn by a rotational injury with the knee flexed and weight bearing. There may be severe pain in the knee radiating down the leg and tenderness along the associated joint margin. An effusion soon forms and the patient is often unable to walk. Locking of the knee may inhibit full extension.

In older patients mucinous degeneration of the cartilage centre may lead to herniation and cystic formation along the joint margin. The process may be symptomless but more commonly it causes localized pain. Patients with cartilage damage should be referred to an orthopaedic surgeon for assessment. These injuries usually lead to early degeneration of the joint.

Loose bodies

These are usually composed of bone and/or cartilage. They form as a result of osteochondritis, osteochondral fractures or synovial chondromatosis.

The loose body, if free in the joint capsule, may lead to locking of the knees which can 'give way'. There is wasting of the quadriceps and perhaps an effusion in the joint. The fragment may be visible on an X-ray. If the condition is causing symptoms the patient should be referred for an orthopaedic assessment.

Swellings

Usually occurs as a result of inflammation or trauma. In knee joint effusion, it is more commonly seen in the suprapatella pouch and either side of the patella.

The prepatellar bursa may become evident as a 'housemaid's knee'. It is limited to the margins of the patella and may become infected.

Cystic swellings may occur over the patellar tendon, in relationship to the semi-membranous tendon at the posteromedial aspect of the knee and at the back of the joint capsule (popliteal cyst).

Treatment depends on the underlying cause. A severe joint effusion or prepatellar bursa is best treated with rest and firm support bandage. If infection is suspected the fluid should be aspirated for culture; referral may be necessary for adequate drainage. Recurrent haemarthrosis are best referred since they may lead to joint destruction. A popliteal cyst may require excision if it interferes with joint functions.

Fracture of the patella

The patella may be fractured by direct or indirect injury. It usually requires operative repair. There may be a delay of several hours before signs develop.

Dislocation of the patella

The patella dislocates laterally with the knee flexed. The patient is usually unable to straighten the knee until it is reduced.

A first dislocation will necessitate referral and subsequent immobilizations to allow the torn retinaculum to heal, followed by physiotherapy. Recurrent dislocation is usually associated with weak quadriceps and there may be a history of 'giving way' particularly when walking downstairs or downhill. Treatment demands vigorous and prolonged physiotherapy, if this fails then surgery would be indicated.

Chondromalacia patellae

This is a condition of softening of the articular cartilage behind the patella found particularly in teenage girls. It is caused by trauma, recurrent dislocation or excessive use during running or cycling. There is pain in the knee on walking up or down hill. The pain is reproduced by stressing the patella. There is associated wasting of the quadriceps. Treatment is with physiotherapy and analgesics since the condition is usually self-limiting, but more severe cases require orthopaedic referral.

Osgood–Schlatter disease

This is an osteochondritis at the epiphysis of the tibial tuberosity which occurs more commonly in boys. Patients present with a painful swelling exacerbated by exercise. The swelling will increase with an excessive traction from the quadriceps muscle until the epiphysis fuses at the end of puberty.

Exercise must be limited to the level of pain. NSAID may relieve symptoms and in some cases immobilization in a full length plaster cylinder is indicated.

'Knock-knees'

Most commonly seen in children who recover spontaneously by the age of 8 years.

Knock-knees can occur in adults as a result of injury or arthritis with damage to the medial collateral ligament or destruction of the lateral tibial condyle. In this later group orthopaedic assessment is necessary.

Bow legs

May be seen in overweight infants, and, in this case, rarely requires treatment. More rarely in children rickets or Blount's disease may be the cause. In more severe cases splinting or tibial osteotomy may be required.

In adults degenerative arthritis of the medial compartment is more commonly the cause, perhaps after medial menisectomy. More rarely Paget's disease underlies the diagnosis.

See also:

Hip (p. 146)
Osteoarthritis (p. 485)

Rheumatoid arthritis (p. 493)
Bone injury (p. 513)

Lethargy

'I'm tired all the time'; 'I need a tonic'; 'I'm tense'; 'I've got no energy'; 'I feel lethargic'; 'I feel washed out' are all presenting symptoms of the familiar state of lassitude. The significance of the symptom is relative to the patient's expectations of health and illness and to the accompanying symptoms and signs and circumstances. The many causes may be physical or psychological or both; they often coincide and are usually interrelated.

Causes

Physical

Pregnancy
Anaemia
Infections
Heart disease
Effects of medication
Problem drinking
Osteoarthritis
Rheumatoid arthritis
Liver disease
Diabetes
Thyroid disorders
Terminal illness

Psychological

Anxiety
Depression
Hypochondriasis
Dementia
Insomnia
Excessive sleep
Excessive dieting

Social

Loneliness
Boredom
Young children at home
Stress at school/college/work
Marital problems
Sexual problems
Bereavement

Rare causes

Narcolepsy
Food allergy
Malabsorption
Addison's disease
Tuberculosis
Ankylosing spondylitis
Osteomalacia
Hyperparathyroidism
Hypopituitarism
Myelomatosis
Porphyria
Polymyalgia rheumatica

History

Duration of symptoms
Associated symptoms
Life-style
Occupation
Associated 'life events'
Weight loss or gain
History of medication
Menstrual history
Sleep pattern
Diet
Depressive symptoms, morale and libido

Examination

Non-verbal clues to undeclared problems
Limited examination relevant to the history
Age and weight
Check for
- thyroid status
- anaemia
- liver or spleen enlargement
- muscle or joint disease

Investigation

FBC
ESR
LFT
Urine (glucose, protein & blood)
CXR

If indicated
- thyroid function
- Fe + TIBC
- B_{12} + folate
- ANF
- ECG
- relevant X-rays to detect arthritic or malignant changes

Options

Treat any underlying physical condition
Discuss
- life-style, expectations, social support
- ability to cope and attitudes to ageing or physical handicap
- relaxation and leisure pursuits
- diet and alcohol consumption

Tonics can occasionally have beneficial placebo effects
Review current medication, particularly
- tranquillizers – major and minor
- diuretics and antihistamines
- β-blockers and methyldopa.

See also:

Depression (p. 63)
Food allergy (p. 113)
Insomnia (p. 170)
Malnutrition and malabsorption (p. 195)
Pallor/anaemia (p. 231)
Psychosexual problems (p. 266)
Stress and anxiety (p. 303)
Diabetes (p. 457)
Heart failure (p. 469)
Hypothyroidism (p. 481)
Osteoarthritis (p. 485)
Pulmonary tuberculosis (p. 492)
Rheumatoid arthritis (p. 493)
Bereavement (p. 505)
Terminal care (p. 506)

Localized rash

In the following group of conditions the rash presents on a localized area of skin. The onset is gradual but the condition may occasionally spread more widely.

Causes

Eczema

Eczema is the response of the skin to a wide variety of challenges which may be manifested in different patterns of presentation. It is usually intensely irritating and itchy.

Pattern of presentation

Atopic This constitutes part of the triad of eczema, asthma and hay fever. It tends to occur in early childhood particularly affecting the flexures of the knees and elbows. It may become generalized and tends to persist through childhood.

Contact The condition results on contact with an allergen. The pattern of distribution depends on the extent of contact. A wide variety of substances have been implicated as allergens. These include rubber, metals, dyes and topical medications.

Irritants Solvents, caustic agents and detergents will produce an eczematous reaction if sufficiently strong, even in apparently normal individuals.

Nummular This form presents as single or multiple disc-shaped lesions on the trunk and distal limbs. It occurs in adults.

Seborrhoeic The rash particularly affects the hair margin, eyebrows, ears, nasolabial folds, sternum, axillae and groins. It is often associated with dandruff.

Pompholyx This is an acute irritant blistering condition which affects the hands and feet. It is more common in hot weather.

Skin lesions

Acute

erythema and swelling
vesicles and blistering
exudation
crusting

Chronic

erythema
dryness and scaling
thickened skin
fissuring.

Options

Avoidance of precipitating factors and soaps

Lotions and saline soaks are soothing in the acute exudative forms

Topical steroids are the mainstay in the treatment of the subacute and chronic forms

Emulsifying ointment helps to keep the dry skin from

cracking and can be applied topically as a soap substitute or put in the bath water

Occlusive dressings help to break the itch-scratch-itch cycle.

Psoriasis

This relatively common condition tends to start in young adults. It is typically chronic or recurrent. Classically the lesions present on the knees, elbows and scalp. It can be a more generalized rash on the trunk with rather small lesions (<1 cm) known as guttate psoriasis. A pustular form may affect the palms and soles.

Skin lesions

Red, raised scaly plaque

Varying sizes which may become more confluent

Sharply defined edges

The silvery scales can be scraped away leaving small capillary bleeding points.

Associated features

Pitting of the nails

Arthritis (particularly hips and spine).

Options

Coal tar preparations for chronic lesions

Dithranol is a more effective but potentially irritant alternative

Steroid creams to the intertriginous areas, and isolated small lesions

Ultraviolet light (PUVA) is helpful in more extensive skin involvement.

Fungal infections

There are a variety of fungal skin infections. They can affect the feet, between the toes (Tinea pedis), the scalp (Tinea capitis) and the groin (Tinea cruris). They can also occur on the trunk and limbs (Tinea corporis) and nails (paronychia).

Skin lesions

Red, slightly scaly patches

Spread circumferentially to form annular lesions

Central clearing

Acute forms can blister leading to superficial ulcers.

Options

Whitfield's ointment

Miconazole cream Clotrimazole cream	for the chronic scaling lesions
Potassium permanganate soaks Castellani's paint	for acute exudative lesions

Oral griseofulvin for the nail and refractory skin lesions.

Moniliasis This is caused by an infection of the skin with the yeast organism *Candida albicans*. It commonly affects moist areas and mucous membranes. It is not always pathogenic and can exist in normal individuals without the presence of the disease. The organism is usually classed as a secondary invader. It occurs particularly in patients with depressed immunity, diabetes mellitus, in pregnant women and in patients taking antibiotics, or the oral contraceptive pill.

Skin lesions

Erythematous macerated areas
Ill-defined edge
Distributed in groin, interdigital webs, mouth and sub-mammary regions
Paronychia (see p. 187)

Options

Careful drying after washing
Topical agents, e.g. nystatin cream
Avoiding prolonged immersion in water and damage to the cuticle helps to prevent and clear paronychia.

Lichen planus A condition of unknown aetiology which affects young and middle aged adults. It particularly affects the wrists, scalp, nails, mucous membranes, palms and soles. If untreated it resolves spontaneously after a few months although hypertrophic forms on the legs and feet may last several years. About one-fifth of affected patients may suffer a recurrence.

Skin lesions

Small, polygonal, flat topped papules with central umbilication
Violaceous colour
White streaks on the surface of papules (Wickham's striae)
On the scalp there may be skin atrophy with hair loss
In the mouth the small papules fuse to give a white lace-like pattern.

Options

No treatment required in minor forms
Topical steroids may alleviate itching and aid suppression of lesions
Occlusive steroid dressings may be necessary in refractory cases
Intralesional triamcinolone may help hypertrophic forms
Oral antihistamines to relieve itching.

Scabies This is sue to an infestation of the skin with a mite (*Sar-*

coptes scabiei). It is passed on by close bodily contact, so other members of the household may be affected.

The female mite burrows into the skin and lays up to 50 eggs. The emergent larvae spread into the surrounding epidermis and subsequently hatch. After mating the cycle continues.

The lesions cause intense irritation.

Skin lesions

Burrows – greyish linear scaly lesions up to 1 cm long
A small vesicle at one end of the burrow represents the gravid female mite just visible to the naked eye
Scratching leads to excoriated papules
Secondary bacterial infection leads to impetigo
Distributed mainly on palms, fingers, interdigital webs, wrists, buttocks, breasts and external genitalia.

Options

Lotions

Benzyl benzoate
Gamma benzene hexachloride
Crotamiton

After a bath the lotion is applied to all skin from neck to feet
The sheets and underwear should be changed
After 24 hours the patient takes a second bath
Advise the patient that the irritation may persist for 2 weeks after treatment due to a persisting allergic reaction even if the mite has been killed.

Rosacea

A disorder of unknown aetiology which affects the young and middle aged adult. The face only is involved, chiefly the forehead, cheeks and chin. It tends to persist for a number of years but rarely beyond middle age.

Skin lesions

Flushing of the skin is exaggerated by heat, emotion and certain foodstuffs
Telangiectasia develops
Ultimately papules and pustules appear.

Associated features

Rhinophyma – thickening of the skin around the tip of the nose due to sebaceous gland hypertrophy
Keratitis of the eye.

Options

Sulphur creams (e.g. 3% sulphur in salicylic acid ointment BNF)
Oral tetracycline 250 mg 12 hourly for several months.
Steroid creams should be avoided

Eye complications should be referred to an ophthalmologist.

See also: Generalized rash (p. 118)
Nail problems (p. 212)

Loss of bladder control

Urinary incontinence or loss of bladder control is a particularly distressing and embarrassing symptom to the patient. The causes are numerous. While only a few cases will be cured a large number may be helped with the aid of physiotherapy or simple appliances.

Enuresis in children (see p. 410).

Causes

Retention with overflow
- Prostatic hypertrophy
- Faecal inpaction
- Autonomic neuropathy

Stress incontinence
- Uterovesical prolapse
- Senile vaginitis

Neurogenic bladder
- Detrusor instability

Cerebral impairment
- Dementia
- Confusional state
- Epilepsy
- Manipulative behaviour

Infection
- Cystitis
- Urethritis

Diuresis
- Renal failure
- Diabetes mellitus

Medication
- Diuretics
- Anticholinergic drugs
- Sedatives

Environmental
- Unfamiliar surroundings
- Too far from toilet

History

Onset and duration of symptoms

Urinary frequency (day and night)
Associated symptoms
- urgency
- hesitancy
- stream
- terminal dribbling
- strangury
- dysuria
- haematuria

Stress incontinence with coughing, laughing and exercise
Awareness of incontinence
General health and recent illnesses
History of medication
Effect on mobility and morale
Domestic support

Examination

Mental state
Mobility
Palpate abdomen (after micturition) for
- bladder
- pelvic masses
- enlarged abdominal organs
- pelvic and rectal examination

Check for
- prolapse
- senile vaginitis
- prostatic hypertrophy
- faecal impaction
- localizing signs of MS, CVA or cerebral tumours
- anal and cremasteric reflexes

Investigation

Urine
- glucose
- protein
- culture

Urea and electrolytes

Options

Treat underlying cause appropriately
- infection – antibiotics according to MSU
- uterovaginal prolapse – trial with ring pessary
- senile vaginitis – course of dienoestrol cream
- faecal impaction
  - manual removal
  - laxatives as required
- drugs
  - flaxovate 200 mg 8 hourly
  - imipramine 25 mg 8 hourly

Review existing drug therapy
Advice on regular toilet
Altered environment
- commode/urine bottles
- grab handles in toilet
- raised toilet seat

Incontinence pants
Penile sheath
Catheterization (a last resort).

Referral

Urodynamic studies
Prostatic or gynaecological surgery
Neurological assessment
Help from continence nurse advisor if available.

See also:

Confusion and dementia (p. 52)
Enlarged prostate (p. 90)
Fits (p. 110)
Enuresis (p. 410)
Chronic renal failure (p. 443)
Diabetes (p. 457)

Male subfertility

10–14% of all couples are unable to conceive without medical intervention. A much larger proportion present for advice on relative delay in conception.

Subfertility in the female is discussed separately (see p. 103), although the couple should be seen and assessed together.

Causes

Psychosexual problems (see p. 266)
Mumps orchitis
Torsion of the testis
Cryptorchidism
Varicocoele
Obstructed vas deferens (trauma, infection, congenital)
Prostatitis
Hypospadias
Medication, e.g.
- hypotensives
- MAOI antidepressants
- sulphasalazine
- phenytoin
- alcohol
- cannabis

Chronic illness

Pituitary/hypothalamic lesions
Intersex states

History

Sexual history and contraception
Previous paternity
Medication
History of venereal disease or mumps
History of genital surgery

Examination

General
- physique
- distribution of body hair
- genital scars

Penis
- hypospadias
- other congenital abnormalities
- Peyronie's syndrome

Scrotum
- varicocoele
- vas deferens
- herniae

Testes
- size and shape
- cryptorchidism

P.R. examination
- prostatitis

Investigation

Semen analysis – fresh sample less than 6 hours old
Normal values
- volume >2 ml
- morphology 60% normal forms
- motility 50%
- count $>20 \times 10^6$ per ml

Options

Discussion
- range of normal time for conception
- sex techniques and timing in relation to ovulation
- cool testes – loose underwear and trousers, avoid hot baths

Review drug therapy
Treat underlying pathology is possible.

Referral

Investigation – after 18 months of attempting conception in a apparently healthy young couple, (earlier if the woman is over 35 years of age)
Surgery – to correct any pathology
In vitro fertilization – assessment and selection

Artificial insemination — consideration and assessment
Adoption as a realistic alternative.

See also:

Enlarged prostate (p. 90)
Female subfertility (p. 103)
Psychosexual problems (p. 266)

Male genital problems

These are relatively uncommon presenting symptoms in general practice. They can be broadly divided into problems relating to the penis and those relating to the scrotum.

Penis

Symptom	Cause	Options
Discharge	NSU	Oxytetracycline 10–14 days
	Gonococcal infection	Ampicillin and probenecid
		Refer for contact tracing
	Prostatitis	Ampicillin or Septrin 10–14 days
	Carcinoma (blood-stained)	Refer to urologist
Injury	Frenular tear	Avoid intercourse until healed
	Bruising	Consider stilboestrol for 5 days
	Crush injuries	Refer to urologist
Swellings	Paraphimosis/phimosis	Refer for circumcision
	Carcinoma	Refer to urologist
	Warts	Solitary–podophyllum 25%
		Multiple–surgical excision
		Diathermy
Pain/itching	Balanoposthitis	Topical antiseptic (circumcision)
	Candidiasis	Anti-candida cream, e.g. nystatin
	Tight frenulum	Refer for surgical release
Ulceration	Herpes simplex	Idoxuridine paint or ointment
	Syphilitic	Penicillin (see p. 302)
	Carcinoma	Refer to urologist
Deformity	Hypospadias	Minimal deformity – no action otherwise refer for surgical correction
	Peyronie's disease	May resolve spontaneously
		Vitamin E
		Refer for surgical opinion
	Priapism	Sedate in acute distress
		Refer for surgical correction

Scrotum

Symptom	Cause	Options
Soreness and itching	Infective (usually fungus)	Nystatin or miconazole cream
	Dermatological	
	psoriasis	Steroid cream
	contact dermatitis	"
Swelling	Haematoma	Refer to surgeon
	Indirect hernia	"
	Hydrocele	"
	Haematocele	"
	Varicocele	"
	Spermatocele	"
	Sebaceous cyst	"
	Seminoma	"
	Teratoma	"
Pain	Torsion	"
	Carcinoma	Refer immediately to surgeon
	Orchitis	Scrotal support and analgesia
	Epididymitis	Treat any underlying UTI Consider gonorrhoea or TB if slow to respond

Malabsorption and malnutrition

Malabsorption is the inadequate absorption by the gut of any constituent of the diet, including fats, carbohydrates, proteins, minerals and vitamins. Malnutrition is the inadequate nutrition of the body as a result of malabsorption and a poorly digested or restricted diet.

In international primary care kwashiorkor and marasmus are far more important than the usual modes of presentation in Britain, which are considered here.

Patterns of presentation

Malabsorption

Weight loss
Failure to thrive in children
Anaemia
Steatorrhoea
Osteomalacia
Food allergy, e.g. milk or sugar

Malnutrition

Weight loss
Failure to thrive
Anaemia

Causes

Pathological
- Obstructive jaundice
- Coeliacs disease
- Tropical sprue
- Cystic fibrosis
- Pancreatic disease
- Zollinger–Ellison syndrome
- Gastric atrophy

Structural
- Surgery
- Strictures
- Crohn's disease
- Fistulae

Infectious
- Tuberculosis
- Intestinal parasites

Medication
- Phenytoin
- Antibiotics, e.g. amoxicillin and clindamycin

Self-neglect
Inadequate diet
Problem drinking

History

Present and previous weight
Bowel habit
Dentures and dysphagia
Diet and alcohol
Medication
Surgical history
Travel
Social and psychological factors affecting food

Examination

Record
- Height and weight in metres and kilos (W/H^2 is proportional to fat content of the body – BMI)
- Skinfold thickness
- Circumference of upper arm

Check for
- Anaemia
- Oedema
- Bruising
- Stomatitis
- Dermatitis herpetiformis
- Abdominal distension
- Muscle wasting
- Peripheral neuropathy

Mental disorder
Ascites and liver disease

Investigation **Consider**
FBC
ESR
Urea and albumin
Calcium, magnesium phosphate
Alkaline phosphatase
Glucose tolerance test
Prothrombin time
Fe+TIBC
Vitamin B_{12} and RBC folate
24 hour creatinine collection
CXR
X-ray wrists and pelvis
Cholecystogram
Barium meal and follow through
Stool for fat and sugar content, and parasites

Options Improve availability, quality and quantity of food
Review financial status
Discuss
- diet
- exclusion diets, e.g. gluten-free
- food fads

Diet supplements
- multiple vitamins
- electrolytes, e.g. potassium
- iron and folate
- pancreatic enzymes

Low allergy diet (see p. 114)

Referral Refer for jejeunal biopsy
Refer for controlled feeding programme if indicated.

See also:
Food allergy (p. 113)
Imported disease (p. 157)
Pallor/anaemia (p. 231)
Problem drinking (p. 261)
Weight loss (p. 337)
Worms (p. 339)
Failure to thrive (p. 413)
Pulmonary tuberculosis (p. 492)

Mania

The affective disorder of mania is distinguished by elevation of mood, increased activity and self-important ideas. It can occur in isolation but is usually associated with depression in an alternating, mixed, or, 'bi-polar' fashion. It appears to be more common in women than in men. The aetiology is obscure; there may be psychological, genetic or biochemical factors; it can occur in association with physical illness such as virus infections, medication (steroids), surgery and cerebral tumour.

The mean age of onset is around 30 years and 90% of cases occur before the age of 50 years. The duration of the illness is variable and often cyclical but nearly all recover eventually.

Manic symptoms

Euphoric mood (but some can become more irritable than euphoric)
Flamboyant dress
Rapid speech
Insomnia
Increased appetite and libido
Expansive ideas of self-importance
Extravagance
Grandiose delusions of special importance (sometimes with a paranoid quality)
Hallucinations – auditory and, less common, visual
Impaired insight

Degrees of severity

Although the distinction between grades is blurred, the following is a useful guide to assessment and management

Mild

Increased activity and speech
Labile mood
Extravagance
Increased libido

Moderate

Overactivity and pressure of speech which may be disorganized
Swinging mood with euphoria, punctuated by periods of irritability and depressive delusions

Severe

Overactivity and incoherent thought
Bizarre delusions and hallucinations

Assessment

Onset, duration and severity of symptoms
Assessment of behaviour as judged by the relatives (the patient may control or play down symptoms during the interview)
Social consequences
Recent life events
Intercurrent physical illness or drug therapy
Past psychiatric illness and pre-morbid personality

Options

Medication with antipsychotic drugs is the mainstay of treatment

Haloperidol

This is probably the drug of first choice in acute mania but control may be followed by a depressive episode
The initial dosage should be adequate to control symptoms quickly
1.5 mg–20 mg daily in divided doses increasing to 100 mg daily.

Chlorpromazine

This is a more sedating alternative
75–300 mg daily in divided doses.

Lithium carbonate

This is usually reserved for prophylactic treatment once the acute episode is controlled
It is a dangerous drug and therapy should be preceded by tests of renal and thyroid functions. During treatment plasma levels should be monitored regularly and the dosage adjusted accordingly. The use of lithium earlier in the course of the illness may leave the patient more alert and less likely to progress to the depressive phase.

Support for the patient's family.

Referral

It is probably wise to refer all but the most minor cases to hospital to initiate management.
Compulsory orders may be required (see p. 527).

See also:

Depression (p. 63)
Mental Health Act 1983 (p. 527)
Psychiatric emergencies (p. 533)

The menopause

The menopause is the cessation of menstruation. The climacteric is the time from the first change in menstruation until 12 months after the menopause. It usually occurs about the age of 50 years.

75% of women have symptoms but only 35–40% will declare them.

A combination of minor symptoms may contribute towards a sense of hopelessness and low self-esteem and an abrupt or unsympathetic response from the doctor can easily exacerbate this 'worthlessness'.

Many symptoms are erroneously ascribed to the menopause (e.g. headaches, stress or urge incontinence, insomnia).

Symptoms of the menopause can be loosely grouped into four different types.

Patterns of presentation

General

Hot flushes
Sweating
Dizziness
Gastrointenstinal symptoms

Psychological

Depression
Loss of confidence
Indecision
Anxiety
Palpitations
Loss of libido

Atrophic

Lax skin
Vaginitis (with or without dyspareunia)
Aching breasts
Musculo-skeletal pain

Menstrual

Irregular periods
Heavy periods

Assessment

Menstrual history
Psychological and social factors
Symptoms and/or history of depression
Contraindications to hormone replacement therapy (HRT)

Absolute contraindications to HRT

Thromboembolism
Oestrogen dependent tumour
Abnormal liver function tests
Abnormal kidney function
Familial hyperlipidaemia

Stroke
Pregnancy
Previous severe complications using the Pill

Relative contraindications to HRT
Obesity
Smoking
Hypertension (untreated)
Diabetes (if poorly controlled)
Endometrial hyperplasia (untreated)

Examination
Weight
BP
Breast examination
Pelvic examination

Investigation
Urinalysis
Cervical smear
FBC
Calcium
Alkaline phosphatase
Phosphate

Options
Information
Sympathetic discussion of the physical, social and psychological factors that can complicate the menopause.

Self-help
Reducing diet
Increase exercise
Keeping a menstrual chart
Reduce alcohol intake and spiced foods.

Hormone replacement therapy (HRT)
For treatment of
hot flushes
vaginitis
musculo-skeletal pain
pyschosexual and psychological symptoms

If the uterus is present oestrogens are best combined with progestogens (to avoid endometrial hyperplasia)

Natural conjugated equine oestrogen, e.g. Premarin 0.625 mg – 2.5 mg for 21 days then 7 days tablet free

Synthetic oestroedial with a progestogen e.g. Cyclo-Progynova; oestradiol valerate 1 mg + norgestrel 0.25 mg for 11 days (oestrogen), then 10 days (combined), then 7 days tablet free

Sequential preparation

Menophase; mestranol 12.5 μg to 50 μg + norethisterone 1 mg in sequential regimen of different dosage

Mefenamic acid, e.g. Ponstan 250–500 mg 8 hourly

This antiprostaglandin agent may alleviate the menstrual and musculo-skeletal symptoms

Clonidine, e.g. Dixarit 50 μg 8–12 hourly

This is useful for hot flushes when HRT is contraindicated

Oestrogen creams, e.g. dienoestrol for atrophic vaginitis

Such creams should only be used intermittently in the lowest effective dosage

Psychotropic drugs

Tranquillizers, e.g. diazepam 2–5 mg 8 hourly

Antidepressants, e.g. amitryptyline 25 mg 8 hourly

These drugs are best reserved until HRT has proved to be ineffective in symptom relief, unless HRT is contraindicated

Vaginal applications, e.g.

'KY-jelly'

'Aci-jel'

These may relieve vaginitis in addition to oestrogens or can be used in cases where oestrogens are contraindicated.

Follow-up

Hormone replacement therapy

(Review at 1 month and then 3 to 6 monthly)

Maintain therapy only while symptoms persist (usually 12–18 months)

Routine check for
- side effects or complications
- BP
- weight
- breast examination

Annual check for
- pelvic examination
- cervical smear
- urinalysis
- D + C should be considered

Complications of HRT – short term
- irregular periods
- breast tenderness
- weight gain
- nausea
- malaise

depression
varicose veins
hypertension
endometriosis
fibroids

Complications of HRT – long term
possibility of endometrial cancer with unopposed oestrogen
breast cancer
thromboembolism

Osteoporosis

Check
X-rays
serum calcium

Consider
long term replacement
calcium and vitamin D
androgens

Persistent symptoms

Consider other causes of symptoms
thyrotoxicosis
depression
psychosexual problems

Referral

Sub-cutaneous oestrogen implant
Investigation of intermenstrual bleeding or flooding in HRT
Suspicions of breast cancer or endometrial cancer
Uncontrolled osteoporosis
Uncontrolled psychological problems.

See also:

Heavy periods (p. 144)
Irregular periods (p. 172)

Migraine

The name migraine is derived from hemi-cranium but the one-sided headache is not a constant feature; migraine has many and varied presentations. In its simplest form it consists of a headache, usually unilateral, and associated nausea and visual disturbance.

The aura and headache are thought to be related to intracranial vasoconstriction and vasodilation respectively.

The onset is usually before 40 years of age and tends to improve with time. There is often a family history of this condition.

Females are affected more than males (3:1).

Patterns of presentation

Classical migraine (10%)

Aura of 15–20 minutes – visual, sensory or motor – resolves before the onset of pain. Headache unilateral (or bilateral) with associated nausea, vomiting, speech disturbance, photophobia, pallor and diuresis. Pain lasts 1–2 hours (may be up to 5 days).

Common migraine (85%)

No aura, headache is often bilateral and onset is more predictable following recognized trigger factors.

Migrainous neuralgia (4%)

'Cluster headaches' or 'Alarm clock headaches'.

Predictable timing of rapid onset. Severe pain, invariably commencing on one side around the eyes and radiating to the forehead, cheek and temple. There is associated lacrimation, flushing, unilateral nasal congestion, red eye and ptosis. It usually occurs at night for anything between 15 minutes and 2 hours, in episodes of 3–6 weeks. It is a recurrent condition, and males are affected more than women (6:1). It can be mistaken for raised intracranial pressure or cranial arteritis.

Other migraine variants

Facial migraine

Vertebro-basiliar migraine

Table 1.9. Migraine trigger factors

Dietary	Environmental/social	Hormonal	Psychological
Cheese	Smells	Menstruation	Exertion
Beans	Noise	The Pill	Excitement
Onions	Sunlight	Puberty	Stress
Wine	Artificial light	Menopause	Anxiety
Dieting	TV	HRT (oestrogens)	Depression
Fried food	Disco lights		Relaxation from stress
Chocolate	Change in climate		Pain
Citrus fruit	Travel		
Alcohol	Irregular meals		
Tobacco	Shift work		
	Excessive sleep		
	Fatigue		

Opthalmoplegic migraine
Hemiplegic migraine
Migraine equivalents
Abdominal migraine ('Periodic syndrome').

History

Onset of migraine
- age
- periodicity
- recent changes in pattern of attack

Aura trigger factors (see Table 1.9)

Headache
- site
- duration
- severity

Associated symptoms
- nausea
- photophobia
- dizziness
- hemiparesis
- lacrimation
- vomiting
- visual changes
- speech changes
- flushing
- congestion

Past and present medication (especially the contraceptive pill)
Menstrual history
Family history
Diet, alcohol and tobacco
Psychological and social factors
Health beliefs

Examination

BP
ENT and eyes
Cranial nerves

Investigation

FBC
ESR
X-ray skull, cervical spine, paranasal sinuses

Options

Prophylaxis/prevention
Avoid triggers listed above
Avoid stress

Consider stopping the Pill
Promethazine (Phenergan) at night for children
Clonidine (Dixarit) 50 μg 2 times daily
Pizotifen (Sanomigran) 0.5–2 mg 3 times daily
Anxiolytics, e.g. diazepam 2–5 mg 1–3 times daily
β-blockade, e.g. propranolol 20–80 mg 3 times daily
Antidepressants – tricylics
Anticonvulsants – phenytoin or carbamazepine

Steroids
Lithium
Methysergide } For prophylaxis of migrainous neuralgia.

During an attack
Rest, supine in a darkened, quiet room
Antiemetic, e.g. (Maxolon) Metoclopramide 10 mg 4 hourly except in young or pregnant women
Analgesic, e.g. aspirin or paracetamol
Anxiolytic diazepam 5 mg
Ergotamine tartate
- oral 1 mg (30 mins)
- inhaled 360 μg (5 mins)
- rectal 0.25 mg (1 hr)
- i.m. 0.25 mg (1 hr)

Contraindicated in
- pregnancy
- hypertension
- peripheral vascular disease

Ergotamine tartrate – caffeine 100 mg, e.g. Cafergot oral or rectal.

Referral

To neurologist or migraine clinic
For failure to control symptoms
Migrainous neuralgia
Ophthalmic, basilar or hemiplegic migraine
Complications of medication, e.g. the Pill, methysergide, ergot
Marked focal symptoms.

See also:

Facial pain (p. 96)
Food allergy (p. 113)
Headache (p. 133)
Vomiting (p. 328)

Mouth symptoms

Symptoms in the mouth may be due to local or systemic conditions, thus examination must be systematic and comprehensive.

Dental problems are best managed by a dentist and will not be considered here.

Ulcers

Aphthous ulcers

Assessment

These occur singly or in crops as papules, then grey/white ulcers with surrounding erythema. Pain is 'burning' and 'raw'. Resolution without scarring, is complete within three weeks.

Options

Viscous Lignocaine 2%
Steroid in pellets or Orabase
Betamethasone spray.

Herpes simplex

Assessment

Acute, isolated vesicles usually along the edge of the tongue

Vesicles soon burst to leave shallow painful ulcers. Fever and malaise are often associated

Viral swab to confirm.

Options

Rest
Soothing antiseptic mouthwash
Orabase as a barrier.

Herpes labialis

Assessment

Also due to H. simplex with lesions on the lips with similar morphology. One third of the population may suffer recurrent lesions which resolve spontaneously in 1 week. Precipitated by stress, sunlight, fever, menstruation and immune deficient states. Risk of secondary bacterial infection.

Options

Explanation and no action
Topical idoxuridine paint (Herpid 5%)
Acyclovir cream
Antibiotic cream when indicated (e.g. Aureomycin).

Hand, foot and mouth disease

Assessment (see p. 405)

Painless grey ulcers with vesicular lesions on hands and feet. Often epidemic.

Options
Explanation
Isolate the patient.

Traumatic ulcers

Assessment
Accidental, chronic or self-inflicted. Usually due to burns, broken teeth, ill-fitting dentures or abrasion.

Options
Orabase as a barrier
Antiseptic mouthwash
Dental care
Refer to exclude carcinoma if the ulcer continues for more than 6 weeks.

Drugs

Assessment
May mimic erythema multiforme (Stevens–Johnson syndrome).

Options
Stop drug
Refer if severe.

Syphilis

Assessment
Atypical (snail track) ulcers on the fauces.
Syphilis serology.

Options
Refer for treatment.

Lichen planus

Assessment
The ulcer is surrounded by characteristic reticular lesions.

Options
No treatment if asymptomatic
Steroid spray or pellets
Follow-up – may be pre-malignant.

Stevens–Johnson syndrome

Assessment
All mucous membranes are affected
Associated fever and arthralgia.

Options
Refer for treatment.

Behçet's syndrome

Assessment
Associated genital ulcers, conjunctivitis, arthritis, erythema nodosum.

Options
Refer for assessment
Analgesia and steroids.

Gingival hypertrophy

Transient

Assessment
Can occur during pregnancy or puberty.
Options
Reassure
Advice about oral hygiene.

Drugs

Assessment
Can occur with drugs such as phenytoin.
Options
Use an alternative drug if possible.

Sore gums

Pericoronitis

Assessment
Decaying food trapped between gums and teeth. Associated halitosis, pain, malaise and lymphadenopathy.
Options
Antiseptic mouthwash
Analgesia
Penicillin and/or metronidazole
Dental care.

Herpes simplex

See above

Vincent's stomatitis

Assessment
Associated with poor diet, smoking and URTI.
Options
Antiseptic mouthwash
Metronidazole
Dental care.

White lesions

Candidiasis

Assessment
White patches on buccal mucosa and gums
Check for predisposing factors
- medicines (antibiotics and steroids)
- diabetes
- depressed immunity
- malignancy.

Options
Nystatin lozenges or suspension
Gentian violet paint.

Koplik's spots

Assessment
Small white spots on erythematous base on buccal mucosa opposite upper molars
Early signs of measles.
Options
No specific treatment
Check complications of measles (see p. 403).

Aphthous ulcers

See above.

Lichen planus

Assessment
Fine reticular pattern, like lace, on buccal mucosa
Associated skin lesions (see p. 188).
Options
No specific treatment.

Tonsillitis

Assessment
May be associated with white exudate on tonsils and soft palate
Throat swab for streptococcus
Glandular fever screening test.
Options
Antiseptic gargles
Analgesia
Soothing lozenges
Penicillin for proven streptococcal infection
Steroids may be helpful in severe cases of glandular fever.

Leukoplakia

Assessment
'Sheet-like' white thickening of mucosa.
Options
Refer for biopsy or cryotherapy
Follow-up – may be pre-malignant.

Sore lips

Lip licking habit

Assessment
Sore cracking lips spreading into surrounding skin. Often worse in cold, windy weather.
Options
Encourage self-control
Barrier creams.

Eczema

Assessment
Usually associated with skin lesions elsewhere (see page 186).

Options
Moisturizing cream or ointment
Hydrocortisone cream.

Systemic lupus erythematosus

Assessment
Associated
- alopecia
- facial 'butterfly' rash
- telangiectasia

Serum antinuclear factor and ESR.
Options
Refer for treatment.

Depressed immunity

Agranulocytosis, leukaemia, cytoxic drugs, AIDS
Check FBC.
Options
Refer for treatment
Treat secondary bacterial or fungal infections.

Angular cheilosis

Assessment
Soreness and cracking at the corners of the mouth
May be associated with malocclusion of dentures and dribbling.
Options
Barrier creams
Refer to dentist to assess dentures.

Swellings

Mucosal hypertrophy

Assessment
Irritation by dentures.
Options
Exclude carcinoma
Refer to dentist.

Pyogenic granuloma

Assessment
Usually on dorsum of tongue
Bleeds readily.
Options
Refer for excision.

Mucocoele or ranula

Assessment
50% occur on lower lip
Ranulae occur mainly on the floor of the mouth.
Options
Refer for excision.

Carcinoma

Assessment
Usually occur on the tongue or floor of the mouth
Insidious onset
Indurated lesion usually painless
May ulcerate.
Options
Refer on suspicion.

Red tongue

Iron deficiency

Assessment
Associated iron deficient anaemia
Check serum iron and TIBC.
Options
Iron supplements.

Vitamin B_{12} or folate deficiency

Assessment
Associated with megaloblastic anaemia
Check serum B_{12} and folate levels.
Options
Give B_{12} and/or folate supplements.

Geographical glossitis

Assessment
Symptomless and benign
Varying pattern of dermoid epithelium
May be associated with illness or surgical operation.
Options
Reassurance
No specific treatment.

See also:

Bad breath (p. 25)
Localized rash (p. 185)
Common infectious diseases in children (p. 402)

Nail problems

Examination of the nails forms an important part of clinical assessment; not only are they involved in disease processes themselves but changes in the nails also occur as a result of generalized disease.

Beau's lines

These are transverse lines and furrows in the nails. They are often a sign of previous or current generalized disease or trauma to the cuticle.

of the

The nails are larger and curved with obliteration of the angle at the nail bed. The soft tissue around the terminal phalanx may be increased giving a bulbous appearance.

It may be congenital or acquired and occurs most commonly in association with
intrathoracic tumours
lung abscess
bronchiectasis
pulmonary tuberculosis
congenital heart disease
cirrhosis of the liver
steatorrhoea
inflammatory bowel disease.

Fungal infection of the nails

The infection is slow in progress with little inflammatory reaction. A yellowish discoloration spreads from the free margin. The nail plate loosens and becomes brittle, sometimes breaking off.

Treatment is with griseofulvin but the drug must be continued for 3–12 months. In addition, a topical antifungal agent (miconazole cream) may be used.

Hypertrophy of the nail bed

This is due to the piling up of keratin under the nail plate and is often associated with psoriasis or fungal infection.

Ingrowing nails

The lateral nail plate grows out pressing into the nail fold. It may cause pain and, later, the formation of reactive granulation tissue with low grade infection. It is usually the result of poor technique in cutting the nails or tight fitting shoes.

Treatment relies on local toilet and surgical excision of part or all of the nail plate and subsequent attention to footwear and nailcutting.

Koilonychia

The nails are brittle and spoon shaped. The condition is usually associated with iron deficiency but is occasionally seen with syphilis and polycythaemia.

Leuconychia

These are white spots or lines seen in the matrix of the nail plate. Leuconychia may be acquired as a result of trauma, fungal infection, lichen planus or cirrhosis of the liver.

Onychogryphosis

This is hypertrophy of the nail plate with horn-like deformity. It is the result of injury, local pressure, poor hygiene or local disease. Chiropody and regular abrasion is usually sufficient therapy.

Onycholysis This is loosening of the nail plate from its bed. A white discoloration spreads proximally in from the free margin until the nail is shed. One or more nails may be affected.

It is associated with psoriasis, arthritis or from the use of strong detergents or nail polish removers.

Paronychia Acutely painful inflammation and swelling along the nail fold is usually the result of staphylococcal infection. Treatment is with hot soaks and magnesium sulphate dressings. If a collection of pus is evident, incision and drainage is indicated.

Chronic paronychia is more commonly due to candida infection after damage to the cuticle by prolonged immersion in water. Treatment is by the avoidance of soaking and the topical application of nystatin or clotrimazole cream. Resolution is very slow.

Pitting The presence of small shallow pits like the surface of a thimble is often the hallmark of psoriasis, but it can occur in isolation. There is no specific therapy.

Sub-ungual haematoma Bleeding under the nail can be extremely painful if a haematoma develops. The haematoma can be drained through a small hole trephined in the nail plate with the tip of a red hot needle. The procedure is painless provided the needle does not penetrate to the periosteum.

See also:

Localized rash (p. 185)
STD (p. 301)
Osteoarthritis (p. 485)
Pulmonary tuberculosis (p. 492)

Nasal obstruction

A 'stuffy nose' or 'blocked nose' due to nasal obstruction may present as catarrh (see p. 38) but since 20% of all adults will develop a deviated nasal septum during their lifetime, nasal obstruction is not an uncommon condition. There are also several other causes.

Causes

Adenoidal hypertrophy (until puberty is reached)
Deviated nasal septum

Trauma
Foreign body
Oedema of inferior turbinates due to infection, allergy or vasomotor instability
Nasal polyp
Ethmoidal polyp
Granulomatous infections, e.g. TB, syphilis, leprosy
Tumours
Choanal atresia in the newborn

History

Onset and duration of symptoms
Bilateral, unilateral or alternating obstruction
Associated symptoms
- mouth-breathing
- loss of taste and smell
- nasal discharge
- snoring
- sneezing
- nosebleeds
- speech difficulties
- headaches

Family history
Occupation
Smoking habits
History of medication

Examination

Inspect nasal mucosa for
- Colour
- Inflammation
- Oedema
- Polyp
- Mass

Check for
- Patency of nostrils
- LAP
- Cranial nerve lesions
- Hearing loss (see p. 137)
- Adenoidal facies in a chronic mouth-breather
- Pharyngitis if mouth-breathing is recent

Investigation

FBC
ESR
Chest X-ray
Lateral X-ray of post-nasal space
Serology for syphilis

Options

Treat underlying chronic infections
For the initial mamanagement of polypi – steroid spray, e.g. betamethasone
For allergic rhinitis
- steroid spray, e.g. betamethasone
- mast cell inhibitors, e.g. sodium cromoglycate.

Complications

Disturbed speech
Snoring
Pharyngitis
Laryngitis
Irritation of gums
Halitosis

Referral

Acute nasal trauma (e.g. septal haematoma)
Foreign bodies in nasal passages
For consideration of
- SMR
- polypectomy
- adenoidectomy.

See also:

Catarrh (p. 38)
Headache (p. 133)
Nosebleed (p. 219)

The neck

A painful neck may be the result of intrinsic locomotor disorders or may be due to referred pain from the ear, throat or the apices of the lungs and associated pleura. Angina pectoris may also be felt in the neck. Only the locomotor disorders are discussed here.

History

Onset, duration and periodicity of symptoms
Exacerbating and relieving factors
Site and radiation of pain
Associated symptoms
- numbness
- paraesthesia and weakness (arms)
- spasticity and clumsiness (legs)
- hoarse voice
- pharyngitis or oesophagitis

History of trauma

Examination

Inspect symmetry of neck and shoulders
Palpate spine and muscles for tenderness

Assess active and passive range of movements
Check for
Limitations of shoulder movements
Scoliosis of dorsal spine
Soft tissue disorders (thyroid, lymph nodes)
Muscle wasting
Sensory loss } in the arms
Reflex changes }
Upper motor neurone signs in the legs

Investigation X-ray cervical spine especially if manipulation is being considered

Patterns of presentation

'Fibrositis'

This is not a pathological entity as such but is a well used lay-term to describe the common clinical condition of acute neck pain with tenderness in the muscles at the base of the neck. The cause is unknown but may be associated with muscle strain or minor injury. Some patients attribute it to 'sitting in a draft'. There are no other associated objective signs and X-rays are usually normal apart from some tilting, presumably due to muscle spasm. Treatment is by rest, local heat and analgesia. Manipulation may provide the quickest relief for some patients.

Cervical spondylosis

This condition is due to degenerative changes in the cervical spine with narrowing of disc spaces and osteophyte formation. The condition may be asymptomatic but is often assocated with
pain radiating to occiput, shoulders and down one arm
stiffness and limited range of movement
tingling, numbness and weakness in the affected arm or hand
'drop attacks' due to transient vertebro-basilar ischaemia
cervical cord compression with symptoms in the lower limbs occurs only rarely.

The course is often episodic and treatment is usually conservative with
immobilization in a collar particularly at night
physiotherapy and local heat
simple analgesia or NSAID (see p. 495)
advice about head posture and working conditions.

In the presence of signs of cord compression or intractible symptoms referral to a specialist is indicated.

Whiplash injuries

This is a hyperextension injury to the cervical spine, most often sustained in a road traffic accident. It may lead to rupture of the anterior longitudinal ligament and cervical disc prolapse. The patient usually complains of pain some hours after the injury with limitation of all movement. There may be objective neurological signs in the upper limbs. The majority of cases can be managed conservatively with immobilization in a firm collar, rest and analgesia.

Manipulation may be appropriate in the absence of neurological signs and with normal X-rays.

Referral to a specialist should be considered if there is obvious nerve root compression or if X-rays suggest an unstable cervical spine.

Infantile torticollis

In this condition the head is tilted to one side and rotated due to ischaemic contracture of the sternomastoid muscle. It occurs in the infant and young child and can be distinguished from occular torticollis or painful cervical glands by the 'cord-like' feel of the sternomastoid muscle. If presenting early the condition can be treated by physiotherapy with stretching exercises. If this fails then surgical correction is necessary.

Ankylosing spondylitis

This may affect the neck after extension or dorso-lumbar disease. It results in aching pain and permanent stiffness (see p. 21).

Prolapsed cervical disc

This is much less common than in the lumbar spine. It causes pain and stiffness, and frequently neurological signs in the upper limbs. Injury is the usual precipitating cause.

Clinically it is often difficult to distinguish a prolapsed cervical disc from cervical spondylosis, but management is similar in both cases.

Referral is indicated for persistent pain or deteriorating neurological signs.

Cervical rib

This is often asymptomatic and is detected as an incidental X-ray finding. It does not, as a rule, cause neck pain. However symptoms may be referred to the upper limb and so mimic cervical disease.

A cervical rib may cause neurological signs in the C8–T1

distribution, and vascular changes in the hand and arm. It is diagnosed by X-ray of the thoracic inlet.

Other causes

Other conditions may present with neurological and muscular disorders in the arms, or with neck pain associated with more distant symptoms and signs.

Carpal tunnel syndrome
Ulnar nerve neuritis
Poliomyelitis
Toxic neuritis
Motor neurone disease
Syringomyelia
Cervical cord tumours
Pancoast's tumour
Cervical spondylolisthesis
Tension headache
Bad posture
Lymphadenopathy
Pharyngeal and oesophageal disorders
Meningitis
Sub-arachnoid haemorrhage
Metastases
Fractured vertebrae

See also:

Backache (p. 18)
Chest pain – angina pectoris (p. 43)
Earache (p. 77)
Headache (p. 133)

Nosebleed

The occasional nosebleed (epistaxis) of short duration, small amount and without other symptoms need not be a cause for concern.

Epistaxis with prolonged and profuse bleeding is alarming to both the patient and attendants, and a doctor usually becomes involved.

First aid

Pressure over cartilaginous part of the nose for a full 10 minutes and repeated as necessary
Sit forward and spit out blood from mouth
When bleeding stops avoid interfering with the nose for 24 hours

Causes

Local
- Rhinitis
- Trauma
- Nose blowing
- Sinusitis
- Foreign body
- Nose picking
- Carcinoma

Bleeding disorder
- Platelet deficiency
- Coagulopathy
- Excessive anticoagulants

Rarer causes
- Adenoid hypertrophy
- Haemangioma
- Telangiectasia
- Liver disease
- Kidney disease
- Tuberculosis
- Syphilis
- Actinomycosis
- Altitude

History

Age
Duration and estimated volume of blood loss
Trauma
Foreign body
History of previous nosebleeds, other bleeding or bruising
Medication

Examination

Estimate volume of blood loss
Locate site of bleeding
Exclude a septal haematoma with a history of trauma
BP
Pulse
Anaemia
Bruising and purpura
LAP

Investigation

FBC film and platelets
Prothrombin time and kaolin-cephalin time
Glandular fever screening test
Nasal swab
X-ray paranasal sinuses

Options

First aid (see p. 219)
Pack the nose – gauze strips impregnated with cocaine or adrenaline
Balloon catheters – indicated for posterior bleeding site
Cautery
  electrical
  chemical, e.g. $AgNo_3$
Investigate and treat the cause if appropriate
Iron supplements, e.g. ferrous gluconate 300 mg 12 hourly
Advice on first aid, nose blowing, etc.

Complications

Shock – especially in the elderly with atheromatous vessels
Obstruction of airways
Anaemia
Gastric irritation and melaena when blood has been swallowed
There is a 2% mortality from posterior epistaxes

Referral

For management of shock
Cases of persistent or recurrent bleeding
For investigation of possible underlying serious cause.

See also:

Sinusitis (p. 287)
STD (p. 301)
Pulmonary tuberculosis (p. 492)

Numbness and tingling

Numbness – loss of sensation, and tingling – altered sensation, are subjective feelings that are described by patients in various terms
  pins and needles
  stiffness
  heaviness
  deadness
  swelling
  'sandpaper'
  'water running down a limb'
  'walking on a sponge'
  most people will have suffered transient tingling last-

ing a few minutes as a result of stretching, pressure on a nerve, or reduced circulation to a peripheral nerve trunk by pressure or posture.

More prolonged or recurrent conditions do occur and the pattern of presentation depends upon the site of the lesion.

Patterns of presentation

Peripheral nerve lesion

Sensory disturbance (with or without wasting of related muscles) in specific nerve distribution
- median nerve – carpal tunnel syndrome
- ulnar nerve (at elbow) – 'funny bone' or ulnar palsy
- lateral cutaneous nerve of thigh – meralgia paraesthetica
- lateral popliteal nerve (at upper fibula) with or without foot drop

Polyneuropathy

Stocking and glove distribution with loss of reflexes
- diabetes
- drugs
- alcohol
- renal disease
- collagen disease
- vitamin B_{12} deficiency
- Guillain–Barré syndrome

Root lesion

Cervical and lumbar root syndrome

Spinal cord lesion

Sensory level on trunk with or without extensor plantars

Spinal cord compression

Multiple sclerosis

Cortical lesions

Associated defects of upper motor neurone weakness, language and visual–spatial disorder.
- cerebrovascular disease
- tumours
- migraine } transient
- epilepsy } transient

Psychosomatic

Bizarre pattern of attention seeking

History

Onset and duration of symptoms

Periodicity and progress of symptoms

Exacerbating and relieving factors
- movements
- posture

- straining
- coughing

Associated symptoms
- pain
- neck pain
- back pain
- mental changes
- loss of sphincter control
- fear of prognosis

Associated pathology
- hypothyroidism
- diabetes mellitus
- vitamin B_{12} deficiency
- acromegaly
- syphilis

Drugs and alcohol

Examination

Mental state
Sensory assessment – stereognosis and all modalities
Motor assessment – weakness and wasting
Reflexes
Gait
General examination to exclude underlying pathology if appropriate

Investigation

FBC
ESR
Urine (sugar)
LFT
Serum B_{12} estimation
Syphilis serology
Antinuclear factor

Options

Reassurance for transient paraesthesia and meralgia paraesthetica
Rest, splints and diuretics may help mild cases of carpal tunnel syndrome
Vitamin B_{12} supplements in proven deficiency states
Advise – reduced alcohol intake if appropriate
rest of cervical spondylosis and prolapsed intervertebral disc
Analgesics for associated pain.

Referral

Suspicion of cord compression
Persistent or progressive symptoms
Pain due to nerve entrapment
Higher function disturbance.

See also:

Elbow (p. 82)
Foot and ankle (p. 115)
Problem drinking (p. 261)
Wrist and hand (p. 341)
Chronic renal failure (p. 443)
Diabetes (p. 457)
Multiple sclerosis (p. 483)
Back injury (p. 512)

Obesity

Obesity results when energy input exceeds output. An individual's ability to control excess input varies enormously and the metabolic factors that determine the storage of energy in adipose tissue is not yet fully understood. The psychological and social causes and effects of obesity are understood and these are increasingly used to good effect in weight control. A change in life-style is the most important factor in a permanent reduction in weight.

Metabolic disorders may result in obesity but associated characteristic symptoms are usually present.

Medical investigation is generally unrewarding.

Ideal weight

Insurance company statistics indicate an optimal range of weight, in relation to height, which is associated with maximum longevity – the Body Mass Index (BMI).

Men $W/H^2 = 20–25$
Women $W/H^2 = 19–24$
when W = weight in kilos and H = height in metres

The range of 25–30 is considered overweight, over 30 obese.

Causes

Familial
Genetic
Environmental
Life-style
Compulsive over-eating
Problem drinking
Hypothyroidism
Diabetes
Polycystic ovary syndrome
Cushing's syndrome

Chromosome disorders
Medication, e.g. the Pill, steroids

Assessment

Diary of diet and appetite
Diary of exercise
Medication
History of obesity
Family attitudes and expectations
Family history of obesity
Social and psychological effects
Associated symptoms
- breathlessness
- skin changes
- arthritis
- immobility

Associated symptoms in metabolic disease
- Hypothyroidism
  - skin and hair changes
  - constipation
  - amenorrhoea
  - myxoedema
  - lethargy
- Polycystic ovary syndrome
  - hirsuitism
  - infertility
  - amenorrhoea
- Cushing's syndrome
  - moon face
  - buffalo hump
  - red striae
  - lanugo hair
  - amenorrhoea
  - hypertension

Examination

Weight
Height
BP
Cardiovascular status
Respiratory status
Thyroid status
Endocrine status
Joints
Skin

Investigation

Consider
- urinalysis

uric acid
blood sugar
T4 and TSH
CXR
ECG

Prevention

Individual and published advice on catering and cooking habits. Plans for exercise; especially for the family with children. Health education (see p. 466)

Options

Medical management when appropriate, e.g. thyroid disorders
Counselling towards a change in life-style
Diet
- appetite trigger factors, e.g. tea breaks
- timing of meals
- fluid intake
- energy content
- fibre content
- palatability
- cost

Positive attitude – to ideal weight, shape or size – help to revise the expectations and rewards of the obese patient
Exercise – planned programme of graduated exercise taking care not to generate an excessive hunger
Bulk agents, e.g. methylcellulose 2–3 tablets 8 hourly
Appetite suppression – short term – taking care to avoid dependence, e.g. fenfluramine initially 20 mg 12 hourly.

Referral

Slimming groups, e.g. 'Weight Watchers'
Endocrinologist only when associated with specific symptoms
Surgeon (in extreme cases) for
- jaw wiring
- vagotomy
- jejunal bypass
- 'apronectomy'

Complications associated with or exacerbated by obesity

Diabetes
Hypertension
Abdominal surgery
Immobility
Arthritis
Backache

Social status and respect
Pregnancy
Ischaemic heart disease
Thromboembolic disease
Gall bladder disease
Accidents
Intertrigo
Hypoventilation – 'Pickwickian syndrome'
Varicose veins

See also:

Problem drinking (p. 261)
The fat child (p. 415)
Diabetes (p. 457)
Hypothyroidism (p. 481)

Obsessions

In patients with an obsessional neurosis, there is a subjective compulsion to carry out some action, to dwell on an idea, to recall an experience or ruminate on an abstract topic. The unwanted thoughts are perceived by the patient as inappropriate and alien, but are generated within his conscious self. Attempts to control the thoughts may lead to intense anxiety.

Intrusive thoughts can be experienced by normal people but it is the frequency, persistence and intensity of these thoughts that distinguish the patient with obsessional neurosis. The aetiology is unclear; genetic, environmental and organic factors have been considered. About two thirds of sufferers improve within a year; the remainder run a fluctuating course.

The obsessional personality is described as a precise, punctual perfectionist who is inflexible to change and sensitive to criticism. This patient does not necessarily develop obsessional symptoms and indeed, is more likely to become depressed under stress. Normal people with an obsessional trait might be considered admirable, dependable and reliable although occasionally given to obstinacy and preoccupation with detail.

Obsessional symptoms

Thoughts and images

Recurrent, repetitive, unacceptable and unpleasant words, ideas, beliefs or images dominate the consciousness. The patient recognizes them as his own and not generated from an external source. They are frequently of a sexual or obscure nature. The intrusions generate anxiety and the patient makes a variable effort to resist them.

Rumination

Endless internal debates about ordinary everyday actions.

Doubts

Failure to adequately perform necessary actions, e.g. turning off the gas, locking the door.

Impulses

Forceful urges to perform acts of a violent or embarrassing kind.

Rituals

Repetitive mental activities such as counting or senseless actions such as frequent hand washing. Occasionally the activities have to be repeated in a complicated way for a certain number of times. If not adequately achieved the sequence has to be started again. The rituals are perceived as illogical and are therefore practised secretly.

Assessment

Onset, nature and progression of symptoms
Associated anxiety and depression
Associated social disruption
Life events and stress factors
Pre-morbid personality

Options

Support

The neurosis follows a fluctuating course often with long remissions. As a result patients are sometimes vigourously overtreated. Support for the patient and family may be all that is required awaiting a natural remission. Give reassurance that it is not a sign of 'madness'.

Medication

Anxiolytic drugs are helpful in the short term (i.e. less than 3 weeks), e.g. diazepam 2–10 mg 8 hourly

Antidepressants are very helpful for associated depression. Effective treatment can also clear obsessional symptoms, e.g. amitryptyline 75–150 mg at night or clomipramine 75–150 mg at night.

Behavioural therapy

Behavioural techniques can improve obsessional rituals in approximately two thirds of patients.

Psychotherapy

Simple supportive psychotherapy may be helpful for reasons already stated – interpretive or exploratory psychotherapy may be harmful by encouraging rumination.

Psychosurgery

There is little controlled evidence that surgery helps in the long term. It should only be considered when the symptoms have persisted unchanged for several years without response to other treatments.

Referral

For psychiatric assessment
For behavioural therapy.

Oliguria and anuria

The passage of little or no urine through the urethra is a cardinal symptom of either urinary retention or acute renal failure.

Urinary retention is primarily a surgical problem that may be complicated by residual urine, infection, detrusor hypertrophy and back pressure on the ureters.

Acute renal failure is a rare medical emergency characterized by sudden deterioration in renal function usually associated with a urine volume of less than 500 ml/day, and the build up of metabolic waste products. The prognosis is poor and early recognition and referral is the crucial role of the family doctor.

Causes

Pre-renal
(poor renal perfusion)
- Hypovolaemic shock (blood or fluid loss)
- Cardiogenic shock
- Septicaemic shock
- Massive pulmonary embolus

Renal
(renal damage)
- Acute tubular necrosis
- Glomerulonephritis
- Papillary necrosis
- Malignant hypertension
- Hyperuricaemia
- Excess bilirubin or porphyrin

Post-renal
(obstruction)
- Prostatic hypertrophy or carcinoma
- Ureteric stones

Pelvic tumour
Urethral stricture
Retroperitoneal fibrosis
Peripheral neuropathy

History

Thirst, polydipsia, ankle swelling
Recent major trauma, burns or diarrhoea
Approximate urine volume
Intercurrent urinary symptoms – particularly pain and frequency
Past history of renal disease or hypertension
Medication (particularly analgesic abuse)
Toxins, e.g. mercury, carbon tetrachloride, *Clostridium welchii*

Examination

State of hydration (skin turgor and mucous membranes)
Fluid overload (JVP and ankle swelling)
BP
Renal masses or tenderness
Palpable bladder
Rectal examination to exclude enlarged prostate or pelvic tumours
Signs of prolapsed intervertebral disc

Referral

If renal failure is suspected patients should be referred to a specialist for investigation and care as a medical emergency
Oliguria due to prostatic obstruction may require catheterization for symptom relief prior to hospital referral.

See also:

Maternal diseases in pregnancy (p. 367)
Enlarged prostate (p. 90)
Chronic renal failure (p. 443)

Painful periods

Dysmenorrhoea is a cramping pain in the lower abdomen radiating to the back and the thighs, and is associated with menstruation. It is often incapacitating. The pain is related to a rise in intrauterine pressure and is probably mediated by prostaglandins. It is commoner in younger women, 5–10% being affected. In older women the pain may be associated with other causes of pelvic pain (see p. 240). Pain is often a predominant symptom of the premenstrual syndrome.

Causes

Physiological
Endometriosis
Pelvic inflammatory disease
Prolapsing intramural fibroid
Premenstrual syndrome

History

Menarche and menstrual history
Onset of dysmenorrhoea
Gynaecological and obstetric history
Contraceptive history
Associated symptoms
Social and psychological factors (especially the opinions and attitudes of the mother)

Examination

Abdominal examination
Pelvic examination when indicated

Options

Sympathy and reassurance
Mild analgesics
  fenamates (e.g. Ponstan 250–500 mg 8 hourly)
  prostaglandin synthetase inhibitors (e.g. aspirin)
B_2 receptor stimulants (e.g. terbutaline 5 mg 8 hourly)
Hormonal
  the Pill
  bromocryptine
  progesterones (after consultation)
Antibiotics for pelvic inflammatory disease.

Referral

Persistent primary dysmenorrhoea for laparoscopy and cervical dilation
Investigation of secondary dysmenorrhoea, when indicated, e.g. fibroids

See also:

Pelvic pain (p. 240)
Premenstrual syndrome (p. 257)

Pallor (anaemia)

Pallor is the pale appearance of poorly perfused skin. It may be transient as in syncope or hypothermia, or more persistent as in hypothyroidism or depression. Classically, pallor is the accepted, if unreliable, indicator of anaemia. If anaemia is discovered then a cause must be sought.

Definition of anaemia

Hb level in women <12
Hb level in men <13

Causes of anaemia

Hypochromic/Microcytic

MCHC <32
MCV <75

- Menstrual loss
  - menorrhagia
  - IUCD
- Bowel loss
  - peptic ulcer
  - oesophageal varices
  - malignancy
  - haemorrhoids
  - medication
- Poor diet
- Pregnancy
- Thalassaemia

Macrocytic

MCV >95

- Vitamin B_{12} deficiency
  - pernicious anaemia
  - bowel surgery
- Folate deficiency
  - malabsorption
  - dietary deficiency
  - problem drinking
  - pregnancy
  - medication
- Vitamin C deficiency
- Hypothyroidism

Normochromic/normocytic

MCHC 32–38 (normal)
MCV 75–95 (normal)

- Acute blood loss
- Haemolytic anaemia
- Medication
- Chronic disease
  - renal failure
  - tuberculosis
  - Crohn's disease
  - malignancy
- Haemoglobinopathies
- Bone marrow infiltration
  - leukaemia
  - myelofibrosis

History

Associated blood loss
- Major trauma (including ruptured spleen or liver)
- Haematemesis
- Melaena
- Menorrhagia

Associated symptoms
- Change in appetite
- Weight loss
- Tiredness and fatigue
- Epigastric pain
- Change in bowel habit, dark stools, bleeding P.R.
- Shortness of breath, ankle swelling, chest pain
- Paraesthesiae, numbness and weakness

Menstrual history
Past history
- recent surgery
- previous anaemia
- chronic illness

Family history of anaemia
Medication
Alcohol and diet
Occupation

Examination

Mucous membranes and palms for pallor
Tongue for glossitis and telangiectasia
Nails for koilonychia and clubbing
Skin for petechiae and bruising
Lymphadenopathy
CVS for cardiac failure and murmurs
CNS for peripheral neuropathy especially in macrocytic anaemia
Abdomen for enlarged liver or spleen
Pelvic examination
Rectal examination (check stool colour)

Investigation

Initially
- Haemoglobin
- MCV
- Blood film
- ESR

Subsequently

Hypochromic anaemia
- Serum iron and TIBC
- Faecal occult blood
- Proctoscopy

Sigmoidoscopy
Barium meal and enema

Marcrocytic anaemia

Serum B_{12}
Serum folate or red cell folate
Thyroid function
Barium meal and follow through

Normocytic anaemia

White blood count
Reticulocyte count
Serum bilirubin (unconjugated)
LFT
Thyroid function
Antinuclear factor
Haemoglobin electrophoresis
Chest X-ray
Barium meal and enema

Options

Treat underlying pathology where appropriate
Iron supplements, e.g.
Ferrous sulphate 200 mg 8 hourly
Ferrous gluconate 300 mg 6–8 hourly
Sometimes troublesome side effects necessitate a change of preparation
Continue treatment for 3 months after the haemoglobin level returns to normal in order to replenish iron stores
Vitamin B_{12}, e.g. Hydroxycobalamin
Initially 1000 μg daily for 5–10 days to replenish stores then a maintenance dose according to need (usually 250 μg–500 μg per month)
Folic acid, e.g.
5 mg 8 hourly for 2 weeks then once daily for 3–4 months. It should not be given in undiagnosed macrocytic anaemia unless vitamin B_{12} is given concurrently.

Referral

Acute severe blood loss
Suspected internal haemorrhage
Haemoglobin less than 7 g per 100 ml with significant symptoms
Underlying surgical pathology for investigation and treatment
Marrow failure and haemoglobinopathies for haematological assessment.

See also:

Anal bleeding (p. 8)
Depression (p. 63)
Faints (p. 101)
Heavy periods (p. 144)
Hypothermia (p. 154)
Malnutrition and malabsorption (p. 195)
Oliguria and anuria (p. 229)
Piles (p. 249)
Problem drinking (p. 261)
Maternal diseases in pregnancy (p. 367)
Chronic renal failure (p. 443)
Contraception (p. 446)
Hypothyroidism (p. 481)
Pulmonary tuberculosis (p. 492)

Palpitations

This is a rather vague symptom, loosely defined as an increased awareness of the heart beat as a result of increased force of action, increased rate or irregular rhythm. The true incidence of this symptom is difficult to ascertain; it would appear to be more common in females (2:1).

Causes

Anxiety
Drugs and coffee
Smoking
Hyperthyroidism
(Rarely true heart disease or phaeochromocytoma)

History

Frequency and duration of the episodes of palpitations
Mode of onset
- sudden (e.g. paroxysmal tachycardia)
- gradual (e.g. anxiety)

Ask patient to tap out the rhythm
Precipitating factors
- drugs and coffee
- emotion
- cigarettes
- exertion

Associated features
- dyspnoea
- dizziness
- pain

syncope
diuresis (during or after)
Past history of ischaemic or rheumatic heart disease

Examination Full CVS examination is helpful mainly as a form of reassurance
Record
pulse rate and rhythm (compare radial with apex rate)
BP
heart sounds
Check for
anaemia
tremor
goitre
level of anxiety
sympathetic activity (e.g. sweating palms)

Investigation Only when specifically indicated from the history or examination
ECG including a rhythm strip in lead II (best taken during the episode)
FBC
T_3

Options Firm reassurance is usually effective since in the vast majority of cases the cause is psychogenic
Advice about smoking and coffee drinking
Propranolol 10–20 mg 8 hourly may help anxiety induced tachycardia
Minor tranquillizers may help occasionally
Induced vagal stimulation by eyeball pressure, valsalva's manoeuvre or cold drink may help paroxysmal atrial tachycardias
Digoxin is helpful in uncontrolled atrial fibrillation
Hyperthyroidism must be treated appropriately.

Referral For urgent control of tachycardia (i.e. <120 per minute) when it is associated with chest pain or marked dyspnoea
For 24 hour monitoring for paroxysmal tachycardias.

See also: Stress and anxiety (p. 303)
Hyperthyroidism (p. 479)

Paranoid ideas

The use of this term is descriptive not diagnostic. It encompasses the symptoms of abnormal ideas or delusions of self-reference with feelings of suspicion, persecution, guilt and jealousy. It should be considered in the context of a spectrum of presentations

Paranoid personality (see p. 242)

Primary paranoid state – a state in which there are well defined delusional complexes without hallucinations in an otherwise normal personality

Secondary paranoid state – paranoid features can occur in association with primary mental disorders
- organic mental state – drug or alcohol involved
  - dementia
- severe depressive illness
- schizophrenia

The spouse or family of the patient may seek help initially since paranoid ideas can be very disruptive and are hard to tolerate. However, the ideas of persecution or jealousy may well be justified.

Social isolation or sensory deprivation (e.g. deafness) can potentiate paranoid ideas.

Assessment

Onset, sequence and content of paranoid ideas
Establish how much the ideas are based on fact
Associated symptoms including confusion, depression or homicidal intent if relevant
Medical history
Psychiatric history
Drugs and alcohol
Social support
Mental state examination
- orientation
- IQ
- memory
- concentration
- clouded consciousness
- hallucinations
- delusions
- thought disorder

Options

Accept patient's perceptions as the basis for discussion without colluding with his or her delusions

Involve friends and relatives whom the patient trusts
Review medication
Deal with any underlying primary mental disorder
Encourage domestic and social contacts and support
Attend to sensory deficits (vision and hearing)
Advise and support family, neighbours, attendants.

Medication

Hypnotics for insomnia
- Temazepam 10–20 mg at night
- Nitrazepam 5–10 mg at night

Antipsychotic medication
- Thioridazine 20–200 mg daily
- Trifluoperazine 2–30 mg daily
- Flupenthixol decanoate 20–40 mg every 2–4 weeks

The dosage and duration of treatment should be titrated to the patient's needs and responses.

Referral

Admission to psychiatric hospital if the delusions are causing aggressive behaviour or social difficulties
Compulsory admission is sometimes justified (see p. 527).

See also:

Personality disorders (p. 242)
Schizophrenia (p. 276)
Mental Health Act 1983 (p. 527)

Pelvic mass

A pelvic mass is a sign which is often detected unexpectedly at routine examination. A pelvic mass can also be found in association with pain, 'bloatedness', urinary or gynaecological symptoms.

Gynaecological causes predominate and if vaginal examination is undertaken (e.g. for HVS or cervical cytology) a full bimanual pelvic assessment should be made to exclude a pelvic mass.

An ectopic pregnancy can present with a pelvic mass as the initial manifestation.

Causes

Uterine mass
- pregnancy
- fibroids
- adenomyosis

- carcinoma
- congenital abnormalities

Adnexal mass
- ovarian tumours
- endometriosis
- pelvic inflammatory disease
- ectopic pregnancy
- hydrosalpinx

Non-gynaecological causes
- full bladder
- constipated rectum or sigmoid colon
- primary cancer of the bladder, rectum or sigmoid colon
- secondary deposits from a distant primary cancer

History

Menstrual history including abnormal bleeding
Vaginal discharge
Dyspareunia
Pelvic or abdominal pain and relationship to masses
Problems with micturition and bowel habit
General health
- weight loss
- appetite

Examination

Bimanual vaginal examination (with empty bladder)
Visualize the cervix
Abdominal palpation for masses and tenderness
Rectal examination

Investigation

Consider
- FBC
- ESR
- LFT
- pregnancy test
- cervical smear
- vaginal smear
- MSU
- stool occult blood
- ultrasound examination of the pelvis
- IVP
- barium enema

Options

Pregnancy – antenatal care (see p. 348)
Ovarian cysts greater than 5 cm diameter should be referred for early assessment and ultrasound

A fibroid uterus which is symptomless and less than '14 weeks' in size requires no treatment
Pelvic inflammatory disease should be treated aggressively with antibiotics. A combination of amoxycillin 250 mg 8 hourly and metronidazole 400 mg 8 hourly would be first choice, amended according to bacteriological results
Endometriosis can be treated conservatively with continuous oral contraceptive therapy or danazol for 6–12 months
Constipation (see p. 55).

Referral

Urgent referral if associated with unilateral pain to exclude
- torsion of ovarian cyst
- pedunculated fibroids
- ectopic pregnancy

Gynaecologist for further assessment
Urologist if bladder pathology is suspected
Gastroenterologist for further investigation of bowel tumours.

See also:

Constipation (p. 55)
Pelvic pain (p. 240)
Diagnosis of pregnancy (p. 346)
Disorders of pregnancy (p. 357)

Pelvic pain

Pelvic pain is a common presenting feature of several gynaecological conditions. The pain may be acute, coincident with periods, may occur randomly or constantly or only during the premenstrual phase of the cycle.

Dyspareunia, pelvic pain during sexual intercourse, is an increasingly common presenting complaint. Women can usually make the distinction between superficial and deep dyspareunia which can help assessment and diagnosis.

Causes

Acute
- Ectopic pregnancy
- Ovulation pain (mittelschmerz)
- Torsion of ovarian cyst
- Pelvic inflammatory disease

Chronic

- Displaced ovary
- 'Pelvic congestion syndrome'
- First trimester pregnancy
- Prolapsed uterus
- IUCD
- Fibroids
- Endometriosis
- Sexually transmitted disease
- Irritable bowel syndrome

History

Menstrual history and LMP
Onset, duration and periodicity of pain
Situation, radiation and severity
Associated symptoms
- dyspareunia
- dysuria
- vaginal discharge
- nausea
- pain on defaecation
- pain on micturition
- rash
- fever

Social and psychological factors

Examination

BP
Temperature
Pulse
Abdominal signs
Pelvic examination
Rectal examination

Investigation

Pregnancy test
FBC
High vaginal swab

Options

Analgesics
Suppression of menstruation
- Danazol 200–800 mg in divided doses 4 times daily
- Norethisterone 5 mg 3 times daily
- Continuous oral contraceptive pill

Antibiotics (having excluded pregnancy)
- Amoxil 250–500 mg 8 hourly
- Metronidazole 200 mg 8 hourly
- Tetracycline 250 mg 6 hourly
- Cephalosporins

Treat co-existing disease, e.g.
irritable bowel syndrome
sexually transmitted disease.

Failure to control Consider more obscure diagnosis
TB salpingitis
mumps oophoritis
endometriosis

Complications Dyspareunia
Heavy periods
Anaemia
Pelvic adhesions
Infertility

Referral Suspected ectopic pregnancy
Pelvic masses or endometriosis for laparoscopy
Associated heavy bleeding
Pelvic inflammatory disease for further bacteriological studies.

See also:
Pelvic mass (p. 238)
STD (p. 301)
Disorders of pregnancy (p. 357)
Contraception (p. 446)

Personality disorders

An understanding of personality types can be a helpful guide in predicting how a patient might behave when ill. Some features of personality produce a vulnerability to neurosis under stress. In patients with personality disorders unusual and maladaptive behaviour occurs even in the absence of stress.

Any classification of personality type carries a risk of giving 'pseudo-insight' through terminology and a tendency to be judgemental. In clinical practice it is better to consider the individual patient's strengths and weaknesses in a descriptive way. The following classification should be considered in the light of these limitations.

Classification **Paranoid**
Suspicious and over sensitive
Problems with making friends

- Little sense of humour or capacity for enjoyment
- Tendency to jealousy
- Overcautious
- Sense of self-importance beyond capabilities
- Tendency to blame others for failings

Affective

- Depressive
  - gloomy in outlook
  - strong sense of duty
  - poor capacity for enjoyment
  - irritable and bad tempered
- Hyperthymic
  - cheerful and optimistic
  - poor sense of judgement
  - uncritical
- Cycloid
  - alternation between the above extremes

Schizoid

(Contrary to the name it does not imply a causal relationship with schizophrenia)

- Introspective and emotionally cold
- Self-sufficient and detached
- Often remain single
- Solitary hobbies and interests
- More concerned with intellectual than practical activities

Explosive

- Poor control of emotions
- Sudden outbursts of anger both verbal and physical

Obsessional

(Contrary to the name there is no direct link with obsessional neurosis see p. 227)

- Lack of adaptability to new situations
- Inflexible and rigid
- Inhibiting perfectionism
- Moralistic
- Indecisive because of fear of making mistakes
- Sensitivity to criticism
- Difficulty expressing emotions

Histrionic

- Self-centred
- Tendency to self-dramatization
- Searches for excitement, novelty and attention
- Short-lived enthusiasm
- Vain and demanding
- Self-deceptive
- Transient swings of emotion

Asthenic
- Passive and dependent
- Unduly compliant and weak-willed
- Poor self-confidence

Antisocial
- Failure to make lasting relationships despite superficial charm
- Cruel and callous
- Indifference to other people's feelings
- Impulsive actions
- Lack of guilt
- Failure to learn from adverse experiences
- Alcohol and drug abuse
- Poor work record

Assessment

- Nature and duration of the personality problem
- Social effects and consequences
- Circumstances which exacerbate symptoms or adverse characteristics
- Childhood history
- Life events
- Stress factors
- Family history
- Career history
- Exclude neurotic and psychotic conditions
- Assess motivation to change

Options

The opportunities for change are limited and so the aims should be modest. Try to build on the strengths and advise avoidance of exacerbating factors or situations.

Medication
- Has little place in the long term management because of dependency
- Anxiolytics in short courses (less than 3 weeks) may be helpful in stressful situations, e.g. diazapam 2–10 mg 8 hourly

Psychotherapy
- Particularly useful for the younger patient who has difficulty forming relationships
- With histrionic personalities limits must be made in order to contain demands.

Supervision and support
- Perhaps involving the social worker or health visitor
- If antisocial behaviour has lead to trouble with the law then the probation service can be approached.

Therapeutic communities
May be helpful for antisocial personalities.

See also: Obsessions (p. 227)

Phobias

Phobic anxiety states are associated with an abnormally intense dread and wish to avoid certain objects or specific situations which would not normally have that effect.

The prevalence is about six in every thousand total population. Agoraphobia and simple phobias are more common in women, while social phobias are equally common in both sexes.

Simple phobias

There are many examples in this category but amongst the more common would be
heights
thunderstorms
enclosed spaces
flying
visiting dentists
spiders
snakes
dogs
using public lavatories

The patient not only feels intense anxiety in the presence of feared objects or situations but also suffers anxious thoughts in anticipation and hence will avoid possible confrontation. The condition may be learnt by imitation of parents or other children or by conditioning in response to a frightening event.

Social phobias

These patients become anxious in situations in which they may be observed by other people, e.g. restaurants, canteens, public transport, hairdressers, theatre, cinemas and parties.

Patients often take alcohol to relieve symptoms and alcohol abuse is more common in this type of phobia.

Agoraphobia

These patients become anxious when they travel away from home or are in situations they cannot easily leave. The association is characteristically allied to ideas of fainting or losing control. Occasionally it is so severe that the patient becomes housebound.

Assessment

Details of phobia
Age of onset
Extent and effect of avoidance behaviour
Symptoms of associated depression
Previous psychiatric illness
Alcohol abuse

Options

Behavioural therapy
Sustained improvement depends on overcoming accompanying avoidance behaviour. Programmes of graded exposure to the situation give best results.
Hypnotherapy
Hypnotherapy has been used with some limited success.
Medication
Anxiolytics produce immediate relief but are of little long term benefit unless avoidance behaviour is dealt with, e.g. diazapam 2–10 mg 8 hourly.
Antidepressants are helpful for treatment of underlying depression and also for the anxiolytic effect in primary phobic states, e.g. imipramine 25–50 mg 8 hourly.

Referral

For behavioural therapy
For psychiatric treatment.

See also:

Problem drinking (p. 261)

Pigmentation

Melanin pigmentation is influenced by genetic and hormonal factors as well as physical and chemical agents. The colour can vary from brown to black (eumelanins). Red and yellow pigments are chemically distinct (phaeomelanins).

Cause of pigmentation problems

Lack of pigment
- Post-inflammatory
  - eczema
  - psoriasis
  - pityriasis versicolor
- Occupational
  - antioxidant in rubber
  - phenolic compounds

- Auto-immune
  - vitiligo
- Hormonal
  - hypopituitarism (lack of MSH)
- Inborn errors of metabolism
  - albinism
  - phenylketonuria

Increase in pigment

- Post-inflammatory
- Varicose pigmentation
- Hormonal
  - pregnancy and the Pill (chloasma)
  - Addison's disease
  - hyperthyroidism
- Nutritional
  - malabsorption
  - vitamin B_{12} deficiency
- Metabolic
  - chronic liver disease
  - renal failure
  - porphyria
- Occupational
  - some chemicals act as photosensitizers, e.g. tar, mineral oil coolants
- Cosmetic
  - bergamot oil act as a photosensitizer
- Other causes
  - neurofibromatosis
  - Peutz–Jeghers syndrome
  - Albright's disease
  - urticaria pigmentosa
  - acanthosis nigricans

Non-melanin pigmentations

- Jaundice (yellow)
- Agyria–silver salts (slate-grey)
- Chlorpromazine (slate-grey)
- Haemachromatosis (bronze)
- Carotinaemia (orange-yellow)
- Tattooing (various colours)

History

- Onset, duration and distribution of pigmentation
- Symptoms of underlying systemic disease
- Past history of inflammatory skin condition, renal or liver disease
- Menstrual history
- Medication
- Occupational and social circumstances

Examination Distribution of pigmentation
Associated skin disease
Signs of underlying systemic disease

Investigation May be necessary when considering underlying systemic disease
- FBC
- ESR
- MCV
- B_{12} & folate
- U & E
- LFT
- thyroid function
- serum iron and TIBC
- hormone assay
- CXR
- barium meal

Options Explanation – may be all that is required
Reassurance – post-inflammatory hypo/hyper pigmentation will often resolve once the skin condition is controlled
Avoidance of sunlight – fair-skinned individuals may look worse when the normal skin is pigmented, highlighting the contrast with depigmented patches. Avoiding sunlight and use of barrier creams may reduce this effect
Avoidance of implicated drugs and photosensitizers
Psoralens – act as photosensitizers. They may be applied topically or systemically and used in conjunction with natural or artificial UV light
Cosmetics – masking creams and powders
Dihydroxyacetone – may be used to 'stain' patches of pigmentation
Hydroquinones – applied topically may help to reduce hyperpigmented patches.

See also:
Generalized rash (p. 118)
Localized rash (p. 185)
Malnutrition and malabsorption (p. 195)
Symptoms in pregnancy (p. 352)
Chronic renal failure (p. 443)
Hyperthyroidism (p. 479)

Piles

Patients occasionally complain of an 'attack of piles' or simply pain, bleeding or anal irritation.

Pathologically the cause is varicosity of the submucous veins in the anal canal.

Internal piles may remain in the anal canal (first degree) or prolapse beyond the anal margin on straining (second degree) and some remain prolapsed (third degree). All are liable to complications of thrombosis, strangulation or infection.

External piles may occur on the outside of the mucocutaneous boundary.

The cause is unknown but may be related to chronic constipation and straining at stool; there may be hereditary factors involved and pregnancy can exacerbate and precipitate piles. More rarely, portal hypertension, pelvic and rectocolonic tumours or local inflammatory conditions may cause venous congestion and so aggravate haemorrhoids.

History

General symptoms – appetite, change in weight or bowel habit

Local symptoms – pain, itching, blood or mucus

Examination

Palpate the abdomen for masses or enlarged liver

Check presence of prolapsing piles in the relaxed state and on straining down – skin tags, external piles and anal fissures

Digital examination to exclude pelvic masses

Proctoscopy to assess the extent of internal piles

Investigation

Usually unnecessary but consider referral for
 sigmoidoscopy
 barium enema – (similarly for rectal bleeding p. 8)

Options

Diet – advise increased roughage in natural diet and supplement with synthetic preparations (Normocol, Isogel) as necessary

Bowel habit – avoid straining at stool and consider laxatives

Local creams – mild astringent antiseptic ointments can be soothing and may be combined with local anaesthetic and/or steroid preparations

Incision and evacuation of external piles will produce rapid relief of pain.

Referral

For sclerosant injection or cryosurgery

For formal excision of haemorrhoids (particularly with third degree piles)

For anal sphincter stretch procedure with anal fissures

For further investigation of possible underlying serious cause.

See also:

Anal bleeding (p. 8)
Anal irritation (p. 10)
Constipation (p. 55)

Pleural effusion

Pleural effusion may present as shortness of breath of gradual onset, tightness in the chest or pleuritic pain. It may be detected by a dullness of percussion or by diminished breath or voice sounds on auscultation. The effusion may be a transudate, exudate or pus, or rarely a chylous pleural effusion, following trauma to the thoracic duct.

Collapsed or consolidated lower lobes of the lungs can mimic the signs of pleural effusion.

Causes

Transudate

Left ventricular failure
Low albumin states

Exudate

Pneumonia
Pulmonary infarction
Primary or secondary cancer
Tuberculosis

Other causes

Systemic lupus erythematosis
Polyarteritis nodosum
Rheumatoid arthritis
Rheumatic fever
Pericarditis
Lymphomas
Ruptured oesophagus
Ascites
Peritoneal dialysis
Meige's syndrome
Trauma

History

Onset and duration of symptoms
- shortness of breath
- pain
- haemoptysis
- fever
- cough
- tightness of the chest
- oedema
- weight loss

Recent trauma
History of contraception

Examination

Cardiovascular status – exclude DVT
Examination of chest
- expansion
- percussion note
- voice sounds
- breath sounds
- respiratory rate
- peak expiratory flow rate

Investigation

CXR and ECG – for signs of pulmonary infarction
FBC
ESR
Serum protein
ANF
LE cells
Rheumatoid factor
Mantoux test
Pleural aspirate for cytology and culture

Referral

Most cases for drainage and futher investigation.

See also:

Ascites (p. 14)
Pulmonary tuberculosis (p. 492)
Rheumatoid arthritis (p. 493)
Respiratory distress – acute left ventricular failure (p. 535)

Polyuria

Polyuria presents as a subjective awareness of the passage of a larger than normal volume of urine. It should not be confused with simple frequency of micturition which is more often associated with a urinary infection or anxiety.

True polyuria associated with organic disease is almost always accompanied by a sensation of increased thirst.

Causes

Early pregnancy
Compulsive drinking
Diuretic therapy
Diabetes mellitus
Chronic renal failure
Hypokalaemia
Hypercalcaemia
Diabetes insipidus

Rare causes

Nephrogenic diabetes insipidus
Fanconi's syndrome
Lesion of the thirst centre
Hypothalamic tumours

History

Presenting symptoms
- weight loss
- diarrhoea
- thirst
- nocturia
- dysuria
- assessment of daily fluid intake

Associated symptoms
- muscular weakness (hypokalaemia)
- nausea
- constipation
- abdominal and bone pain (hypercalcaemia)
- headache and failing vision (hypothalamic tumours)

Past medical history
- renal disease
- recent head injury or CVA
- diabetes mellitus
- hypertension

Family history
- renal disease
- diabetes mellitus

Medication
- diuretic therapy
- steroids

Examination

General
- weight
- anaemia

BP
breath (ketolic smell)
Eyes
corneal calcification (hypercalcaemia)
visual fields
funduscopy for retinopathy
Abdomen
palpate for renal masses
exclude pregnancy
CNS
mental state
tendon reflexes (diminished in hypokalaemia)

Investigation

Assessment of daily fluid balance
Urine
proteinuria
glycosuria
specific gravity
culture
U & E and calcium
Random blood sugar
Chest X-ray
IVP

Options

Specific therapy will depend on the underlying cause
Reassure the patient with polyuria in early pregnancy
Reconsider diuretic therapy
Correct hypokalaemia
Psychotherapy for compulsive drinking
Diabetes mellitus (see p. 457)
Renal failure (p. 443)

Referral

Further investigation – a water deprivation test under hospital supervision may be necessary to distinguish between diabetes insipidus and compulsive drinking
For correction of hypercalcaemia
For assistance in management of renal failure or diabetes mellitus.

See also:

Problem drinking (p. 261)
Symptoms of pregnancy (p. 352)
Chronic renal failure (p. 443)
Diabetes (p. 457)

Poor circulation

'Poor circulation' is the commonest presenting complaint associated with peripheral vascular disease. The majority of cases are functional and an exaggeration of physiological control of skin temperature, whereas some cases are progressive and benefit from careful assessment and review. Occasionally poor circulation and pain are indicative of arterial occlusion requiring urgent surgical intervention.

Causes

Raynaud's disease (primary)
Raynaud's phenomenon (secondary)
- oral contraception
- β-blockade
- vibration trauma
- scleroderma or SLE
- protein disorders
- rheumatoid arthritis

Arteritis
- Buerger's disease
- giant cell arteritis

Livedo reticularis
- physiological
- PAN

Cold trauma
- frostbite
- hypothermia
- chilblains
- acrocyanosis

Ischaemia
- atherosclerosis
- thrombosis
- embolism
  - diabetes
  - myocardial infarction
  - aneurysm
  - sub-acute bacterial endocarditis
  - atrial fibrillation

History

Onset, duration and progress of symptoms
Precipitating, exacerbating and relieving factors
Associated symptoms
- claudication
- rest pain
- chest pain

- palpitations
- lethargy
- malaise
- arthritis
- shortness of breath

Medication, e.g. OC pill, β-blockers, ergot derivatives
Occupation
Family history

- Raynaud's phenomenon
- migraine
- vascular disease
- IHD

Smoking habits

Examination

Record

- Core temperature
- Colour, texture and appearance of skin
- Capillary filling
- Peripheral pulses
- BP
- Pulse

Check

- Heart sounds
- Arterial bruits
- Abdominal aorta
- Splinter haemorrhages
- Fundi
- Localizing neurological signs

Investigations

FBC & ESR
U & E
Blood glucose
Cholesterol and triglycerides
Urinalysis
ECG & CXR
Consider

- ANF and rheumatoid factor
- syphilis serology
- cervical spine X-ray

Options

Advice

- Information on transient forms of ischaemia
- Protection from cold
- Avoid trauma
- Stop smoking

Stop any offending drugs
Skin care

Chiropody

Medication

Anticoagulants
Antibiotics – (as indicated)
Steroids – (only when indicated)
Vasodilators – (of dubious benefit)

Surgery

To release pus
Sympathectomy
Endarteriectomy
Bypass grafts.

Follow-up

Claudication distance
Peripheral pulses
Skin condition
Temperature
Review medication

Complications

Necrosis, gangrene and amputation
Deformity of digits
Sub-cutaneous calcification

Referral

Arterial occlusion requires urgent referral
Persistent symptoms – for surgical assessment.

See also:

Chest pain – myocardial infarction (p. 46)
Hypothermia (p. 154)
Contraception (p. 446)
Diabetes (p. 457)
Rheumatoid arthritis (p. 493)

Post-menopausal bleeding

Vaginal bleeding occuring more than six months after the cessation of periods at the menopause is a cardinal feature of carcinoma of the body of the uterus. This diagnosis must be excluded in all cases, even when some other source of bleeding is evident. In up to one-third of all cases no diagnosis can be made.

Causes

Atrophic vaginitis with
uterine prolapse
pessary

or post-traumatic/coital
Infective vaginitis
Urethral caruncle
Haematuria
Rectal bleeding
Carcinoma of the body of the uterus
Cervical carcinoma
Cervical polyp
Endometrial polyp
Ovarian tumour
Hormone replacement therapy
Blood clotting defect

History

Menopause – date
Menstrual and obstetric history
Associated vaginal symptoms
Associated general symptoms – malaise, weight loss

Examination

BP
Anaemia
Abdominal examination
Pelvic examination
Rectal examination

Investigation

Cervical smear
FBC
ESR
Urinalysis

Options

Oestrogens – local and systemic preparation in short course
Ring pessary
Treat any other cause of bleeding.

Follow-up

Follow-up all cases – especially when no diagnosis is made
Advise immediate reporting of any further bleeding.

Referral

Refer all cases for D & C.

See also: Menopause (p. 199)

Premenstrual syndrome

The collection of symptoms that may occur in the premenstrual phase of the cycle is being increasingly recognized by women as a clinical entity amenable to medical treatment. It is a common condition occurring predominantly in the 30–40 year age group and is of variable severity. Cultural background, personality and the life circumstances of the woman may all affect the mode of presentation. Irrationality and poor insight are features of the condition and it may be helpful to consult with the woman and her partner between the episodes of distress.

The pathophysiology of the premenstrual syndrome is not yet fully understood and the options in management are still 'empirical'.

Presentation

Bloatedness
Weight gain
Breast engorgement
Oedema
Backache
Joint pains
Tension
Aggression
Depression
Lethargy
Irritability
Change/loss of libido
Fainting
Change of sleep pattern
Boils
Herpes simplex
Styes
Sore throat
Conjunctivitis
Rhinitis
Sinusitis
URTI

Assessment

Weight chart/calendar
Menstrual chart/calendar
Symptom chart/calendar (may also have a therapeutic effect)
Life style and health beliefs
Exclude contraindication to hormone therapy
Exclude breast disease

Options

The 'placebo effect' – sympathetic discussion of symptoms, the condition and range of management
Pyridoxine 50–100 mg daily

The Pill (unless contraindicated by age)
Progesterone or synthetic equivalent, e.g. dydrogesterone 10 mg 12 hourly
Fluid restriction
Diuretics – potassium sparing, e.g. spironolactone 25–100 mg daily
Bromocryptine 2.5 mg tablet daily (initial dose quarter or half tablet daily)
Sedation, e.g. diazepam 5 mg 8 or 12 hourly
Antidepressants, e.g. amitriptyline 25 mg 8 hourly.

Follow-up

Plan 3 monthly follow-up
Wait 3 months before changing options or combination of options

Complications

Exacerbation of co-existing condition
- asthma
- glaucoma
- migraine
- acne
- cardiac failure
- epilepsy
- depression
- urticaria

Behaviour changes during premenstrual phase result in a higher rate of
- suicides
- alcohol abuse
- child abuse
- absence from work
- psychiatric admissions
- crime
- child accidents
- examination failure

Primary amenorrhoea

Menstruation is a later feature of puberty in a girl and amenorrhoea may merely indicate a delay in puberty. In the absence of other symptoms or signs amenorrhoea itself need not be fully investigated until the age of 16.

Causes

Chromosomal
- male intersex, e.g. Turner's syndrome
- ovarian agenesis or disgenesis

Anatomical
- imperforate hymen
- absent uterus
- underdeveloped genitalia

Hormonal
- adrenal hyperplasia

Ovarian
- polycystic ovaries
- hypogonadism

Hypothalamic
- anorexia nervosa
- malnutrition
- craniopharyngioma

Pregnancy

History

Growth
Secondary sexual characteristics
Social and psychological factors
Trauma
Galactorrhoea
Family history
- late development
- infertility
- hereditary disease

Examination

Height
Weight
Growth and pubertal changes
Breasts
Pubic, axillary, body and facial hair
Genital examination
Rectal or pelvic examination (if indicated)

Investigation

X-ray to assess bone age
Karyotyping

Options

Education in range of 'normal puberty'
No action in absence of pathological signs or if bone age is within 2 years of chronological age
Referral
Advice on diet – if indicated.

Follow-up

Height
Weight
Secondary characteristics
Avoid the contraceptive pill

Referral

Before 16 years
Intersex states
Symptoms or signs of associated pathology
After 16 years
All cases for further investigation.

See also:

Anorexia (p. 12)
Malnutrition and malabsorption (p. 195)
Secondary amenorrhoea (p. 279)

Problem drinking

The term alcoholism is an evocative label which invites patient denial; the euphemism of problem drinking is generally more acceptable, but the risk factors and complications remain the same.

Heavy drinking and problem drinking presents most often in primary care and increasingly the recognition, prevention, assessment and management of the condition are the responsibility of primary care teams.

An individual's level of alcohol consumption is not fixed but alters throughout his life. This consumption is determined by various balancing factors such as age, money, friends, employment, status and self-respect. To help an individual find new levels for his drinking doctors must understand and discuss these factors. Throughout the intervention the individual's autonomy must be respected.

Alcohol consumption (in the UK)

'One drink' (unit of alcohol)
$\frac{1}{2}$ pint of beer or lager
1 tot of spirit
1 glass of wine or fortified wine

Social drinking

Men: 0–20 drinks per week (74%)
Women: 0–13 drinks per week (87%)
No long term health risks

Heavy drinking

Men: 21–50 drinks per week (21%)
Women: 14–35 drinks per week (12%)
Symptoms may be denied and signs undetectable. Social and psychological effects may become established. Legal and financial problems and accidents are common

Problem drinking

Men: more than 50 drinks per week (6%)
Women: more than 36 drinks per week (1%)
Physical, social and psychological complications are almost inevitable

Recognition of problem drinking

Symptomatic
- Obesity
- Epigastric pain
- Vomiting
- Diarrhoea
- Collapse and blackout
- Recurrent trauma or accidents
- Non-specific symptoms in patient, spouse or family

Psychological
- Anxiety
- Depression
- Insomnia
- Memory lapses
- Psychosexual problems
- Inappropriate behaviour

Social
- Drug abuse
- Family violence
- Money problems
- Job problems and absenteeism
- Crime
- Loss of friends

Risk factors
- Alcohol related offences
- Gastritis or peptic ulceration
- Alcohol related employment
- Separation or divorce
- Marital problems
- Single women over 40 years old
- Family history of problem drinking

History

Alcohol intake
- times of drinking
- quantities consumed and balancing factors
- frequency of drinking
- intervals without alcohol and intervening symptoms
- maximum alcohol intake

Onset and duration of physical symptoms

Risk factors

Medication

Social circumstances (independent account from family if permitted)
- domestic
- financial
- employment
- litigation

Examination

Breath smell
Social skills
Demeanour
Dress

Skin
- Palmar erythema
- Injected conjunctiva
- Signs of trauma
- Spider naevi
- Jaundice

Abdomen
- Enlarged liver

Cardiovascular
- Enlarged heart
- Tachycardia

Endocrine
- Gynaecomastia
- Testicular atrophy

Nervous system
- Mental impairment
- Tremor
- Peripheral neuropathy

Investigation

Hb
MCV
γ GT and AST
Alkaline phosphatase
Albumin
Alcohol level
- <50 mg % safe
- legal limit 80 mg % – Road Traffic Act

Prevention

Health education
- National – mass media coverage
- Personal – primary care teams, hospitals

Political intervention
- Alcohol taxation
- Licensing laws
- Advertising restrictions
- Alcohol related accidents and crime

Improved detection
- In primary care
- In hospitals
- In place of work

Options

Information

Discussion of drinking habit, risks and complications and the likely developments for patients and their families.

Motivation

Assess and encourage self-confidence, self-respect, self-discipline, the expectations for the future and the will to change.

Stop drinking

Total abstinence may occasionally be indicated in the early months of changing the drinking habit.

Social drinking with a non-harmful alcohol intake can be agreed if the patient is aware of the facilitating and inhibiting controls to his drinking.

Family support

Often the major factor in returning to acceptable social drinking. Health beliefs must be appropriate and the importance of their support must be acknowledged.

Behavioural therapy

Counselling and support

Sedation

In short courses of 10–14 days only to minimize withdrawal syndrome

e.g. diazepam 5–10 mg 8 hourly

e.g. chlormethiazole 500 mg 6 hourly.

Vitamin supplements

For presumed vitamin B deficiency, e.g. i.m. 'Parentrovite'.

Antidepresants

e.g. amitriptylline 25 mg 8 hourly.

Referral

Medical supervision of complicated withdrawal symptoms, e.g. fits

For liver biopsy report if liver function remains abnormal

Psychiatric supervision

- Failure of primary management
- Inadequate social skills
- Severe personality disorder
- Unsupportive social environment
- Psychosis or dementia

Organization for alcoholism

- National Council on Alcoholism
- 'Alcoholics Anonymous'
- 'Accept' Alcohol counselling service
- 'Al – Anon' Family groups.

Follow-up

Check accuracy of the initial assessment
Check progress of any physical signs
Repeat abnormal investigations
Detailed record of
- alcohol intake
- change in medical state
- change in social predicament

Random blood alcohol levels

Complications

Alcohol withdrawal
- delirium tremens
- hallucinations
- raised temperature
- unsteady gait
- anxiety
- convulsions
- tachycardia
- sweating
- fatigue
- withdrawn demeanour

Alcohol and drug interaction

Alcohol related conditions
- peptic ulceration
- cirrhosis and hepatitis
- pancreatitis
- peripheral neuropathy
- minor brain damage
- cardiomyopathy
- gonadal malfunction
- malnutrition
- anaemia
- TB
- hypoglycaemia
- hypothermia
- depression and suicide
- marital breakdown
- job failure
- trauma, e.g. RTA and domestic accidents
- excessive smoking (often associated)

Alcohol and the fetus
- abnormal facies
- growth retardation *in utero*
- delayed CNS development
- major anomalies more likely

Uncontrolled drinking ranges from
- antisocial behaviour
- memory lapses
- surreptitious drinking

to
- inability to abstain
- collapse of self-care
- decreased tolerance for alcohol

See also:
Depression (p. 63)
Psychosexual problems (p. 266)
Stress and anxiety (p. 303)

Psychosexual problems

Patients will only seldom declare a psychosexual problem as a primary complaint. Usually a psychosexual problem will underly an apparently trivial complaint. It is therefore important for the doctor to be sufficiently sympathetic to help the patient overcome his or her embarrassment and inhibitions and talk freely about the symptoms and anxieties. Usually the assessment and management is completed over several consultations and in the majority of cases it is best to involve both partners from the start.

Flexibility in assessment and management is essential in order to accommodate the wide range in concepts of normality of both the doctor and the patients.

The objective of management is to identify and then modify the causes, either physical or psychological, that lead to the anxieties which manifest themselves as sexual symptoms.

Symptoms of sexual dysfunction are conveniently grouped using Kaplan's concept of three phases in the sexual sequence:

I desire
II excitement
III orgasm

To these three can be added the symptoms relating to pelvic muscle spasm and sexual phobias.

Causes

Psychological

Sexual anxieties can interfere with any phase in the 'sequence of sex'

Ignorance

Distorted concept of normal sex

Fear of erection, erotic sensations, penetration

Table 1.10. Presentations

I Disorder of desire	Male and female	Inhibition of sex drive or loss of libido
II Disorder of excitement/arousal	Male	Impotence or erectile failure
	Female	Failure to lubricate
III Disorder of orgasm	Male and female	Anorgasmia
	Male	Premature ejaculation
		Retarded ejaculation
	Female	Coital anorgasmia
Muscle spasm	Male	Ejaculation pain
	Female	Vaginismus
		Dyspareunia
Sex phobia, e.g.		
nudity		
oral sex		
semen		
masturbation		
anal sex		
lubrication		

Fear of failure, commitment or rejection
Performance anxiety
Self consciousness
Unrealistic expectations
Suppressed aggression or jealousy
Premenstrual tension
Depression
Menopause
Physical
Congenital
- spina bifida
- intersex state
- mental handicap

Systemic disease
- TB
- carcinoma
- anaemia
- rheumatoid arthritis
- Still's disease
- Sjogren's syndrome
- senility
- thyroid disorder
- myocardial infarction

Neurological disease
- diabetes
- multiple sclerosis

- epilepsy
- stroke

Surgery
- colostomy
- ileostomy
- hysterectomy
- mastectomy
- prostatectomy
- renal failure

Trauma
- vertebrae
- pelvis

Medication
- alcohol
- sedatives
- the Pill
- antidepressants
- hypotensives
- steroids

Assessment

Identify the symptoms and the 'phase' of dysfunction

Identify the anxieties and their mode of interference in the different phases

Sexual function
- desire/libido
- excitement/arousal
- orgasm
- fantasies
- masturbation
- variations

Sexual history
- sex education
- family and religious attitudes
- puberty
- homosexuality/homosexual phase
- onset and frequency of intercourse
- number of sexual partners
- marital history
- extra-marital history
- contraception

Medical history

Exclude a physical cause (see above)

Examination

General physical examination – as indicated

Full neurological examination – as indicated

Examination of pelvis and genitalia (observe the patient's reaction to examination which may reflect sexual attitudes)

Options

Education – by discussion, diagrams, books, films or video.

Treatment – of any underlying physical cause and consideration of relevant medication being used.

Psychotherapy – to modify the causes of any sexual anxieties. The style of psychotherapy is dictated by the needs of the couple and must be an integral part of any behavioural therapy.

Behavioural therapy – planned programmes of graduated 'exercises' should be modified to the needs of each couple.

'Start–stop' or 'squeeze' (for premature ejaculation)

The woman stops stimulation or squeezes the penis during activity at a level of excitement decided by the man. She restarts the stimulation when excitement has waned. The cycle is repeated until adequate control of the excitement phase is reached.

'Orgasm inhibition' (for anorgasmia)

Sexual anxiety inhibited by fantasy or auditory or visual distraction while orgasm is reached first by masturbation then mutual masturbation and finally by penetration.

'Sensate focus' (for both desire and excitement phase disorders)

Non-genital caressing progresses to genital caressing. Genital contact is forbidden until both partners are ready as judged by the therapist. The next phase is to allow penetration without orgasm and finally penetration with orgasm.

'Gradual vaginal dilation' (for vaginismus)

Self-examination of vagina with mirror

Self-exploration with 1, 2, then 3 fingers (or graduated dilators)

Partner explores with 1, 2, then 3 fingers with lubrication (e.g. KY jelly). Partner penetrates without thrusting. Partner penetrates with thrusting.

Drug therapy – is very rarely of value. Anxiolytics are of no proven benefit but antidepressants may help with phobic anxiety states or in the presence of an underlying depression. Testosterone is only rarely justified when there is evidence of hormonal abnormality.

Referral

For treatment of physical cause if appropriate
For further therapy if symptoms are persistent
Consider
- Family Planning Association
- Marriage Guidance Council
- psychiatric units
- homosexual organizations.

Other conditions which may present as sexual problems

Homosexuality
Transvestitism
Transexualism
Exhibitionism
Voyeurism
Paedophilia
Rape

See also:

Chest pain – myocardial infarction (p. 46)
Depression (p. 63)
Fits (p. 110)
Menopause (p. 199)
Premenstrual syndrome (p. 257)
Contraception (p. 446)
Diabetes (p. 457)
Multiple sclerosis (p. 483)
Pulmonary tuberculosis (p. 492)
Rheumatoid arthritis (p. 493)
Stroke (p. 497)

Ptosis

In ptosis the upper eyelid reaches the upper margin of the pupil in the resting state.

Comparison with an old photograph may be helpful to deduce the degree of change.

Sudden onset of ptosis must be investigated as this can be a sign of intracranial pathology.

Causes

Congenital (often bilateral)
Acquired
- mechanical, e.g. trauma to eyelid
- neurogenic, e.g. Horner's syndrome – 3rd nerve lesion
- myogenic, e.g. myasthenia gravis

History

Onset and duration of ptosis
Variation throughout the day
History of trauma to the eye or head injury

Associated symptoms
- headache
- interference with vision
- general weakness or difficulty swallowing

Examination

Unilateral/bilateral ptosis
Voluntary control (elevation is present in Horner's syndrome and absent in 3rd nerve lesions)
Eye movements
Pupil sizes
Examination of fundi for papilloedema if of sudden onset
Evidence of other cranial nerve lesions

Investigation

Chest X-ray – to exclude lesions in lung apex on affected side
'Tensilon test' for myasthenia gravis – Edrophonium 3 mg is given i.v. as a very short acting anticholinesterase
Skull X-ray
Serology for syphilis

Options

Congenital ptosis needs no treatment unless it interferes with vision
Myasthenia gravis can be treated in the usual way with neostigmine and possibly steroids.

Referral

Sudden onset unilateral ptosis with associated dilated pupil may require urgent referral to exclude rising intracranial pressure
Congenital or mechanical ptosis may need plastic surgery
For further investigation of possible intracranial lesions.

See also:

Difficulty in swallowing (p. 71)
Headache (p. 133)
Visual loss (p. 325)

Red eye

This is a relatively common presentation in primary care and the cause is usually benign. Some causes can lead to visual failure and these require urgent referral to an ophthalmologist.

Causes

Conjunctivitis
- bacterial

viral
allergic
Dry eye – keratoconjunctivitis sicca
Acute glaucoma
Episcleritis and scleritis
Keratitis
dendritic
marginal
corneal ulcer
Anterior uveitis
Foreign body
Trauma
Sub-conjunctival haemorrhage
Blepharitis
stye
chalazion
dermatitis

History Onset and duration of red eye
Associated symptoms
discharge
pain
photophobia
rhinitis
irritation
watering
visual failure
Recent trauma or foreign body
Previous history of allergy
Family history of glaucoma
Medication
topical
systemic

Examination Distribution of redness
generalized – conjunctivitis
circumcorneal – uveitis, glaucoma
localized – corneal ulcer, sub-conjunctival haemorrhage
Colour
red – conjunctivitis, iritis
purple/red – glaucoma
Pupil
size and regularity
constricted – uveitis
dilated + oval – glaucoma

Cornea
ulcers, exudate and precipitates in anterior chamber
cloudy in acute glaucoma
Occular pressure
clinical assessment

Investigation

Fluorescein stain – check for abrasions or ulcers on the cornea
Swab discharge

Options

Reassurance – all that is required in sub-conjunctival haemorrhage
Antibiotic drops – e.g. chloramphenicol or framycetin every 2 hours for infective conjunctivitis or corneal ulcers
Astringent drops – zinc sulphate 0.25 will decongest and dry an inflamed eye
Steroid drops – helpful in allergic conjunctivitis, iritis, episcleritis – *must* be avoided in glaucoma and dendritic corneal ulcers
Atropine drops 0.5% – useful mydriatic in iritis to rest the iris and ciliary muscle and to prevent posterior synechiae
Pilocarpine drops 1–4% to constrict the pupil and aid aqueous drainage from anterior chamber in glaucoma
Acetazolamide tablets 250 mg 8 hourly to inhibit aqueous humour production in glaucoma
Eye pad – helps to relieve photophobia in iritis, glaucoma and corneal ulcer but best avoided in conjunctivitis
Warmth – relieves pain of iritis and glaucoma.

Follow-up

Iritis should be followed regularly until settled – an underlying cause should be sought but is rarely found
Glaucoma must be reviewed at three to six monthly intervals for life, to check visual fields and compliance with treatment

Referral

Iritis and glaucoma for specialist assessment
Persistent corneal ulceration or conjunctivitis – for tarsorrhaphy when corneal ulcers are due to over exposure (e.g. facial palsy or exophthalmos).

See also:

Imported disease (p. 157)
Visual loss (p. 325)

Retinopathy

Inspection of the retina with an ophthalmoscope should be part of routine examination of a patient presenting with
- symptoms of failing vision
- head injury
- headaches
- cranial nerve lesions
- eye trauma

Causes

Diabetes
Hypertension
Renal failure
Familial conditions
- glaucoma
- retinitis pigmentosa

Patterns of presentation

Abnormal findings may present in a variety of different patterns but for simplicity may be considered under the following headings.

Haemorrhages

These are usually distinguished by their shape
- 'Flame' – superficial layers of the retina (hypertension)
- 'Dot and blot' – deeper retinal layer (diabetes mellitus)
- 'Bundles of straw' – central retinal vein occlusion
- Vitreous haemorrhage – injury, haemorrhagic disorders, anaemia.

Exudates

Hard-yellowish-white patches with a clear outline (diabetes mellitus).

Fan shaped hard exudates around the macula that are described in renal retinopathy are very rare and are probably due to associated hypertensive changes.

Soft-white patches with blurred outline (cotton wool spots) – hypertension.

Pigmentation

This is sometimes a normal finding with streaks of pigment between the vessels, and when it is not associated with visual impairment.

Inflammatory changes in the choroid retina may lead to pale irregular patches with surrounding pigmentation.

Retinitis pigmentosa is recognized by spider shaped patches of pigmentation which resemble 'bone corpuscles'. The central retina is spared. It leads to peripheral visual failure and night blindness.

Oedema

Oedema of the optic nerve head, papilloedema, occurs with raised intracranial pressure, malignant hypertension and optic neuritis. The disc is elevated and its edges are blurred and pale.

More generalized oedema of the retina can occur with occular injuries, retinal vein occlusion, diabetes mellitus and hypertension.

Cupping

There is usually a small central pit in the optic disc, which may be deeper in myopic patients and associated with a paler crescent around the temporal margin of the disc.

In glaucoma the cupping is more obvious and may extend beyond the disc margin – if the 'cup-disc' ratio is more than 0.6 it is an important diagnostic indicator.

Hypertensive retinopathy

This is usually graded according to its severity
- arterial narrowing
- arteriovenous nipping
- haemorrhages and exudates
- papilloedema in addition to the above changes (malignant hypertension).

Diabetic retinopathy

Background retinopathy
- microaneurysms – dots
- haemorrhages – blots
- hard exudates
- maculopathy – exudates and haemorrhages affecting central vision

Preproliferative retinopathy
- venous beading
- venous reduplication
- soft exudates – cotton wool spots

Proliferative
- new vessel formation
- vitreous haemorrhage
- fibrous proliferation
- retinal detachment.

Retinal detachment

The patient senses flashes and floating spots followed by the apparent rising or falling of a curtain with sudden loss of central vision if the macula is involved

The detachment appears as a ballooning sheet in the vitreous usually with a visible tear.

History

Associated symptoms
- failing vision

eye injury
occular pain
bruising and bleeding

Past history of hypertension, diabetes and previous eye problems

Family history of glaucoma, retinitis pigmentosa

Examination
Visual acuity
Visual fields
Occular pressure
Blood pressure

Investigation
Urine for sugar and protein
FBC
Coagulation studies

Referral
Failing vision
Consideration for blind register
Treatment of proliferative retinitis in diabetes (see p. 462)

See also:
Diabetes (p. 457)
Hypertension (p. 475)

Schizophrenia

Schizophrenia is a mental disorder which defies adequate definition. It should, perhaps, be considered as a group of conditions in which there may be severe disorder of thought, perception, feelings and behaviour.

The aetiology is obscure but there is a strong suggestion of a genetic element. Stress may provoke exacerbations. Biochemical factors have been considered.

The prevalence is 0.5–1.0% and in 75% of cases the onset is in the 15–30 year age group.

Table 1.11. Characteristics of schizophrenia in order of frequency (WHO 1973)

Acute	Frequency (%)	Chronic	Frequency (%)
Lack of insight	97	Social withdrawal	74
Auditory hallucinations	74	Underactivity	56
Ideas of reference	70	Lack of conversation	54
Suspiciousness	66	Few leisure interests	50
Flat affect	66	Slowness	48
Voices speaking to patients	65	Overactivity	41
Delusional mood	64	Odd ideas	34
Delusions of persecution	64	Depression	34
Thought alienation	52	Odd behaviour	34
Thoughts spoken aloud	50	Neglect of appearance	30

There have been many attempts to classify this disorder. None are universally accepted without qualification.

A very simple and practical approach is to consider schizophrenia in separate acute and chronic forms as judged by the quality of symptoms expressed. This distinction is not always clear in practice; in the individual patient a few symptoms may predominate.

Differential diagnosis

Drug induced
- LSD
- Mescaline
- Amphetamines
- Phenytoin
- Primidone
- Carbamazepine

Alcohol
Sleep deprivation
Post-traumatic
Temporal lobe epilepsy
GPI
Depressive illness
Dementia with persecutory delusion
Paranoid personality
Autism in children

Assessment

It is not easy to elicit the symptoms of a schizophrenic disorder in a withdrawn and suspicious patient. It is helpful to involve a relative or friend.

The following are an indication of symptoms encountered which may be present in various combinations. Schneider's 'first rank' symptoms are marked *; these are probably the clearest indications of diagnosis.

Thought
- *Ideas of passivity and external influence
- *Thought withdrawal and broadcasting
- *Delusions
- Ideas of reference
- Loosening of association ('knight's move' in thought)
- Confusion between fact and fantasy
- Thought blocking

Perception
- *Auditory hallucinations (particularly third person or running commentary)
- Visual hallucinations
- *Somatic, tactile and olfactory hallucinations

Emotion
- Extreme lability of mood

Flattened affect
Inappropriate expressions

Behaviour

Withdrawn and preoccupied
Sudden unexpected changes in behaviour
Automatic obedience
Personal neglect
Catatonic symptoms – alternating stupor and excitement, waxy flexibility of muscle tone, odd physical posture maintained

History

Onset, sequence and progress of symptoms and events
Recent change in
- personality
- attitudes
- behaviour
- efficiency
- sleep pattern
- mood

Symptoms of depression
History of epilepsy or sleep disorder
Premorbid personality and achievements
Childhood development
Family history
History of medication and alcohol intake
Social circumstances and support

Prognosis

Good	Bad
Acute onset	Insidious onset
Short duration	Long episode
Late age of onset	Early age of onset
Good premorbid personality	Repeated relapses
Obvious precipitating factors	Blunted affect
Higher IQ	Low resistance to symptoms
Good career record	Poor career record
Good social support	Social isolation

Options

Acute care

Medication

Major tranquillizers, e.g.
- Chlorpromazine 50–500 mg daily
- Thioridazine 150–600 mg daily
- Trifluoperazine 28–30 mg daily

Anticholinergics for extra-pyramidal side-effects, e.g.
- Benzhexol 5–15 mg daily
- Benztropine 1–4 mg daily.

Family support

Schizophrenics can cause great disruption in families with increased risk of neurosis or depression in the relatives.

Aftercare **Medication**

Major tranquillers, e.g.

Fluphenazine 25 mg 2–4 weekly

Flupenthixol 20–40 mg 2 weekly

Anticholinergics (as above).

Supportive psychotherapy in conjunction with a psychiatrist.

Education and employment

Social skills

General education

Sheltered workshops

Sheltered social contacts

Training for employment.

Social support

At home

'Group homes'

Hospital

Flats

Hostels.

Liaison

Relatives

Health visitor

Occupational therapist

Teachers

Voluntary organizations

Psychiatrist

Community Psychiatric Nurse

Social workers

Educational psychologist

Schizophrenia Fellowship.

Referral All cases for psychiatric assessment on reasonable suspicion of diagnosis to

confirm diagnosis

plan management

shelter environment during the acute phase.

See also: Mental Health Act 1983 (p. 527)

Psychiatric emergencies (p. 533)

Secondary amenorrhoea

The commonest causes of a missed period are pregnancy or the menopause. These conditions must be excluded before investigating further. In the absence of associated symptoms or signs no further action may be necessary except to emphasize a continuing need for contraception.

Causes

Pregnancy
Menopause
Weight related – excessive loss or gain, e.g. anorexia nervosa
Hypothalamic
- trauma
- emotional strain
- physical stress
- change in life-style

Pituitary failure
Hyperprolactinaemia
Ovarian – tumours, polycystic ovaries
Tuberculosis
Thyroid disorder

Other causes

Systemic disease
Endocrine disease
- Cushing's disease
- acromegaly
- pituitary tumours

Radiotherapy effect
Effect of medication
- metoclopramide
- phenothiazines
- haloperidol
- tricyclic antidepressants
- methyldopa
- the Pill

Premature menopause (confirm by increased FSH levels)

History

Menarche
Menstrual history
Contraceptive history
Obstetric history
Gynaecological history
Social and psychological factors
Health beliefs
Medication

Examination

Signs of endocrine pathology including
- galactorrhoea
- virilism
- hirsutism
- pigmentation
- thyroid disorder

Pelvic examination

Investigation

Pregnancy test
Skull X-ray
Prolactin level
FSH/LH levels

Options

No action – if no associated symptoms or signs
Advice on contraception
Advice on diet
Advice on life-style
Treat underlying disease
Review medication
Treat menopausal symptoms (see p. 199)

Follow-up

Menstrual history
Assess any new symptoms or signs
Contraceptive advice
Regular pregnancy tests

Referral

After more than 12 months amenorrhoea
Infertility/subfertility
Associated galactorrhoea – unless drug induced.

See also:

Anorexia (p. 12)
Menopause (p. 199)
Pelvic mass (p. 238)
Primary amenorrhoea (p. 259)
Weight loss (p. 337)
Symptoms of pregnancy (p. 352)
Hyperthyroidism (p. 479)
Hypothyroidism (p. 481)
Pulmonary tuberculosis (p. 492)

Shortness of breath

There are many causes of shortness of breath. It can occur in a perfectly fit person during strenuous exercise. It should be related to the expected normal exercise tolerance adjusted for age, physique and fitness.

Causes

Pulmonary

Acute obstruction (foreign body, croup, diphtheria)
Infective (bronchitis, bronchiolitis, pneumonia)
Chronic obstructive bronchitis
Emphysema
Asthma
Pneumothorax

Pulmonary embolism
Large pleural effusion
Sarcoidosis
Pulmonary fibrosis

Cardiac
LVF
Uncontrolled tachycardias
Cardiac tamponade

Haematological
Anaemia

Psychogenic
Anxiety state
Hyperventilation

Obesity – Pickwickian syndrome

Metabolic – acidosis or uraemia or diabetes

Neuromuscular
Myasthenia
Motor neurone disease

History

Onset – sudden, insidious or progressive
Precipitating and relieving factors
Associated features
- cough
- sputum
- chest pain
- haemoptysis
- orthopnoea
- paroxysmal nocturnal dyspnoea

Exercise tolerance
General health – weight loss and fever
Past history of pulmonary or cardiac disease
Environment – occupation, smoking and hobbies (e.g. bird fancier)

Examination

Pallor, cyanosis and finger clubbing
Record weight and temperature (if relevant)
Cardiovascular and pulmonary assessment
CNS and mental state assessment (if relevant)

Investigation

FBC
ESR
Urinalysis
Peak expiratory flow (before and after bronchodilator)
Chest X-ray
Sputum culture } (when indicated)
Urea and electrolytes } (when indicated)

Emergency care

Laryngeal obstruction – tracheostomy or large bore needle through the cricothyroid ligament

Asthma Acute LVF	It is often difficult to distinguish between these two conditions therefore try aminophylline 250 mg i.v. slowly and frusemide 20–40 mg i.v. (in preference to adrenaline and diamorphine)

Tension pneumothorax – large bore needle through an intercostal space on the affected side

Oxygen therapy is helpful but a 24% ventimask should be used for the long standing respiratory cripple

Options

Bronchodilators, sodium cromoglycate and steroids
Diuretics and digoxin
Antibiotics
Chest physiotherapy
Domiciliary oxygen therapy
Mucolytics (evidence of efficiency is tenuous)
Steam inhalation
Haematinics as appropriate
Advise against smoking and environmental factors.

Failure to control

Review diagnosis
Check drug dosage and compliance
Reconsider rarer causes.

Referral

Continuation of emergency care
Severe incapacitation by breathlessness
Marked anaemia (Hb <8 g% may require transfusion)
Further investigations of underlying cause
Failure to control symptoms.

See also:

Asthma and wheezing (p. 15)
Chest pain – pulmonary embolism (p. 50)
Nasal obstruction (p. 214)
Obesity (p. 224)
Pallor/anaemia (p. 231)
Pleural effusion (p. 250)
Stress and anxiety (p. 303)
Chronic bronchitis (p. 440)
Diabetes (p. 457)
Respiratory distress – acute left ventricular failure (p. 535)

Croup (p. 537)
Pneumothorax (p. 538)

The shoulder

The painful shoulder is a relatively common complaint in primary care.

It may be due to intrinsic pathology in the shoulder or referred from lesions in a phrenic nerve distribution such as basal pleurisy, free blood in the absomen, chole-cystitis, sub-phrenic abscess or myocardial ischaemia.

Local pain in the shoulder may arise from the glenohumeral or acromioclavicular joints or the surrounding muscles, tendons or ligaments.

History

Onset, duration and timing of symptoms
Exacerbating and relieving factors
Site and radiation of pain
Associated symptoms
- stiffness
- neck pain
- paraesthesiae in arms
- cardiovascular
- abdominal symptoms (or signs)

History of trauma

Examination

Inspect symmetry of shoulders
Palpate bones, muscles and the axillae
Assess active and passive range of movements distinguishing glenohumeral from scapulothoracic ranges
Check for
- muscle wasting
- neurological signs
- chest signs
- skin lesions

Investigation

X-ray cervical spine and shoulders
Chest X-ray

Patterns of presentation

Arthritis

(See pp. 485, 493)

Trauma

This may be caused by a fall onto the outstretched hand or a direct blow to the shoulder. In the elderly the neck of the humerus can fracture with relatively minor injury.

It may result in simple sprains, fractures or dislocations.

It is occasionally subject to recurrent dislocations especially with congenital laxity of the joints when other joints will also be affected.

If a fracture or dislocation is suspected. It is wise to refer to the accident service in hospital for immediate attention.

Painful arc syndrome

There is pain on abduction of the shoulder joint between 60 and 120 degrees of movement from the neutral position. There is limited clearance between the humeral tuberosity and the acromion. It may be caused by

injury to the greater tuberosity
minor tear of the supraspinatus tendon
supraspinatus tendonitis
calcification in the supraspinatus tendon
sub-acromial bursitis.

Treatment is with analgesia, heat and gentle exercise. Local injection may help supraspinatus tendonitis. If the pain is very severe or persists after three weeks of simple measures an orthopaedic opinion should be arranged.

Frozen shoulder

This is characterized by pain and uniform limitations of movement in all directions. It is sometimes associated with previous mild trauma. Spontaneous but slow recovery occurs over 6–24 months.

The underlying pathology is poorly understood.

In the acute phase the joint should be rested in a sling but passive and assisted exercises should be performed as early and regularly as possible to avoid permanent joint stiffness. As pain subsides more active exercises should be introduced.

Heat treatment and ultra-sound therapy may be helpful for the pain. Analgesic drugs do not appear to be very useful.

Polymyalgia rheumatica

Causes bilateral shoulder pain and stiffness. There is local tenderness in the shoulder girdle and upper arm muscles. It may occasionally also affect the pelvic girdle muscles. The onset is fairly rapid.

The morning stiffness may last more than an hour. Characteristically the ESR is over 40mm/hr; other symptoms include weight loss, fever, night sweats, malaise and depression.

It particularly affects those of 60 years of age and more.

The response to steroids is dramatic. The initial dose should be quite high e.g. 30–60 mg prednisolone per day. This is reduced to the minimum dose which will control symptoms (often less than 5 mg per day). After 1–2 years the steroid can gradually be withdrawn while monitoring symptoms and the ESR. Relapse can occur and care should be taken to avoid the precipitation of hypoadrenalism.

There may be associated cranial arteritis.

'Fibrositis' This is a rather vague diagnostic label that has little to do with inflammation in fibrous tissue, but it is commonly a presenting complaint in primary care. It presents as a painful and stiff shoulder unrelated to injury or underlying joint disease. Spontaneous recovery usually occurs within two weeks. There is often tenderness in localized muscle groups with pain on active but not passive movement of the shoulder joint.

Treatment is with analgesia, heat, massage and gentle exercise.

Bicipital tendonitis Tendonitis may cause pain over the bicipital groove on lifting or pulling with the arm, or supination of the forearm against force.

Complete rupture of the tendon is not especially painful but will produce an obvious bulge in the muscle belly of the long head of biceps.

Treatment is conservative with analgesia. Surgical intervention is rarely necessary.

Nerve root pain Pressure on the brachial plexus or nerve roots sometimes causes pain referred to the shoulder, arm, and hand. The precise distribution depends on the site of the lesion, but consider

cervical disc prolapse
cervical spondylosis
cervical rib
osteophyte formation
Herpes zoster
apical lung tumours

Angina pectoris This is usually easily distinguished by associated exercise induced chest pain with radiation to the neck, shoulder and arm. In a small proportion of cases it may present with pain in the shoulder alone.

See also:

Chest pain – angina (p. 43)
Osteoarthritis (p. 485)
Rheumatoid arthritis (p. 493)

Sinusitis

Sinusitis implies inflammation of the paranasal sinuses which consist of
- maxillary – most commonly affected
- ethmoidal
- frontal
- sphenoidal – most likely to become complicated

The acute condition is usually benign and many cases are never seen by a doctor.

However, with malignant tumours and infections that are complicated by intracranial thrombophlebitis sinusitis can be fatal.

Chronic sinusitis is often very resistant to treatment.

Causes

Viral infection
Bacterial infection, e.g. *Streptococcus pneumoniae* and *Staphylococcus aureus*
Allergy
Foreign body
Trauma
Dental sepsis and extraction of upper wisdom teeth
Congenital malformation
Tumour and granulomas

History

Onset, duration and nature of symptoms
- congestion
- facial pain
- headache

Associated symptoms
- URTI
- loss of taste and smell
- purulent post-nasal discharge

Precipitating factors
- drugs (e.g. hypotensives)
- stooping
- supine posture
- altitude changes

Examination

Facial swelling and inflammation
Facial tenderness on palpation over sinuses

Temperature
Nasal inflammation
Dental examination
Signs of local spread of malignant tumours into jaw, cheek or orbit

Investigation

ESR and differential white cell count
Nasal swabs
X-ray paranasal sinuses
Skin tests for allergy

Options

Self-help
- inhalation, e.g. 'Karvol' capsules
- avoid dust, alcohol, tobacco smoke
- simple analgesics

Decongestants, e.g.
- topical – oxymetazoline drops or spray
- systemic – pseudoephedrine 60 mg 8 hourly

Antihistamines, e.g. promethazine 10–25 mg 8 hourly
Antihistamine/decongestant combinations, e.g. 'Actifed', 'Triominic'
Antibiotics, e.g.
- amoxycillin 250 mg 8 hourly
- tetracycline 250 mg 6 hourly.

Referral

ENT specialist
- signs of rising intracranial pressure – urgent
- local spread of inflammation to orbit – urgent
- chronic sinusitis for sinus washout and/or bilateral intranasal antrostomy

Dentist on suspicion of dental sepsis.

Complications

Sphenoidal and frontal sinusitis may progress to abscess formation and thrombophlebitis resulting in raised intracranial pressure
Septicaemia
Osteomyelitis of frontal or maxillary bones (especially in children)
Bone necrosis – pressure effect. Direct spread of infection to the orbit
Nasal obstruction
Anosmia
Chronic malaise
Recurrence of symptoms – review antibiotic sensitivity

See also:

Facial pain (p. 96)

Headache (p. 133)
Nasal obstruction (p. 214)

Sore throat

There are many causes of sore throat but acute follicular tonsillitis is the most common. It occurs most commonly between 3–8 years of age and in the late teens and early twenties. The condition is self-limiting – a consideration that is relevant when assessing the options of management.

Scarlet fever and post-streptococcal nephritis are now rare and much less troublesome than they were, and the classical recommendation of throat swab, MSU and ASO in every case is now rarely justified.

Causes

Acute follicular tonsillitis – haemolytic *Streptococcus* in about one-third of cases
Glandular fever
Oral candidiasis
Apthous ulcers
URTI
Pharyngitis – including Herpes simplex
Laryngitis

Other causes

Foreign body
Mouth breathing
Shouting
Smoking
Peritonsillar abscess/quinsy
Vincent's angina
Diphtheria
Hand, foot and mouth disease
Actinomycosis
Agranulocytosis
Aplastic anaemia
Lymphoma
Leukemia
Carcinoma of
- tonsil
- larynx
- pharynx

Radiotherapy

History

Onset, duration and nature of sore throat
Associated symptoms

fever
rhinitis
snoring
dysphagia
weight loss
hoarseness
cough
halitosis

Family history of tonsillitis
Social and psychological factors
Attitudes to tonsillectomy

Examination

Inspect

Gums – gingivitis
Soft palate – petechiae, vesicles, ulcers and swelling
Tonsils – pitting, injection, swelling, exudate, follicles, vesicles
Pharynx – injection, vesicles, ulcers
Cervical glands – enlargement, tenderness
Skin – rashes

Record

Temperature
Pulse
Hydration

Investigation

Throat swab in equivocal or severe cases to differentiate between bacterial and viral infection
If no improvement after one week
FBC and ESR
Glandular fever screening test
MSO

Options

Self-help

Simple analgesics (aspirin or paracetamol)
Gargles (antiseptic, salt water or soluble aspirin)
Soothing lozenges
Advice on mouth breathing
Stop smoking.

Medication

Streptococcal infections

It is impossible to distinguish, on clinical grounds, between streptococcal and viral infections. Both are usually self-limiting illnesses and the exhibition of antibiotics in bacterial infection probably only limits the illness by less than 24 hours. If this illness is particularly severe or a positive throat swab is obtained then treatment may be indicated with

Penicillin 250 mg 6 hourly for one week or
Erythromycin 250 mg 6 hourly for one week

Candida – nystatin suspension 1 ml 6 hourly for one week
Vincent's angine – metronidazole 200 mg 8 hourly
Apthous ulcers (see p. 207)
Glandular fever (see p. 122)
For incision peritonsillar absess.

Referral

For tonsillectomy
There are no absolute indications for tonsillectomy. When assessing the merits of referral the following factors might be considered
six weeks off school or work in one year
six episodes of confirmed tonsillitis
peritonsillar enlargement
persistent asymmetrically enlarged tonsils for biopsy.

For further investigation

For further investigation
suspected immune deficient state
suspected leukaemia or neoplasm

See also:

Glandular fever-like illness (p. 122)
Hoarseness (p. 151)
Mouth symptoms (p. 207)

Speech disorder

Speech disorders may present in a multitude of ways but can be divided into two basic difficulties in phonation or neurological control.

An anxious parent may present a child with delay in acquiring speech. Most children start using words by one year, and phrases by two years of age. Mental retardation and deafness are the commonest causes of delayed speech. The older child may also develop altered speech sounds in association with nasal stuffiness or laryngitis with croup (see pp. 38 and 537).

In adults the vast majority of cases occur in a self-limiting hoarseness associated with laryngitis. If the disorder lasts more than four weeks then further investigation is necessary to exclude more serious damage to the vocal cords, or the recurrent laryngeal nerve. Dysarthria may occur in association with more general conditions of Parkinsonism, cerebrovascular accidents, multiple sclerosis and myxoedema.

Causes

Children
Hoarseness with laryngitis
Nasal stuffiness

- Palate deformities
- Stammer and lisps
- Delayed speech in
  - deafness
  - neurological disorders
  - mental retardation

Adults

- Laryngitis
- Voice abuse
- Laryngeal tumours
- Laryngeal nerve palsies
  - thyroid surgery
  - carcinoma of the bronchus
- Myxoedema
- Cerebrovascular accident
- Parkinsonism
- Multiple sclerosis
- Hysterical aphonia

History

- Onset and duration
- Recent upper respiratory tract infection
- Voice misuse
- Symptoms of generalized disease (CVA, Parkinsonism, carcinoma bronchus, MS)
- Past history of thyroid surgery
- Associated dysphagia or nasal regurgitation
- In children consider
  - developmental milestones
  - behavioural/social problems
  - hearing
  - birth trauma
  - congenital infections (rubella) deformities (palate)
  - perinatal hyperbilirubinaemia

Examination

- Nasal passages
- Palate
- Throat
- Ears and hearing
- Cervical glands
- Ability to cough
- Mental assessment } in children
- Developmental assessment } in children
- Thyroid status
- Signs of neurological disease

Investigation These are usually unnecessary but consider

- FBC
- ESR
- Thyroid function tests
- Audiometry
- CXR

Options Reassurance may be all that is necessary if underlying pathology can be excluded. Stammering and lisping almost always improves with time and only needs referral if persistent after six months, or parental anxiety is high

Hot drinks and steam inhalation may help in acute laryngitis

Decongestant preparations (oral and topical) may help nasal stuffiness and secretory otitis media with conductive deafness.

Referral Speech therapy is useful in persistent stammering and delayed speech after three years of age. It may be of limited value in adults with neurological disease

Clinical psychologists can provide a more accurate developmental assessment

Neurological referral is appropriate and early assessment is merited in children with mental retardation or cerebral palsy

ENT referral is indicated if laryngoscopy is necessary or laryngeal tumour is suspected. In children the presence of unexplained deafness requires further investigation

Surgical assessment may be required if carcinoma of the bronchus is the underlying cause.

See also:

Catarrh (p. 38)
Hearing loss (p. 137)
Hoarseness (p. 151)
Nasal obstruction (p. 214)
Sore throat (p. 289)
Hypothyroidism (p. 481)
Multiple sclerosis (p. 483)
Parkinsonism (p. 487)
Stroke (p. 497)
Respiratory distress – croup (p. 537)

Spots

In this group of conditions the patient presents with small skin lesions either solitary or few in number. The conditions are usually easy to recognize and of little clinical importance but, to the patient, particularly women, they may be of major cosmetic importance.

Viral warts Warts are the result of viral infection of the skin. They are relatively common, particularly in children. Contrary to popular belief they are only mildly contagious. The vast majority undergo spontaneous resolution in a matter of months or years and because of this a profusion of 'folk-lore' treatments have arisen. It is important to stress this point to the patient because medical treatments are not consistently successful. It is also helpful to stress that when they do resolve spontaneously they leave no scars. They are usually asymptomatic apart from plantar warts which may be very painful.

Skin lesions

Depend on the site infected

The virus causes epidermal cell proliferation

Capillary loops extend into the hyperkeratotic tumour and may bleed if traumatized or appear as small black dots if thrombosed

Hands – small, rough hyperkeratotic papules of 2–5 mm on the palmar surface; flat brown 'plane' warts occur on the backs of the hands

Feet – the papule is driven into the sole of the foot (verruca) thus appearing flat. They may be grouped into a confluent area (mosaic wart)

Face and body – usually seen as flat (plane) warts or small white papules

Genitals – rough fleshing and rapidly growing lesions.

Options

Salicylic acid preparations with or without occlusion are a palliative keratolytic treatment

Podophyllin is applied topically to destroy the hyperkeratotic epidermis and is particularly useful for genital warts. It should be avoided during pregnancy

Formalin soaks can be used for plantar warts but the interdigital webs should be protected with vaseline

Curettage and cautery is useful for larger solitary warts

Cryotherapy with liquid nitrogen or carbon dioxide snow will destroy the local epidermis but should be used with care to avoid damage to surrounding normal skin.

Molluscum contagiosum

This is another viral infection of the skin usually seen in children but occasionally also in adults. It spreads locally by auto-innoculation but it is not very contagious since rarely more than one member of the household is affected.

Skin lesions

Pearl coloured, umbilicated papules
Multiple and grouped in an area of skin
May be secondarily infected with surrounding erythema.

Options

Phenol 1% on a sharp orange stick, pricked into each lesion
Cryotherapy with liquid nitrogen spray
Natural resolution may occur after trauma or secondary infection.

Insect bites

These are relatively common lesions which produce intense irritation but usually subside within a few days. Occasionally the papular variety persists due to a local allergic reaction which may lead to residual scarring.

Skin lesions

Urticarial papule (2–3 mm) with a central punctum and surrounding flare
Blistering may occur
Distributed in clusters usually on exposed areas of distal limbs.

Options

Avoidance of the source of insects (fleas, flies, lice etc.)
Insect repellants are of limited value
Oral antihistamines help to relieve itching
Phenol 1% in calamine lotion is soothing.

Acne

This is an extremely common condition particularly during adolescence. It is very variable in duration and severity. The cause is not known but may be related to hormonal or dietary factors.

Sebum is prevented from escaping from the pilosebaceous unit due to excess keratin production at the opening (comedone). The contained sebum leaks into the surrounding dermis causing an intense local reaction and sometimes cyst formation. The cystic lesions can be very unsightly and lead to scarring and much embarrassment.

Skin lesions

Comedones are the hallmark of acne
Red papules and pustules then form
Cysts up to 2 cm diameter may develop
Fibrosis and scarring ultimately occur in severe cases
Distribution over the face, shoulders and upper trunk.

Options

Dietary manipulation has not proved to be an effective treatment
Mild soaps remove excess keratin
Comedone extraction may prevent pustule formation
Ultraviolet light (natural and artificial) is helpful in some cases
Benzoyl peroxide application acts as a dekeratinizing preparation and is useful for superficial lesions
Various combinations of abrasives, antiseptics keratolytics, peroxide, sulphur, salicylic acid or tretinoin are available and effective
Oral tetracycline 250 mg/12 hourly for 8 weeks reducing dosage according to activity of lesions. Particularly useful for inflammatory pustules (avoid during pregnancy)
Intralesional triamcinolone is used for treating cysts and helps to reduce subsequent scar formation.

Boils

A boil starts as an infection of a hair follicle which develops into pustulation with central necrosis. The resulting abscess comes to a head and discharges leaving a scar. Some patients suffer recurrent boils. These patients usually harbour the germ *Staphylococcus aureas* in the nares, axillae and/or the perinum. Recurrent boils are also more common in patients with diabetes mellitus, reticuloses and altered immune states.

Skin lesions

Initially a small red nodule
Abscess formation causes painful induration
A yellow 'head' appears when the abscess becomes fluctuant
Sometimes ulceration develops when the abscess discharges.

Options

Hot compresses and magnesium sulphate dressings accelerate resolution
Incision and drainage releases the pus when the abscess becomes fluctuant

Topical antibiotics or antiseptics help to clear sites where the germ may be harboured (see above)
Oral antibiotics may suppress an early boil or help to limit spreading cellulitis.

Folliculitis

Folliculitis is a local inflammation in the hair follicles. It may be due to infection, irritation with lubricating oils or in association with seborrhoeic eczema. It commonly occurs in areas where the hair is shaved (sycosis barbae).

Skin lesions

Small red nodules at the site of hair follicles
Pustules may develop.

Options

Antiseptic preparations (chlorhexidine) may clear surface infection
Avoiding shaving allows the inflammatory process to clear
Avoiding immersion in oil or the topical application of greasy agents.

Impetigo

Impetigo is a common epidermal infection with mixed bacterial growth of *Staphylococcus aureas* and β-haemolytic *Streptococcus*. It often occurs as a secondary infection of an underlying skin disease such as eczema. It is contagious. Sometimes family members harbour the germ in the nares, axillae or perineum and can cause recurrent infection in close contacts. The carriers can be identified by swabbing the suspected sites.

Skin lesions

Initially a purulent blister
Yellow crusting develops when the blister bursts
Satellite lesions develop by local spread
Distribution anywhere on the skin but typically face and hands.

Options

Careful toilet to remove crusting
Topical antibiotic preparations (neomycin or Fucidin ointment)
Careful hygiene to avoid contagious spread
Treatment of carriers with antiseptic baths and topical antibiotics.

Moles

These are papular or macular lesions usually containing brown/black pigments due to overgrowth of melanocytes and neural elements in the skin. They are developmental defects which become apparent during childhood or pregnancy. They are clinically important because they may, albeit rarely, undergo malignant change. More commonly they are presented by patients who want them removed for cosmetic reasons.

Skin lesions

May be one of three types

Flat macular pigmented lesions of varying size and irregular outline

Papular cellular naevi

Verrucous lesions with fissuring of the surface

Hairs sometimes grow in the lesions

Malignant change is characterized by

itch

size < 1 cm

increasing size

irregular shape

varying pigmentation

inflammation and satellite lesions

bleeding, crusting and ulceration.

Options

Reassurance for benign lesions

Surgical removal for cosmetic reasons

Urgent referral if malignancy is suspected, to a plastic surgeon for wide excision and grafting.

Seborrhoeic warts These commonly occur in the middle aged and elderly. They are *not* due to viral infection. They do not resolve spontaneously or undergo malignant change

Skin lesions

Oval raised and lightly pigmented papules

The surface is fissured

'Greasy' appearance.

Options

Reassurance

Curettage under local anaesthetic if removal is necessary.

Spider naevi These are common vascular lesions. They can occur at any age but are occasionally associated with liver disease. Sometimes they appear during pregnancy but disappear after delivery.

Skin lesions

Small central, red, vascular papule

Radiation of superficial venules from central point

Distribution on face, arms and upper trunk.

Options

Reassurance

Cautery to the central vessel obliterates the lesion.

Campbell de Morgan's spot

These are superficial angiomas which appear in middle aged and elderly patients. They are of no clinical significance.

Skin lesions

Small, bright red, raised vascular papule.

Options

Reassurance

Cautery if necessary for cosmetic reasons.

See also:

Bites and stings (p. 26)
Common infectious diseases in children (p. 402)

Squint

A squint (strabismus) is represented by an incoordination of the visual axes leading to the loss of stereoscopic or binocular vision. That is to say the eyes do not seem to be straight. The vast majority of squints occur in children.

There are two types of squint.

Paralytic squint

This occurs when there has been damage to muscular or nervous control of eye movements. The eye is restricted in movement in the direction of pull of the paralysed muscles, i.e. diplopia will be greatest on gaze in that direction. This may lead to torticollis to avoid diplopia.

Concomitant squint

This can be present in the first year of life. The visual axes deviate at a constant angle in any direction of gaze. It may be precipitated by visual failure in one eye or poor development of the reflex arc co-ordinating the visual axes. In the latter, the child learns to suppress vision in the squinting eye to avoid diplopia (called amblyopia). Treatment is usually successful before seven years of age but rarely after 10 years.

Visual failure in one eye later in life may lead to a squint, as coordination of the visual axis in that one eye is lost.

History

Age and onset

Presence of diplopia – direction of maximum divergence

History of

- skull trauma
- vascular disease
- neuritis
- myasthenia
- hyperthyroidism
- cerebral tumour

Examination **Paralytic squint** – assess the relative positions of the eyes in the cardinal directions of gaze.

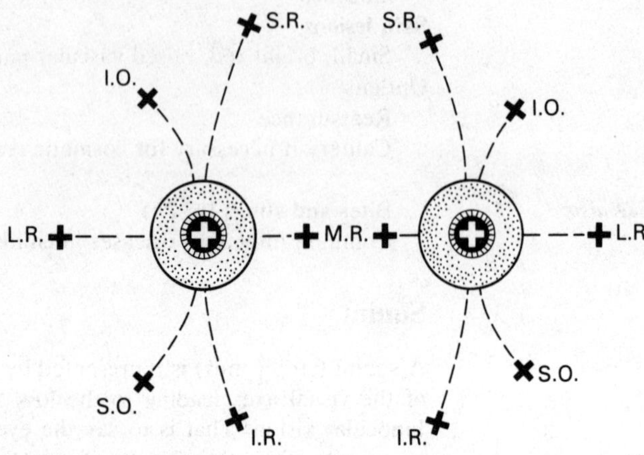

Fig. 1.3. The lines of action of the extra-occular muscles

Concomitant squint

Check symmetrical light reflections on the cornea from a light shone at least 18 inches away.

Cover test.

Options Treatment depends on the underlying cause but usually requires hospital assessment.

Referral All cases of childhood squint should be referred as early as possible if amblyopia is to be prevented.

For cosmetic surgery in the presence of visual failure or paralytic squint.

Complications Amblyopia

Diplopia

Failure of stereoscopic vision

Torticollis – compensatory

Sexually transmitted diseases (STD)

While the incidence of syphilis has remained at a fairly constant low level, gonorrhoea has increased steadily, and recently non-specific genital infection has increased dramatically, and AIDS alarmingly.

Attendances at special clinics have doubled to 400,000 per year in the last ten years. Of these about two-thirds have been found to have a sexually transmitted disease.

Causes

Syphilis
Gonorrhoea } legally defined as venereal disease
AIDS
Non-specific genital infection
Trichomonas
Candidiasis
Scabes
Pediculosis
Herpes simplex
Genital warts
Molluscum contagiosum } other more common sexually transmitted diseases

History

Fever
Rashes
Dysuria
Urethral and vaginal discharge
Genital ulcers and lumps
Contraception
Sexual contacts – heterosexual and homosexual
Drug abuse contacts
Joint pains
Conjunctivitis/uveitis
Frequency
Health beliefs and factual knowledge

Examination

Skin – rashes and subcutaneous gumma
Oropharynx – snail track ulcers and mucosal gumma
Joints – arthritis
Genitals – urethral and vaginal discharge, lumps and ulcers, epididymitis
Nodes – inguinal and generalized
P.R. – prostatitis
CNS
CVS } if indicated in later stages of syphilis

Investigation

Probably more effectively carried out in special clinic but if necessary consider
Swabs – urethral, cervical, os and anus for

Gonorrhoea (charcoal swab and Stuart's transport medium)

Trichomonas } (plain swab)
Candida }

NSU – usually sterile on routine testing

Herpes – virus transport medium necessary

Blood – serum tests for syphilis – HIV (in appropriately labelled container)

MSU

Microscopy

of ulcer serum under dark ground illumination for syphilis

of urethral discharge with Gram stain for gonococcus

Referral

Refer all suspected cases of AIDS, syphilis or gonorrhoea to a specialist clinic

Several sexually transmitted diseases may coexist and so all cases should be considered for referral.

Options

Explain the importance of contact tracing.

Syphilis

Procaine penicillin 600,000 units daily i.m. for 10–14 days

or Erythromycin 500 mg 6 hourly for 14 days.

Gonorrhoea

Amoxycillin 3 gm and probenecid 1 g orally stat.

or Septrin 4 tablets 12 hourly for 2 days.

NSU

Oxytetracycline 250 mg 6 hourly for 10–21 days.

Trichomonas

Metronidazole 200 mg 8 hourly for 7 days.

Candidiasis

e.g. Nystatin pessaries 2 at night for 14 nights

or Clotrimazole pessaries 1 at night for 6 nights

and Nystatin cream for penis and vulva.

Scabes and pediculosis

Gamma benzene hexachloride 1% painted on the whole body from neck down and left overnight

In pediculosis it should be applies locally to hairy areas.

Herpes simplex

Idoxuridine paint or ointment locally to lesion until clear.

Genital warts
Podophyllin 25% in spirit applied to lesion and left for 6 hours before washing off. Repeat weekly until clear
Diathermy under anaesthesia.
Molluscum contagiosum
Electrocautery.

Follow-up

All cases should be followed-up until clinically asymptomatic *and* repeated investigations are cleared
In cases of AIDS and syphilis follow-up should be continued for life because of complications
Patients should be advised to encourage known sexual contacts to attend their own doctor or nearest special clinic for check-up
In simple cases of candidiasis and trichomoniasis offer treatment to the sexual partner where ethically possible.
Counselling and education for HIV carriers.

See also:

Localized rash (p. 185)

Stress and anxiety

Anxiety presents in many of our daily activities and may become a significant factor in any episode of illness. This section is confined to stress related and non-specific, 'free-floating' anxiety. Phobic states, obsessive-compulsive neurosis and hypochondriasis are considered separately.

Anxiety may be expressed through psychological and physical symptoms (see Table 1.11). It becomes significant when it is not attributable to any real danger. The presentation may be complicated by various psychological defence mechanisms or the anxiety may be 'free-floating'. The illness may be of short duration, episodic or protracted over many years.

The lifetime prevalence of anxiety neurosis is very difficult to estimate and figures vary between 3–17 per 1000 men and 1–38 per 1000 women. Family and twin studies would indicate a genetic element.

Symptoms **Psychological**

Alarm
Tension
Insecurity
Restlessness
Irritability
Fatigue
Panic
Depression
Apprehension
Insomnia
Sensitivity to noise
Loss of concentration

Physical

Increased tension in skeletal muscles
Fronto-occipital headaches
Neck stiffness
Aching limbs
Tremor

Table 1.12. Increased sympathetic activity

Cardiovascular	Gastrointestinal	Respiratory
Palpitations	Dry mouth	Shortness of breath
Chest pain	Dysphagia	Chest constriction
Throbbing in the neck	Epigastric discomfort	Hyperventilation
Awareness of ectopics	Flatulence	
	Diarrhoea	
Genito-urinary	**Nervous**	
Frequency	Blurred vision	
Urgency	Tinnitus	
Failure of erection	Dizziness	
Lack of libido	Paraesthesia	
Dysmenorrhoea	Faintness	
Amenorrhoea		

Defence mechanisms

Denial – rejection of reality by suppressing significant events and facts

Compensation – overreacting to imposed limitations by inappropriate or excessive behaviour

Rationalization – plausible but inaccurate explanations that underestimate the significance of events or facts

Intellectualization – often expressed in the third person, a 'matter of fact' and detached discussion of the minutiae of a problem evading the central issue

Dependency – abdication of all responsibility by helpless and passive attitude to attendants. Often a regression to child-like attitudes and behaviour

Displacement – strong emotions of fear or anger are redirected away from the source of anxiety onto inappropriate but less threatening persons or activities

Projection – wishes and beliefs are attributed to others

Fatalism – suppression of any emotions from grief to frivolity, in the face of provocative circumstances – 'stiff upper lip'.

Stress factors

Illness

Disability

Threatened loss or conflict arising in
- Schooling
- Employment
- Housing
- Relationships
- Marriage
- Finances

Personal life events
- Pregnancy
- Engagement
- Separation
- Illness
- Bereavement
- Birth
- Marriage
- Divorce
- Menopause

Career
- New school
- New job
- Unemployment
- Litigation
- Change within a job
- Retirement

Family
- New home
- Family disagreements
- Member leaving or rejoining the home

New community
Family illness

Differential diagnosis

Hyperthyroidism
Diabetes
Drug abuse
Problem drinking
Premenstrual syndrome
Menopause
Depression
Psychotic illness
Carcinoid syndrome
Phaeochromocytoma

History

Onset and duration of symptoms
Patient's perception of his condition
Stress factors and life events
Previous personality
Previous reaction to stress
Social factors
Menstrual history
Drug, smoking and alcohol use
Medical and psychiatric history

Examination and investigation

As appropriate for exclusion of differential diagnosis and reassurance.

The appearance of the patient is often characteristic
- face looks strained
- brow furrowed
- tense posture
- restless and tremulous
- sweating and pale
- close to tears

Prevention

Anticipation by recognizing significant life events, stress factors and their implications

Early detection of symptoms and signs of stress and anxiety

Support both during and after a crisis

Options

Counselling: just listening or a comprehensive initial explanation may help the patient to clarify the problems and re-establish the perspectives

Behavioural techniques including muscle relaxation and hyperventilation control to encourage independent self-help for anxiety reactions

Reassurance: should be used with caution, too much may exacerbate the anxiety

Psychotherapy

Social support: adjustment of life style or social circumstances with advice and support of social worker, health visitor and other family members

Drugs: benzodiazepines at a fixed dose for an agreed time (2–3 weeks) e.g. diazepam 2–10 mg 8 hourly

Tricyclic antidepressants have an anxiolytic as well as anti-depressant effect. They are sometimes used in primary anxiety states when medication is required beyond three weeks in place of a benzodiazepine.

Referral

Psychiatric assessment
Clinical psychologist for behavioural training
Counselling service
Social worker
Marriage guidance
Complementary therapy
- acupuncture
- meditation
- yoga
- keep-fit classes.

See also:

Depression (p. 63)
Food allergy (p. 113)
Hypochondriasis (p. 153)
Menopause (p. 199)
Obsessions (p. 227)
Phobias (p. 245)
Premenstrual syndrome (p. 257)
Problem drinking (p. 261)

Suicide

Of all patients who deliberately harm themselves only a small minority intend to take their lives. In general this minority is usually male, in an older age group, and possibly suffering from psychiatric illness. The suicide is carefully planned, and care is taken to avoid discovery.

The majority are not psychiatrically ill, and are usually facing social difficulties; the act is usually impulsive and invites discovery. This group is often distinguishable from true suicides and is termed 'parasuicide' or 'deliberate self-harm'. The motives involved are mixed and difficult to identify with any certainty. Some wish to die; others are uncertain and leave it to fate; others admit to an attempt to influence someone in what is described as a 'cry for help'.

The distinction between suicide and deliberate self-harm is unclear since patients who intend to die may be revived while those who have no intention of dying may succumb to the act.

The incidence of suicide is difficult to determine and is probably underestimated because apparent accidents may have been deliberate.

The methods involved are many and variable but include

Drug overdose

60% of female suicides
30% of male suicides
e.g. analgesics (aspirin or paracetamol)
antidepressants
anxiolytic agents (benzodiazepines)

Carbon monoxide poisoning

30% male suicides
5% female suicides

Physical means

Hanging
Shooting
Wounding
Drowning
Falling in front of moving vehicles
Jumping from high places
Car accidents

Assessment

It has been noted that the patient often gives a warning of suicidal thought or intent before committing the act. Indeed a reasonable proportion present to the doctor some time before the event. It is therefore the doctor's role to identify the suicidal inclination by recognizing intent and considering the risk factors involved.

Grades of suicidal intent

Future seems bleak
Future is a blank
Patient just wants to sleep
Patient avoids morning activity
Activities become futile
Suicidal thoughts intrude and are declared
Suicidal plans evolve and are rehearsed

Risk factors

Age

More common in the older age group

Declared suicidal intent

Should be taken seriously but is more difficult to assess for people who repeatedly talk of suicide

Depression

With change in vitality, mood or function, especially
- weight loss
- insomnia
- self-neglect
- low self-esteem

Medical history

- Previous overdose
- Problem drinking
- Drug abuse
- Epilepsy
- Chronic painful illness
- Dementia

Social factors

- Bereavement
- Redundancy
- Loss of social status
- Breakdown of a relationship
- Deprived environment

Prevention

- Recognition of risk factors
- Accessibility
- Sympathetic response to presenting problems
- Counselling through life events
- Restricted prescribed habits
- Regular contact
- Improving social circumstances
- Samaritans

Options

Emergency care (see p. 530 for overdose and self injury)

- Try to negotiate a 'contract of care'
- Identify the underlying physical, psychological and social problems
- With the family co-operation consider the possible solutions
- Offer personal support
- Involve the family where possible
- Involve other support groups
- Drugs are of very limited value and can provide the means to future suicide.

Referral For emergency treatment
When risk of suicide is high or the associated depression severe enough to merit urgent, supervised therapy
Where there is little domestic support or understanding.

See also: Overdose and self-poisoning (p. 530)
Sudden unexpected death (p. 543)

Sweating

Sweating is a physiological process, occasionally a pathological sign, and when excessive it is often a presenting symptom much prejudiced by the pressures of commercial perfumiers.

Perspiration is the constant and insensible loss of water through the epidermis by evaporation.

Apocrine 'sweat' is excreted from vestigial scent glands situated in the axillae and perineum which exude the familiar odour.

Eccrine sweat is secreted from sweat glands all over the skin but especially on the palms and soles. Excretion is under sympathetic control and serves to regulate body temperature.

Causes
Foods – especially hot or spicy foods and alcohol
Anxiety
Exertion
Obesity
Environmental temperature and humidity
Fever
Vasovagal attacks and arrhythmias
Blood loss and shock
Hypoglycaemia
Thyrotoxicosis
Menopause
Cholinergic drugs and aspirin

Other causes
Carcinoid syndrome
Phaeochromocytoma
Intracerebral lesions
Post-trauma

History
Onset and duration of symptoms
Precipitating factors, e.g. climatic changes, trauma

Associated symptoms
- cardiovascular
- Raynaud's phenomenon
- thyroid
- sympathetic nervous system activity

Social and psychological factors
Menstrual history
Family history
Medication

Examination

Record
- Temperature
- Weight
- BP and pulse

Check for
- Shock
- Hypoglycaemia
- Infectious disease
- Thyroid state
- Cardiovascular state
- Skin disease
- Carcinomatosis
- Mental state

Investigation

FBC
ESR
Blood glucose or urinalysis
Thyroid function tests
Screen for fever – if indicated
ECG – if indicated

Options

Treat shock or hypoglycaemia if present
Advise on clothing and footwear
Advise on diet and exercise in obesity (see p. 224)
Astringents, e.g. 20% aluminium chloride hexahydrate ('Anhydrol Forte')
Formaldehyde 2% solution alternate days
Powder, e.g. 'Zeasorb'
β-Blockers, e.g. propranolol 20–40 mg 8 hourly
Anticholinergics, e.g. propantheline bromide 15 mg 8 hourly taking care to recognize side effects
Surgery – sympathectomy or axillary skin disc excision.

Complications

Dehydration
Cramp
Secondary bacterial and fungal infections

Intertrigo
Hyperkeratosis
Social disruption

Referral

Cardiovascular investigation
Neurological assessment
Sympathectomy
Excision of sweat glands in the axillae.

See also:

Fever (p. 106)
Menopause (p. 199)
Obesity (p. 224)
Stress and anxiety (p. 303)
Hyperthyroidism (p. 479)
Hypoglycaemia (p. 525)
Shock (p. 540)

Swollen legs

To the patient swollen legs are unsightly, uncomfortable and sometimes worrying.

Physiologically it is a condition of increased extracellular fluid due to increased vascular fluid pressure, decreased colloid osmotic pressure, vessel wall damage or lymphatic obstruction.

It is more common in females up to the age of 65 years.

Causes

Constitutional
Fluid retention in heart failure
Postural obstruction (immobility)
Varicose veins
DVT
Drugs, e.g. steroids, indomethacin, corbenoxalone

Rarer causes

Hypothyroidism
Renal failure
Liver failure
Protein-losing enteropathy
Pelvic tumours
Lymphatic obstruction (Milroy's disease, filiariasis)
Local inflammation, allergy

History

Onset and duration
Relationship to posture

Unilateral or bilateral
Associated symptoms
- pain
- breathlessness
- orthopnoea and PND
- chest pain
- abdominal pain or swelling
- bowel symptoms

Past history of heart, liver or kidney disease or DVT
Menstrual, contraceptive and obstetric history

Examination

Record extent and type of swelling
- brawny (lymphoedema)
- pitting (fluid retention)

Unilateral or bilateral
Superficial veins
Local tenderness and Homans' sign

Record
- Pulse
- BP
- JVP

Check for
- Enlarged liver, spleen or kidneys
- Ascites
- Pelvic masses
- Local locomotor causes

Investigation

U & E
Urinalysis
ECG and CXR
Thyroid function tests

Options

Advice on posture
- avoid standing immobile
- sit with legs elevated

Advice on diet and sodium restriction
Review drug therapy
Support stockings
Diuretics if required.

See also:

Deep vein thrombosis (p. 62)
Varicose veins (p. 324)
Chronic renal failure (p. 443)
Heart failure (p. 469)
Hypothyroidism (p. 481)

Tinnitus

Tinnitus is a noise originating within the patient's ear which is inaudible to an observer. Because the sensation is subjective there is no consistent description of the noise. It is likened to a wide range of everyday noises.

The patient's suffering is often considerable and referral to a specialist clinic should be considered because some can offer help with techniques of 'masking' the noise.

Causes

High tone deafness
Drugs, e.g. salicylates, streptomycin
Menière's disease
Labyrinthitis
Chronic otitis media
Otosclerosis
Wax
Foreign body
Eustachian tube dysfunction

Other causes

Paget's disease
Space occupying lesion in the temporal lobe and cerebellopontine angle
Temporal lobe epilepsy
Auditory hallucinations in psychotic illness
Vascular bruits
Hypotension or hypertension

History

Onset, duration and nature of tinnitus
Precipitating factors
Subjective hearing loss
Occupation
Medication

Examination

Inspection of ears
Tuning fork test
Cardiovascular examination
- BP
- search for bruits in the neck and skull

Investigation

Audiogram
Hb
X-ray internal auditory meatus

Options

Discussion of the symptoms – frequency and associated hearing loss

Reassurance about the benign nature of tinnitus
Night sedation
Treat any associated depression
Consider tranquillizers, muscle relaxants, vasodilators or carbamazepine
Hearing aid with masking tone – usually fitted in an ENT clinic.

Referral Persistent or progressive tinnitus.

See also:

Fits (p. 110)
Hearing loss (p. 137)
Hypertension (p. 475)

Tremor

A tremor is caused by involuntary, alternating muscular contractions in opposing muscle groups. It can occur in many diseases and also in healthy individuals. It may lead to much social embarrassment and handicap but it is not always amenable to treatment.

There are basically five types of tremor.

Physiological (essential) tremor

This is a fine tremor most commonly seen in the hands but also occasionally in the head
It is best demonstrated by placing a sheet of paper on the outstretched fingers
Embarrassment may be caused by interference with fine movements
It can occur in healthy individuals at any time of life but tends to increase with age and may be associated with
- exhaustion
- drugs (salbutamol, tricyclic antidepressants)
- anxiety states
- thyrotoxicosis
- alcoholism (withdrawal states)
- familial tendency
- lead poisoning

Tremor may be helped by alcohol, β-blockers and minor tranquillizers but reassurance regarding its benign nature may be sufficient

Parkinsonian tremor

This is a rhythmical oscillation of 4–6 cycles per second. It is usually unilateral and frequently affects the hand but may also include the head, jaw, lips, tongue and legs.

It is described as a 'pill-rolling' tremor which is characteristically seen in the stasis or resting state. It is inhibited by voluntary movements and disappears during sleep. It can be precipitated by anxiety or by muscular activity in the contralateral limb.

The tremor is present to a varying degree in paralysis agitans but may be absent if the other features of the triad (rigidity and akinesia) dominate. It is not exclusive to paralysis agitans and may be seen in other diseases of the basal ganglia

- tumours
- vascular occlusions
- carbon monoxide poisoning
- manganese poisoning

Its response to L-dopa is disappointing but the addition of an anticholinergic or β-blocking agent may be useful.

Intention tremor

This is a coarse irregular oscillation of a limb seen during voluntary movement. It may also be associated with titubation (nodding) of the head particularly in older patients.

It is best demonstrated by finger-nose or heel-shin testing of co-ordination which exaggerates the movements of 'past-pointing').

It is a common feature of

- cerebellar disease (particularly multiple sclerosis)
- alcohol intoxication
- familial ataxias

Treatment is very limited but β-blocking agents may be helpful. If this fails referral to a neurosurgeon for consideration of a stereotactic operation on the thalamus.

Flapping tremor

This is an apt description for a tremor seen in the outstretched hand with the wrist extended. It is seen in patients with hepatic or respiratory failure.

Associated features

Hepatic failure

- Liver palms
- Spider naevi
- Gynaecomastia
- Drowsiness
- Testicular atrophy
- Confusion
- Exaggerated reflexes
- Extensor plantar response

Respiratory failure (CO_2 retention)

Vasodilation
Headache
Confusion
Drowsiness
Cyanosis
Cor pulmonale
Papilloedema

Hysterical tremor This is a bizarre and complex tremor seen as a manifestation of psychological problems. The movements may be exaggerated and violent and can mimic myoclonic convulsions.

See also:

Problem drinking (p. 261)
Stress and anxiety (p. 303)
Hyperthyroidism (p. 479)
Parkinsonism (p. 487)

Ulcers

Skin ulcers occur in a wide variety of conditions. Usually there are three underlying aetiological factors which may occur individually or in combination.

- Nutritional defect
  - dietary
  - circulatory
- Trauma
  - injury
  - local pressure
  - in association with sensory neuropathy
- Infection
  - primary
  - secondary

Varicose ulcers These ulcers commonly occur above the medial malleolus. There is usually a history of deep vein thrombosis or varicose veins. The chronic venous stasis leads to poor skin nutrition. Minor trauma leads to breakdown of the superficial layers and ulcer formation. By the same token healing is slow and secondary infection is common, often leading to subsequent scarring. The ulcer may be painful and is often associated with varicose eczema.

Options

Prevention in 'at risk' cases by dealing with varicose veins, advising against prolonged periods of standing, protective padding over malleoli and control of ankle oedema and eczema.

Elevation of the leg improves skin blood flow and nutrition

Compression bandaging } in co-operation with
Antiseptic dressings } nursing staff

Topical antibiotics (may cause sensitization)

Desloughing agents (hydrogen peroxide, Aserbine, Debrisan)

Non-adhesive dressings protect the newly forming epiderimal layer

Consider referral to a plastic surgeon for skin grafts if there is no response to the above treatment.

Pressure sores

Pressure sores are usually painless and can enlarge rapidly before they are presented to a doctor. They occur at sites of pressure on the heels, buttocks, and sacrum. The resultant ischaemia leads to tissue anoxia.

The skin becomes indurated and red. A black necrotic area develops in the centre and is shed to form an ulcer. There is often considerable damage to the underlying subcutaneous tissue.

Pressure sores tend to occur in immobile patients particularly when the skin is macerated and wet with urine.

Options

The immobile patient should be turned regularly with skin care to the pressure areas

Prevention – ripple beds, ring cushins and sheepskins for the 'at-risk' patient

Desloughing agents should be used to clear the necrotic debris

Topical antiseptics and antibiotics for secondary infection

Non-adhesive dressings should be used to protect the newly forming skin layer

Plasti film, e.g. 'Op-site'.

Ischaemic ulcers

Ulcers can develop in the presence of local vascular damage due to poor skin nutrition. There are many causes including
- peripheral vascular disease
- diabetes mellitus
- allergic vasculitis
- connective tissue disorders

rheumatoid arthritis
sickle cell disease.

Options

Control the underlying condition if possible
Prevention by avoiding local trauma, stopping smoking, keeping the limb in a dependent position
Antiseptic dressing to the ulcer
Avoid compressive bandaging and elevation.

Aphthous ulcers

Apthous ulceration is an extremely common and particularly painful condition in the mouth. The ulcers arise spontaneously or after local trauma but usually heal within two weeks. The condition is often recurrent.
The ulcers are shallow and small (up to 1 cm in diameter)
Differential diagnosis
Herpes simplex infection
Coxsackie virus infection (hand, foot and mouth disease)
Erythema multiforme
Beçhet's syndrome.

Options

Antiseptic mouth washes
Topical anaesthetic preparation ('Bonjela')
Steroid ointment or pellets applied topically
Tetracycline suspension as a mouth wash may help in some cases.

Trophic ulcers

Trophic ulcers result from neurological diseases which cause sensory loss
Diabetic neuropathy
Syringomyelia
Myelitis
Leprosy
Tabes dorsalis.

Options

Attention to the underlying cause
Local toilet to the ulcer to prevent secondary infection
Appropriate dressings—see above.

Malignant skin ulcers

The most common malignant ulcer is the basal cell carcinoma or rodent ulcer. Squamous cell carcinoma can also ulcerate but this is comparatively rare in primary care. These malignant skin conditions develop insidiously and grow very slowly. They appear to be induced by over exposure to ultra violet light.
Rodent ulcers tend to occur on the upper face and ears.

They start as a small papule which develops a rolled edge and ulcerates centrally. If untreated the ulcer destroys adjacent structures. They do not metastasize and so are eminently treatable.

Squamous cell carcinoma affects similar areas but can also affect the lips, mucous membranes and back of the hands. It develops as a small papule which scabs and ulcerates. They can metastasize but prognosis is excellent if they are treated early.

Referral All cases should be referred to a dermatologist or plastic surgeon for biopsy and treatment.

Syphilitic ulcers (See p. 301)

See also:

Deep vein thrombosis (p. 62)
Poor circulation (p. 254)
STD (p. 301)
Varicose veins (p. 324)
Diabetes (p. 457)
Rheumatoid arthritis (p. 493)

Vaginal discharge

Vaginal discharge and vaginitis are the commonest conditions of the lower genital tract that present in primary care.

Soreness and itching in the perineum can occur in the absence of vaginitis but are often associated with a discharge.

Swelling and ulceration of the lower genital tract can also cause distress and these are considered briefly.

Causes

Physiological discharge
Post-coital (and during the arousal phase)
Pregnancy
Infection
- *Candida*
- *Trichomonas*
- *Gardnerella*
- *Chlamydia*
- *Neisseria gonorrhoae*
- Non-specific

Foreign body (including retained tampon)
Cervical erosion or polyp
Cervical cancer
Vaginal fistula

History

Description of the amount, consistency and odour
Onset and duration of symptoms
Associated urinary symptoms, pelvic pain or fever
Exacerbating and relieving factors
Menstrual history
Contraception
Medication

Examination

Full pelvic examination

Investigation

High vaginal swabs
MSU
Cervical smear
(Consider pregnancy test)

Options

Reassurance if the discharge is considered physiological
Treat infection
- *Candida* – nystatin or clotrimazole pessaries and cream
- *Trichomonas*, *Gardnerella* } metronidazole 200 mg 8 hourly for ten days
- *Chlamydia* – oxytetracycline 250 mg 6 hourly for ten days
- *N. gonorrhoeae* – see p. 302

Remove retained tampon and give a short course of antiseptic pessaries (e.g. Betadine)
Consider removing IUCD if there is associated salpingitis
Refer to a gynaecologist if cervical cancer or vaginal fistula are suspected.

Vulvo-vaginal soreness and itching	**Causes**	**Options**
Infective	Candidiasis Trichomonas	see above
Dermatological	Contact dermatitis Eczema Psoriasis Lichen planus	avoid sensitizing agents steroid creams consider dermatological referral
Atrophic vulvo vaginitis		dienoestrol cream systemic oestrogens

Soreness and itching cont.	**Causes**	**Options**
Pediculosis pubis	See p. 28	gamma benzene hexachloride
Psychosexual		reassurance and explanation antihistamines
Incontinence	See p. 190	
Tender episiotomy scar		reassurance foam ring to sit on
Generalized itching	See p. 174	
Diabetes	See p. 457	

Vulvo-vaginal swellings	**Causes**	**Options**
Cysts	Sebaceous cyst Bartholin's cyst Lateral vaginal wall cysts	antibiotics and analgesics for acutely inflamed and infected cysts refer for surgical drainage or repair
Boils		magnesium sulphate dressings incision and drainage antibiotics (e.g. Flucloxacillin)
Episiotomy scar	Inclusion dermoid Stitch abcess	refer for excision
Urethral caruncle		reassure if symptomatic refer for excision

Swellings	**Causes**	**Options**
Genital warts		apply podophyllin 25% in spirit and advise to wash it off after 6 hours or sooner if the skin is burning. repeat weekly until cleared electrocautery
Prolapse	Urethrocele Cystocele Enterocele Rectocele	pelvic floor exercises ring pessary consider referral for surgical repair
Vulval varices		support with elasticated pants refer to surgeon for excision or local ties
Vulvo-vaginal cancer		refer to gynaecologist

Vulvo-vaginal ulceration	**Causes**	**Options**
Trauma	Physical Chemical	antiseptic toilet remove irritant
Herpes genitalis		idoxuridine (40%) paint or ointment
Lichen sclerosis et atrophicus		refer to biopsy
Beçhet's syndrome		local antiseptic toilet
Cancer		refer to gynaecologist
Syphilitic chancre	See p. 301	

See also:

Itch (p. 174)
Loss of bladder control (p. 190)
Psychosexual problems (p. 266)
STD (p. 301)
Cervical cancer screening (p. 438)
Diabetes (p. 457)

Varicose veins

The prevalence of this condition has been estimated at over 60% of adults in developed Western societies. The incidence increases with age and it is more common in females. Only a small proportion of patients with varicose veins present to the doctor, usually with associated symptoms of aching and ankle swelling or purely for cosmetic reasons.

Causes

The cause of valvular incompetence in lower limb veins is unclear and is probably multifactorial including
- obesity
- diet
- pregnancy
- family history
- occupation
- lack of exercise
- oestrogen therapy
- past history of DVT

History

Onset and distribution of varicosities
Associated symptoms
- aching on standing
- night cramps
- ankle swelling
- local skin lesions

History of DVT
Previous therapy for varicosities
Obstetric and contraceptive history
Family history
Social history
- occupation
- attitudes about cosmetic appearance

Examination

Weight
Extent of long and short saphenous involvement

Sapheno-femoral incompetence (Trendelenburg's sign)
Ankle oedema
Skin changes
  discoloration
  eczema
  ulceration

Options

General advice regarding posture, exercise, weight
Consider change of contraception
Support hose
Sclerotherapy with ethanolamine oleate 5% injection
Surgery.

Complications

Thrombophlebitis
Eczema
Ulcers
Painful blanche-atrophy
Haemorrhage
DVT

See also:

Deep vein thrombosis (p. 62)
Ulcers (p. 317)

Visual loss

In a practice of 2,500 one would expect about forty consultations per year for failing eyesight. There are many causes with varying degrees of severity. Patients may present with unilateral or bilateral, sudden or gradual, partial or total loss of sight.

Causes

Gradual loss of vision

Occular
  Chronic glaucoma
  Refractive error
  Cataract
  Corneal damage
  Diabetic retinopathy
  Hypertensive retinopathy
  Retinitis pigmentosa
  Macular degeneration
  Choroiditis
Optic nerve
  Optic nerve compression

Optic neuritis
- alcohol
- tobacco
- drugs (ethambutol, chloroquine)
- severe anaemia
- avitaminosis A and B_{12}

Transient loss of vision

Cranial arteritis
Migraine
Glaucoma
Transient ischaemic attacks

Sudden loss of vision

Occular
- Cranial arteritis
- Retinal vein occlusion
- Retinal artery occlusion
- Acute glaucoma
- Vitreous haemorrhage
- Retinal detachment
- Dislocated lens
- Occipital head injury

Optic nerve
- Stroke
- Optic neuritis
- Retrobulbar neuritis

Double vision

Squint – congenital or acquired
Multiple sclerosis
Myasthenia gravis
Intracerebral tumour
Post-traumatic (head injury)

History

Mode of onset – sudden or gradual

Extent of visual loss
- partial or total
- unilateral or bilateral
- transient, worse at night

Extent of incapacity
- difficulty reading
- bumping into people and objects
- interference with career or activities of daily living

Associated symptoms
- headache
- pain in eye
- visual 'haloes'
- trauma to the eye or head

Medical history
- hypertension
- diabetes
- heart murmurs

Family history
- glaucoma
- retinitis pigmentosa
- diabetes

Drug history

Alcohol and tobacco consumption

Examination

Eye
- Visual acuity
- Visual fields
- Ptosis
- Proptosis
- Ocular movements
- Pupil reflexes
- Light reflexes
- Circum-corneal vascular flare
- Corneal ulceration, damage or oedema
- Compare eyeball tension
- Pus or blood in anterior chamber

Ophthalmoscopy
- Retinopathy
- Cupping of the optic disc
- Papilloedema
- Optic atrophy
- Retinal detachment
- Macular degeneration

General examination
- Anaemia
- Pulse rhythm
- BP
- Heart sounds
- Carotid bruits
- Palpate temporal arteries for tenderness
- CNS for localizing signs

Options

Treat underlying conditions
- diabetes (see p. 457)
- hypertension (see p. 475)
- migraine (see p. 203)
- giant cell arteritis (see p. 134)

Specialist referral.

Referral

Papilloedema with visual impairment Suspected temporal (giant cell) arteritis for biopsy	urgent referral to neurologist
Episodic visual loss Progressive visual loss without occular pathology	to neurologist
Further assessment Consideration for blind register	to ophthalmologist
Refractive errors	to optician.

See also:

Migraine (p. 203)
Retinopathy (p. 274)
Squint (p. 299)
Diabetes (p. 457)
Hypertension (p. 475)
Stroke (p. 497)
Head injury (p. 523)
Sudden loss of vision (p. 542)

Vomiting

This is a commonly presented symptom with many causes, The majority of cases are due to self-limiting gastrointestinal infections or dietary indiscretion. These usually settle in 48–72 hours.

If the symptoms persist for three or more days it requires more careful consideration.

Causes

Gastrointestinal

Acute and chronic gastritis
Intestinal obstruction
Acute appendicitis
Gall bladder disease
Gastric ulcers
Oesophageal abnormalities
Gastrointestinal tumours

General

Pregnancy (see p. 352)
Motion sickness
Migraine (see p. 203)
Vertigo (see p. 73)
Urinary tract infection (see p. 76)
Renal failure/renal colic

- Hepatitis (see p. 161)
- Diabetes (see p. 457)
- Raised intracranial pressure
- Drugs – alcohol, opiates, digoxin
- Septicaemia
- Carcinomatosis
- Self-induced vomiting (including bulimia nervosa)

Children

- Feeding problems
- Possetting
- Acute infections (ear, throat, chest, urine, meningitis)
- Gastrointestinal infections
- Pyloric stenosis
- Lead poisoning

History

- Infective contact
- Suspicious foods
- Recent travel – details of itinerary
- Onset of vomiting – acute, chronic, recurrent
- Nature of vomit – undigested food, bile content, blood
- Character of vomiting – projectile, effortless, associated with retching
- Associated symptoms
  - abdominal pain
  - nausea
  - diarrhoea
  - headache
  - urinary symptoms
- Menstrual history
- Past history of gastrointestinal disease or operations
- History of medication
- Alcohol intake
- Patient's health beliefs and explanation

Examination

General

- Temperature
- Hydration
- Fetor
- Jaundice
- Pallor
- Tongue

Abdomen

- Masses
- Hernia

Distension
Visible peristalsis

CNS

Neck stiffness
Nystagmus
Fundi (papilloedema)
Ataxia

Check sites of possible infection in children (ears, throat, chest)

Test feed infants for congenital pyloric 'tumour'

Investigation

These are usually unnecessary in acute self-limiting cases

Consider

haematocrit
LFT
U & E
digoxin level
MSU
pregnancy test
stool for pathogens or parasites
stool occult blood
barium meal
chest X-ray

Options

'Push fluids' and starve

The vast majority will settle on this regimen within 48–72 hours. Water and dilute fruit juices are best but alternatives include flat 'Coca-Cola', or sugar, salt and water mixture (a teaspoon of sugar to a pint of boiled water with a pinch of salt). Conveniently packaged, proprietary preparations are now available on the market. Avoid milk if possible in babies (or dilute the strength).

Antiemetics

Prochlorperazine 12.5 mg i.m. (or suppositories 5–25 mg)

Metoclopramide 10 mg i.m. or orally 6–8 hourly (avoid in puberty or pregnancy)

Meclozine 25 mg 8–12 hourly (would appear safe in pregnancy).

Diet

In early pregnancy small frequent meals are beneficial. In infants, feeding problems due to poor technique may be the cause. The health visitor may be most helpful in these cases.

Drug therapy

Review existing medication.

Alkali preparations
e.g. magnesium trisilicate mixture B.P. 10 ml 6–8 hourly
'Asilone' 10 ml 6–8 hourly.

Antibiotics

Only use when indicated (not as routine).

Referral

Surgical assessment of the acute abdomen demands urgent referral

Neurological / ENT assessment } if such an underlying case is suspected

For nursing in isolation if a more serious infective cause is suspected

Gastroenterological assessment including endoscopy

i.v. rehydration if the oral route is inadequate.

See also:

Dizziness (p. 73)
Dysuria and frequency (p. 76)
Imported disease (p. 157)
Migraine (p. 203)
Symptoms in pregnancy (p. 352)
Feeding problems (p. 417)
Diabetes (p. 457)

Vomiting blood

Haematemesis or vomiting blood can be an alarming occurrence. Whether the blood is fresh and bright red, or 'altered' like coffee grounds, the majority of patients will require urgent admission to hospital.

Causes

Upper gastrointestinal bleed

Duodenal ulcer
Gastric erosions (often drug induced)
Gastric ulcer
Oesophageal varicies from portal hypertension
Tumours
Anticoagulant overdose
Bleeding disorder of haemostasis
Mallory–Weiss syndrome
Aortic aneurysm

Swallowed blood

Epistaxis
Haemoptysis

Tooth extraction
Black puddings

History

Estimate volume of blood loss
Previous episodes of haematemesis
Associated epigastric or chest pains
Colour of stools (melaena)
Recent nosebleeds or tooth extraction
Past history of peptic ulceration, liver disease or clotting disorder
Drugs – particularly NSAID, steroids or anticoagulants
Alcohol intake and recent diet

Examination

Assess for shock
Pulse and BP
Skin – anaemia, bruising, jaundice or spider naevi
Abdominal tenderness
Enlarged liver or spleen or epigastric masses
Rectal examination for melaena

Investigation

Usually done on admission to hospital but consider
- FBC
- platelet count
- ESR
- clotting studies
- U & E (N.B. urea may rise after a Gl bleed)
- LFT
- barium swallow and meal

Options

Emergency treatment
After discharge from hospital consider:

Diet
Should be controlled by patient's needs and symptoms
Small frequent meals are better than prolonged fastings
Severe dietary restrictions are unnecessary.

Drugs
Anti-ulcer treatment – antacids – 50% Aludrox/magnesium trisilicate mixture 10 ml 6–8 hourly
Cimetidine 1000 mg daily in divided doses, then 400 mg at night
Ranitidine 150 mg 12 hourly
Bismulhate (De-Nol) 5 ml 6 hourly
Carbenoxolone – one tablet 8 hourly
Sucralfate 1 g 6 hourly
Iron supplements – may be necessary after a major bleed.

Advise against
Alcohol
Smoking
NSAID.

Life style
Regular hours
Avoid stress and tension where possible
Encourage relaxation technique.

Follow-up

Repeat endoscopy or barium X-ray studies to assess ulcer healing after 2–3 months

Patients with portal hypertension will need regular follow-up at 3–6 monthly intervals to monitor liver function

Referral

All patients should be referred initially for endoscopy and/or emergency barium studies

Failure to heal ulcer

Liver failure

Endoscopy follow-up for gastric ulcer biopsy.

See also:

Haemoptysis (p. 129)
Indigestion (p. 163)
Nosebleed (p. 219)
Problem drinking (p. 261)

Weakness and clumsiness

The complaint of being weak and clumsy is unusual but it is significant as it is often associated with a bad prognosis.

The age and mode of presentation is dependent on the underlying pathology but the doctor should be alert to weakness as a significant sign in the young and the old. The hypotonic or 'floppy' infant for example may have cerebral palsy, and the pensioner with shuffling gait and characteristic facies may have treatable Parkinson's disease.

Patterns of presentation

Extrapyramidal

Tremor, general retardation, shuffling gait, small writing, 'useless hand' if unilateral
Parkinsonism

Pyramidal

Loss of dexterity, dragging feet, legs 'won't go', stiffness and spasticity, muscle spasms

Cerebral lesions
- cerebral palsy
- tumour
- stroke

Cord lesions
- compression
- multiple sclerosis
- motor neurone disease
- spondylosis

Cerebellar Slurred speech, double vision, unsteady gait
- Tumour
- Multiple sclerosis
- Alcohol
- Vascular

Nerve Distal weakness and wasting with associated sensory loss
- Diabetes
- Trauma
- Alcohol

Muscle Wasting, rapid fatigue, difficulty rising from chair or climbing stairs, tender muscles

Neuromuscular
- myasthenia gravis
- motor neurone disease

Myopathy
- hereditary
- acquired

Metabolic
- steroids
- lithium
- β-blockade
- Cushing's syndrome
- hypothyroidism
- diabetes
- Addison's disease
- polymyalgia rheumatica
- carcinomatosis

Joints Weakness and associated symptoms in or around specific joints

History Onset and duration of weakness

Severity and progress of weakness

Associated symptoms
- speech disorder

sensory loss
weight loss
thyroid symptoms
Precipitating and exacerbating factors
Family history
Past history of neurological symptoms
Medication
Psychological factors
Social effects
dressing
cooking
transferring
walking distance
climbing stairs
co-ordination

Examination

Record
Strength and tone in all limbs
Wasting, fasiculation and gait
Weight
BP
Retinopathy
Check for
Joint disease
Thyroid status
Cardiovascular signs
Neurological signs
localizing signs
cerebellar signs
peripheral nerves

Investigation

ESR and FBC
U & E
Liver function tests including γGT
B_{12} and folate
CPK and aldolase
Urinalysis
Chest X-ray

Options

Appropriate management
Stroke (see p. 497)
Parkinsonism (see p. 487)
Multiple sclerosis (see p. 483)
Thyroid disease (see p. 481)
Diabetes (see p. 457)
Discussion of diagnosis and prognosis with patient and his family

Support and co-operation with
- voluntary organizations
- self-help societies
- day care and clubs
- holiday and holiday admissions
- accommodation and supervision

Financial benefits, e.g.
- attendance allowance
- mobility allowance

Physical aids for eating, cooking, bathing, dressing and walking, e.g. chair, hoists, grab rails, splints and 'possum'.

Follow-up

Regularly review
- progress of disease
- emotional factors
- drugs
- social and functional ability

Full assessment of new symptoms

Review of available resources and aids

Referral

Occupational therapist and physiotherapist in rehabilitation

Surgeons for laminectomy and other orthopaedic problems

Physicians or neurologists for EMG studies and confirmation of suspected multiple sclerosis or other more rare diseases.

Complications

Social disadvantages

Depression

Progress to terminal illness

See also:

Elbow (p. 82)
Foot and ankle (p. 115)
Knee (p. 179)
Problem drinking (p. 261)
Wrist and hand (p. 341)
Clumsy children (p. 401)
Diabetes (p. 457)
Hypothyroidism (p. 481)
Multiple sclerosis (p. 483)
Parkinsonism (p. 487)
Stroke (p. 497)

Weight loss

When there is measurable weight loss the metabolic needs, either physiological or pathological, are in excess of the effective absorption of nutrients. This weight may be lost as fluid, fat or muscle bulk.

Weight loss may be a *symptom*, e.g.
- TB
- diabetes
- hyperthyroidism

It may be a *sign*, e.g.
- depression
- fear of cancer
- anorexia nervosa

It may alternatively be a *therapeutic option*, e.g.
- osteoarthritis

Ideal weight

Insurance company statistics indicate an optimal range of weight in relation to height which is associated with maximum longevity – the 'Body Mass Index'

Men (W/H^2) = 20–25
Women (W/H^2) = 19–24
(when W = weight in kilos and H = height in metres)

Causes

Depression
Cancers – especially of the upper gastrointestinal tract
Acute infections
Diabetes
Hyperthyroidism

Other causes

Malnutrition } major causes world wide
Malabsorption }
Tuberculosis
Chronic infections and infestations
Chronic hypoxia
Chronic renal disease
Hepatitis
Glandular fever
Duodenal ulcers
Digoxin toxicity
Anorexia nervosa
Drinking problems
Anxiety
Confusion

Psychosomatic – when there is no objective evidence of a subjective weight loss

History

Weight – present and previous and duration of loss
Appetite – increased, unchanged or lost
Diet – quantity and quality
Associated symptoms
- weakness
- thirst
- sweating and fever
- tremor
- depression
- dysphagia
- cough
- urinary symptoms
- indigestion
- change in bowel habit

Health beliefs and fears
Medication
Alcohol and smoking
Travel
Social and psychological factors
Family attitudes and conflicts

Examination

Record
- Height
- Weight
- General demeanour

Check
- Thyroid state
- Lymph glands and temperature
- Chest and breast examination
- Abdomen and rectal examination

Investigation

Urinalysis
FBC
ESR
U & E and LFT
Serum acid phosphatase (in men)
Blood glucose and serum albumin
Protein electrophoresis
Digoxin level
T_3 and TRH test
CXR
Barium swallow, meal and enema

Stools for occult blood, parasites and faecal fats
Cervical cytology

Options

Treat pathological conditions as appropriate
Monitor weight
Dietary advice
Counselling and psychotherapy as appropriate
Antidepressant therapy as appropriate
Co-operation with dietician.

See also:

Anorexia (p. 12)
Confusion and dementia (p. 52)
Depression (p. 63)
Glandular fever (p. 122)
Imported disease (p. 157)
Malnutrition and malabsorption (p. 195)
Problem drinking (p. 261)
Stress and anxiety (p. 303)
Chronic renal failure (p. 443)
Diabetes (p. 457)
Hyperthyroidism (p. 479)
Pulmonary tuberculosis (p. 492)

Worms

The six varieties of worms affecting man can cause some confusion. The following descriptions may help to differentiate them.

Thread worm or pin worm

Enterobius vermicularis – widespread distribution
Transmission by contact
A visible white worm 3–10 mm long appearing around the anal margin especially in the morning. Anal itching is intense
Diagnosis is by clinical recognition and may be confirmed by 'sellotape slide' and microscopy
Treatment is by piperazine in 2 doses 2 weeks apart and special attention to personal hygiene. If the infestation recurs the whole family should also be investigated.

Round worm

Ascaris lumbricoides – Far East and tropical Africa
Transmission by eggs in human faeces.

In the larval phase symptoms are due to a transient involvement of liver and skin and a more established pneumonitis

In the adult worm phase symptoms include anorexia, weight loss, malabsorption, abdominal distension, pain and occasional intestinal obstruction. Appendicitis, pancreatitis and jaundice also occur

Diagnosis is by stool microscopy and by eosinophilia in the blood film.

Treatment is by piperazine.

Hook worm

Ancylostoma duodenale – tropics and subtropics

Transmission in the soil

Infestation starts with a dermatitis usually limited to the feet. There follows weight loss or growth, retardation, bloody diarrhoea, cough, haemoptysis and shortness of breath

Diagnosis is by stool culture and microscopy and may be suspected if blood loss anaemia and eosinophilia are found

Treatment under specialist care is advisable.

Whip worm

Trichuris trichiura – Far East and tropics

Transmission in the soil

A gut parasite that may remain symptomless or present with weight loss, chronic diarrhoea with blood, abdominal pains and tenesmus

Diagnosis is by stool microscopy and may be suspected if blood loss anaemia and eosinophilia are found.

Treatment is by mebendazole.

Tape worm

Taenia saginata – Middle East and tropical Africa

Taenia solium – widespread distribution and more important since larvae can thrive in man

A gut parasite that may remain symptomless or present with weight loss and anal itching. Segments of the worm may appear in the stool. The infestation can be complicated by cysticercosis

Treatment under specialist care is advisable

Avoid undercooked beef or pork.

Ringworm

Ringworm is not a true worm. *Microsporum*, *Epidermophyton* and *Trichophyton* are fungi that present as ring shaped scaly lesions in the feet, groins, trunk, beard or scalp.

Treatment is effective with any local or systemic antifungal preparation.

See also: Imported disease (p. 157)

The wrist and hand

The proper functioning of the wrist and hand is very important in work and in many activities of daily living. It is thus a particularly important region as regards disability and the maintenance of optimal function is imperative.

Many joints respond well to rest and immobilization but the hand is an important exception. If a finger is immobilized for more than two or three weeks it may lead to permanent stiffness. However, extensor tendon injuries may require more prolonged splintage. In this case the hand should be immobilized with the MCP joints at 90° and the IP joints in full extension in order to minimize subsequent stiffness.

History

Onset and duration of pain and stiffness
Site and severity of symptoms
Exacerbating and relieving factors
Associated symptoms
- paraesthesiae
- weakness
- swelling
- deformity
- nail changes

History of trauma
Social and psychological factors
- employment
- ADL

Immunization state (tetanus)

Examination

Inspect
- deformity
- muscle wasting
- scars
- ganglia
- skin colour

Palpate
bones and tendons
site of maximal pain (including the anatomical snuff box)
temperature, tremor, sweating and radial pulses
active and passive movements
sensation and power

Patterns of presentation

Arthritis

Heberden's nodes over the distal interphalangeal joints may help to differentiate osteoarthritis from rheumatoid arthritis. In this latter condition the characteristic signs are ulnar deviation and swelling at the metacarpal phalangeal joints which can, when associated with wrist involvement, cause considerable disability. Isolated osteoarthritis of the carpometacarpal joint of the thumb is not uncommon.

Psoriatic changes in the nails may point to the diagnosis of a psoriatic arthropathy but septic arthritis, gout and other secondary arthritic conditions are unusual in the hands, with the exception of post-traumatic arthritis.

Infection

Infection of the fingers and hands may require hospitalization for sugical drainage and intravenous antibiotics. Complications include septacaemia, local spread to tendon sheaths and permanent deformity. None of these need occur if primary care is adequate and immediate.

Appropriate antibiotics (e.g. flucloxicillin or clindamycin) rest, splintage, elevation and analgesia are usually sufficient measures to control simple infection. Daily review is essential to detect abscess formation.

When an abscess is diagnosed – it is wise to first exclude gout and orf – incision and drainage under local anaesthetic is essential. During recovery use dry dressings, mobilize the hand and review regularly.

To avoid tetanus excise all necrotic tissue and check immunization state.

Trauma

Abrasions, lacerations, burns, sprains, dislocations, fractures and amputations can all affect the hand. If the injury is severe or if there is a suspicion of a foreign body or damage to nerves, tendons, arteries or bones, then referral to an accident unit is essential.

Pain and loss of mobility, swelling and change of skin colour are all suspicious signs. In particular, pain in the scaphoid fossa after a fall onto an out-stretched hand must be considered as a fractured scaphoid and necessitates immobilization until exclusion by X-ray two weeks later. Intra-articular fractures of the proximal interphalangeal joint may present as sprains.

Less severe injuries can be treated in the usual way with special attention to infection risk, tetanus immunity and early mobilization.

Ganglia

These are degenerative cystic lesions associated with joints or tendon sheaths. They are most commonly found over the dorsum of the wrist. While there may be a fibrous connection with synovial space there is clinically no demonstrable fluid flow between the structures.

The lesions are ussually asymptomatic but if causing pain or particularly unsightly they can be excised. The cyst may rupture either spontaneously or with the aid of the well-loved family bible, but after this will commonly recur.

Carpal tunnel syndrome

In this condition the median nerve is compressed as it passes under the flexor retinaculum. It most commonly occurs in middle aged females. In the majority no cause is found but it may be associated with

fluid retention (pregnancy, the premenstrual phase and menopause)
rheumatoid arthritis
hypothyroidism
Colles' fractures
flexor ganglia

The patient complains of pain in the wrist and hand possibly extending up the forearm also. There is numbness and tingling in the median distribution. The pain is characteristically worse at night and may be relieved by hanging the affected hand out of the bed. On examination there is generally little to find. The paraesthesia may be reproduced by tapping over the median nerve with the wrist extended. In severe cases there may be wasting of the thenar eminence. It is important to exclude symptoms referred from a cervical spine lesion.

In the initial stages, and particularly in pregnancy, treatment is conservative with diuretics and night splints. If this fails, steroid injections or operative decompression of the flexor tunnel is more beneficial and is necessary when sensory loss and muscle wasting are present.

Ulnar nerve compression may also occur in its relationship with the hook of the hamate. Symptoms are similar to the carpal tunnel syndrome but in the ulnar side of the hand. Treatment is best effected by operation.

Tenosynovitis 'canoeist's wrist'

This is a painful condition of the extensor tendons around the wrist. Excessive use results in inflammation around the tendons and there may be associated synovial tendon sheath thickening. Palpable and audible crepitus may be present over the tendon.

Treatment is with rest in a splint and analgesia. Occasionally a local steroid injection will help.

Dupuytren's contracture

In this condition with hereditary and hepatic aetiology there is fibrosis and thickening of the palmar aponeurosis at the base of the ring and little fingers. It particularly affects middle-aged and elderly men. Ultimately it may lead to irreparable contraction of the fingers. It is best to refer to a surgeon to consider excision of the palmar fascia at an early stage. Later, severely contracted fingers may warrant amputation.

Kienbock's disease

Osteochondrosis of the lunate bone results in avascular necrosis. It occurs after injury or repeated minor trauma. It leads to pain and swelling in the wrist after exercise. Referral is necessary to consider replacement with a prosthesis or wrist arthrodesis.

Volkmann's contracture

This results from damage to the brachial artery after a displaced supracondylar fracture of the elbow. The ischaemia leads to a fibrous contracture of the forearm muscles and damage to the median nerve. It causes severe contracture of the fingers and thumb.

Treatment is difficult and surgery not very successful.

Trigger finger

This is due to a thickening of the flexor tendon in the proximal part of the flexor sheath. A tender nodule may be felt at the distal palmar crease below the middle and ring fingers or at the base of the thumb. The digit will flex but then extension is inhibited unless it is performed passively with a notable and painful click. Treatment, where necessary, consists of surgical division of the proximal tendon sheath under the care of a specialist.

Mallet finger The extensor tendon is damaged over the distal interphalangeal joint leading to a flexion deformity. The joint can only be extended passively. In the acute case treatment is by splinting the finger with the proximal IP joint flexed and the distal IP joint extended. However, it is best to X-ray before splinting to exclude an avulsion fracture which may require surgical reduction.

See also:

Elbow (p. 82)
Localized rash (p. 185)
Nail problems (p. 212)
Osteoarthritis (p. 485)
Rheumatoid arthritis (p. 493)

2 Maternity Care

Pre-conception check

Increasingly doctors are taking the opportunity for health education about pregnancy and related topics during consultations and other patient contacts. Many of the symptoms and complications of pregnancy can be anticipated by a 'pre-conception check'. In some centres the opportunity for such checks is offered as a special service. Indeed some investigations – rubella titre and syphilis serology are more appropriately tested before rather than during a pregnancy.

Discussion

Family planning – contraception before and after pregnancy
Fertility and infertility – the patient's expectations and the range of normal
Genetic counselling services – when there is a significant family history of hereditary disease
Smoking
Alcohol
Drugs
Dietary advice – both quality and quantity
Financial advice – maternity grant and allowances
Books about pregnancy, parenthood and childhood

Assessment

BP
Urinalysis
Weight
Rubella titre
Hepatitis B antigen
Blood group
Rhesus antibodies
Syphilis serology
FBC
Cervical cytology

See also Contraception (p. 446)

Diagnosis of pregnancy

Two months amenorrhoea and associated symptoms of pregnancy are adequate grounds for making the diagnosis of pregnancy. The pregnancy can be confirmed clinically by examination at 10–12 weeks of amenorrhoea. Earlier confirmation of pregnancy at 6–8 weeks by urine testing may be helpful.

History

LMP
Menstrual history
Obstetric history
Contraception, especially when the Pill has been used
Symptoms of pregnancy
Attitude towards pregnancy

Examination

Breasts
Engorgement of veins
Pigmentation of areolae
Montgomery's tubercles (8 weeks)
Pelvis – uterine size equivalents
'Hen's Egg' (7 weeks)
'Orange' (10 weeks)
'Grapefruit' (12 weeks)
Abdomen
Palpable uterus (12–14 weeks)
Fundus mid-way to umbilicus (16 weeks)

Investigation

Early morning specimen of urine for HCG (Human Chorionic Gonadotrophin), appropriate for women with prolonged subfertility
irregular periods
indefinite dates
'at risk pregnancy'
for women who are considering termination

Complications of early pregnancy

Uncertain dates
Multiple pregnancy
Abortion
Ectopic pregnancy
Hydatidiform mole
Pelvic tumour
Retroverted uterus

The first antenatal visit

The antenatal clinic is a screening clinic. By careful enquiry and regular examination the doctor and midwife can identify a pregnancy at risk; not only for early detection and intervention in medical complications but also for the recognition of adverse social or psychological factors. The clinic also provides opportunities for health education and advice on birth, parenthood, exercise and relaxation, diet and smoking and maternity benefits.

The first assessment should be made around the twelfth week of pregnancy.

History

Present pregnancy

- Age
- Menstrual history
- Contraceptive history
- LMP
- EDD
- Symptoms of pregnancy

Obstetric history

- Parity
- Pregnancy
- Labour
- Puerperium
- Infant (alive or stillborn)
- Weight
- Sex
- Gestation
- Feeding

Contraceptive history

- Method used
- Date discontinued

Gynaecological history

- Abortion
- Termination
- Subfertility
- Pelvic or abdominal infections
- Pelvic or abdominal surgery

Medical history

- Hypertension
- Diabetes
- Tuberculosis
- UTI
- Varicose veins
- Anaemia
- Liver disease

Cardiac disease
Thyroid disease
Chronic respiratory disease
Thrombosis
Haemoglobinopathy
Autoimmunic disease

Family history
Multiple pregnancy
Malformation or hereditary disease
Diabetes
Renal disease
Tuberculosis
Hypertension

Social history
Smoking and alcohol
Marital status
Housing
Postnatal support
Socio-economic grouping
Employment

Medication
Current therapy
Allergies
Transfusions

Examination

Record
BP
Height
Weight

Check for
Anaemia
Varicose veins
Breasts
Dental care

Auscultation of heart and lungs
Abdominal examination
height of fundus
abdominal masses
Pelvic examination
uterine size
pelvic shape and size
pelvic masses

Investigation

Urine for albumin and glucose
MSU for microscopy and culture

Blood for
- haemaglobin
- blood group
- syphilis screening
- Rhesus antibodies
- rubella antibodies
- hepatitis B antigens
- haemoglobin electrophoresis if indicated

Cervical smear if indicated (see p. 438)
Ultrasonic scan if indicated

Discussion

Symptoms in pregnancy
The respective roles of doctor, midwife, health visitors, father and relatives
Drugs in pregnancy
Smoking and alcohol
Dietary advice
Maternity benefits

Referral

All patients at risk should have an early assessment in an obstetric unit. Those at special risk include

Primipara
- More than 30 years of age
- Less than 5 feet tall
- Low socio-economic grouping
- Significant medical or gynaecological history
- Complications in pregnancy
- Abnormal pelvis
- Abnormal fetal presentation.

Multipara
- More than 35 years of age
- Low socio-economic grouping
- More than four previous pregnancies
- Bad obstetric history.

Subsequent antenatal visits

'Shared care' between the family doctor and the obstetrician implies shared information; full and accurate recording is of vital importance. All observations made by doctor, midwife or obstetric unit should be clearly recorded on the same cards or notes. In the UK the 'Co-op Card' is now very widely used.

The frequency of antenatal visits will be determined by the progress of the pregnancy and the presence and severity of any risk factors. The traditional arrangement is monthly until 28/52 weeks then fortnightly until 36/52 weeks, and then weekly until term.

History

Confirmation of dates
Symptoms or complications of pregnancy
Fetal movements

Examination

Record
- Weight
- BP
- Urinalysis
- Oedema
- Height of fundus
- Lie
- Position
- Presentation
- Engagement of head in pelvis
- Fetal heart rate

Pelvic examination
At 36 weeks – obstetric diameters
At term – assessment of cervix
- length
- position
- dilatation
- consistency

Investigation

At 16–20 weeks AFP after a full discussion of the implications of an abnormal result

At 28 weeks
At 32 weeks
At 36 weeks
} Hb and Rhesus antibodies in 'Rh −ve' mothers

Confirmation of fetal heart beat after threatened abortion

Ultrasonic scan
- serial BPD for dating
- location of placenta
- multiple pregnancy
- fetal activity
- fetal lie and presentation

Urea and uric acid – suspected PET or hypertension
LFT – pruritis of pregnancy

MSU – proteinuria or symptoms of UTI
GTT – glycosuria (see p. 459)
HVS – vaginal discharge (see p. 320)

Continuing discussion

Iron and folate therapy
Other drug therapy
Diet, alcohol and smoking
Exercise and relaxation
Sexual intercourse
Symptoms in pregnancy
Labour and puerperium
Analgesia in obstetrics
Attitudes to feeding and infant care
Role of midwife and health visitor
Maternity benefits, dental care, prescription exemption and free milk (depending on family circumstances)

Reasons for referral

Disease or complications in pregnancy
Hospital investigations, e.g. amniocentesis, fetal monitoring
Effective bed rest in PET and hypertension
Abnormal presentation at term.

Symptoms in pregnancy

Nausea and vomiting

This symptom occurs in about 50% of pregnancies and is usually self-limiting.

Enquire about associated symptoms and check for signs of dehydration and ketonuria. Exclude a urinary infection.

Reassurance and advice on diet is usually sufficient, but when the symptom is disruptive antihistamines may be prescribed.

In refractory cases hospitalization may be necessary.

If the onset of vomiting occurs late in pregnancy, consider causes other than the pregnancy itself. However, late vomiting associated with proteinuria and raised BP is a sign of progressive PET.

Urinary frequency

This symptom is associated with rise in renal blood flow and pressure on the trigone of the bladder.

In early pregnancy this is due to the growth of the uterus and in later pregnancy is due to the descent of the fetal head.

Take MSU if there is associated proteinuria, fever, nausea, urinary symptoms or if the frequency is persistent.

Vaginal discharge

In every pregnancy there is an increase in vaginal secretion due to increased activity in the mucus secreting cells in the cervical columnar epithelium. There is an associated rise in alkalinity and these conditions are conducive to infection.

Causes

Physiological changes
Monilial infection
Trichomonas infection
Other STD

Assessment

Nature of the discharge
Associated symptoms
Symptoms in sexual partner
HVS and cervical smear if indicated
Urinalysis to exclude glycosuria

Options

Advise on hygiene and clothing
Antimicrobial therapy, as indicated by HVS
(Avoid metronidazole before the 12th week).

Constipation

In pregnancy this symptom is exacerbated by the reduced muscle tone of the colon and the mechanical effect of the expanding uterus.

Advise on diet and high roughage intake
Consider withdrawal of prophylactic iron
Consider use of fibre preparations, lubricants (e.g. glycerine, suppository) or colonic stimulant (e.g. Senna).

Piles

'Piles' are exacerbated by the mechanical effects of the pregnant uterus on the pelvic vasculature. They become more common with each successive pregnancy.

Advise on

high fibre diet
regular bowel habit
avoidance of constipation and straining

Symptoms and signs usually resolve in the puerperium but if persistent, surgery may be necessary.

Abdominal pain

Suprapubic pain in early pregnancy may be related to growth of the uterus. Ectopic pregnancy and impacted uterus must be excluded.

In later pregnancy consider the usual differential diagnosis of abdominal pain (see p. 1) and exclude:

concealed abruption of placenta
red degeneration of fibroids
rectus sheath haematoma
Braxton Hicks' contractions
early labour.

Heart burn

This common symptom is caused by reflux of gastric contents into the oesophagus and is exacerbated by a relaxation of the cardia, reduced gastric motility and the mechanical effects of a large uterus.

Options

Advice on diet – 'little and often'
Posture – avoiding stooping and bending
Withdrawal of prophylactic iron
Antacids.

Fainting

In early pregnancy fainting is a feature of rapid changes in haemodynamics with the rise in circulating volume and cardiac output.

In later pregnancy uterine compression of the inferior vena cava may cause the supine hypotensive syndrome.

Explanation of the mechanism of this syndrome and advice on posture is usually sufficient.

Support hose may be helpful.

Breast discomfort

The early symptoms of heaviness, tenderness and sensitivity in the breasts may continue throughout pregnancy.

Early examination to exclude breast disease, including carcinoma, is essential.

Advise on

maternity bras
washing off the crusted secretions from the nipples
massage of nipples with lanolin may help as a preparation of breast feeding.

Sweating

Little can be done for the minor vascular changes of pregnancy.

Sweating is only one of the manifestations of the vasodilation of pregnancy, other features include

- palmar erythema
- spider naevi
- telangiectasia
- haemangiomata
- varicose veins
- Raynaud's phenomenon (which is improved)
- nasal congestion and epistaxis
- breast and pelvic engorgement.

Skin changes

Striae occur on the abdomen, thighs and breast and there is no effective prevention or cure. They fade gradually in the puerperium but may increase with successive pregnancies.

Hirsutism also increases with successive pregnancies. Electrolysis may be indicated in extreme cases.

Pigmentation of the face (chloasma), the abdomen (linea nigra) and of the nipples is common and usually resolves spontaneously. Pigmented naevi may become darker and malignant change must be excluded.

Itching may be due to iron deficiency or cholestatic jaundice; investigation with FBC and LFT may be indicated. Itching usually responds to calamine lotion and/or antihistamines. Spontaneous resolution in the puerperium is the rule. Patients with liver disease should be referred to the specialist unit.

A **rash** may be self-inflicted, secondary to itching.

A **papular rash** maximal over the the abdomen is peculiar to pregnancy (prurigo gestationis). The less common herpes gestationis or erythema multiforme will resolve spontaneously at term but may require steroid therapy. Acne, alopecia and Beçhet's syndrome improve with pregnancy. Psoriasis is unpredictable.

Varicosities

The development of varicose veins in pregnancy is related to peripheral vasodilatation, increased circulating volume and uterine pressure on the inferior vena cava. Phlebitis and broken superficial veins are often associated as are vulval varicosities, but these are seldom declared by the patient.

Advise on rest, elevation and support hose.

Support tights with elasticated gusset or 'panty girdle' should give adequate relief for vulval varicosities.

Cramps

This very common symptom may be related to the physiological fall in serum sodium concentration.

There is no specific treatment but a DVT should be excluded.

Ankle swelling

This is a cardinal sign of PET if associated with raised BP and proteinuria. There may also be swelling of the face and fingers.

In isolation swelling is a manifestation of peripheral vasodilation and increased cardiac output.

Advise on rest and elevation of legs and removal of rings.

Carpal tunnel syndrome

Symptoms in the hands with radiation up the arm may result from compression of the median nerve under the flexor retinaculum at the wrist.

Advise splintage and elevation of the hand.

Associated sensory or motor deficit is an indication for urgent referral.

Exclude hypothyroidism and arthritis of the wrist if symptoms persist in the puerperium.

Bell's palsy

Pregnancy is a precipitating factor in this classical neurological syndrome. Resolution is complete in the puerperium.

Meralgia paraesthetica

Compression of the lateral cutaneous nerve of the thigh at the point of penetration of the fascia lata causes paraesthesiae in the sensory distribution of the nerve.

Pregnancy and obesity are the only causes and resolution is complete in the puerperium.

Backache

Causes

- Compression of the sciatic nerve
- Lax ligaments of pregnancy
- Prolapsed intervertebral disc
- Traumatic neuritis
- Coccidynia may cause persistent pain after delivery.

Options

- Rest and relaxation
- Posture and footwear
- Avoidance of exertion
- Care while lifting (especially if a previous child is of toddler age)
- Consider total bed rest and traction if neurological signs are present.

See also:

Abdominal pain (p. 1)
Constipation (p. 55)
Vaginal discharge (p. 320)

Varicose veins (p. 324)
Wrist and hands (p. 341)

Disorders of pregnancy

Ectopic pregnancy This life threatening condition should be suspected in every woman of child bearing age who complains of abdominal pain. The diagnosis should be confirmed or excluded in all cases of recurrent low abdominal pain in early pregnancy with or without bleeding.

An ectopic gestation occurs in 1 in 250 pregnancies, it can recur in about 10% and infertility follows in 30–60% of cases.

Patterns of presentation

Vaginal bleeding preceded by pain
Lower abdominal pain
Pain radiating to loins and shoulder tips
Suspected pregnancy even before a missed period
History of pelvic surgery, pelvic sepsis, IUCD *in situ* or progesterone-only Pill

Examination

Patient in shock
Signs of guarding and rebound tenderness in either iliac fossa
Cystic mass in either fornix on pelvic examination

Emergency care

Arrange immediate transport to hospital
Establish i.v. line
Maintain circulating blood volume

Differential diagnosis

Abortion
Salpingitis
Appendicitis or diverticulitis
Ovarian cyst

Pre-eclamptic toxaemia (PET) Pre-eclamptic toxaemia can be recognized by the association of three cardinal signs: oedema, proteinuria and elevated BP above 140/90. PET occurs in 6% of all pregnancies and 12% of first pregnancies. There are wide ranging physiological and biochemical changes with a significant association with perinatal and maternal mortality.

Risk factors

Young mothers
Primigravidae and multigravidae
Previous PET
Multiple pregnancy

Diabetes
Pre-existing renal disease
Hypertension
Hydatidiform mole
Hydramnios

History Age, parity and obstetric history
Confirmation of dates
Oedema, headache, visual symptoms, nausea
Enquire about risk factors

Examination **Record**
BP
Urinalysis
Weight
Check
Oedema
Fundi
Fetal size and relation to dates

Investigation MSU (if proteinuria present)
Urea and uric acid
24 hour urine collection for oestriol estimations
Ultrasound scan to monitor fetal growth

Referral All cases with BP 140/90 or more
All cases with a rise in BP 10 mm (diastolic)
All cases with association of oedema and proteinuria and excessive weight gain.

Options Home care should only be undertaken after a period of stable observations in an obstetric unit
Bed rest
Frequent monitoring of BP, weight, urinalysis and fetal movement.

Eclampsia

Emergency treatment Confirm first that the patient is convulsing, is pregnant and is hypertensive
Record BP (and the time) and the state of reflexes
Control
Convulsion diazepam 5 mg i.v. (and repeat if necessary)
Hypertension diamorphine 5 mg i.v. (and repeat if necessary)

Contact

Obstetric Flying Squad
Monitor BP and fetal heart rate
Transfer to an obstetric unit

Bleeding in pregnancy

Abortion

The termination of pregnancy before 28 weeks gestation.

Threatened abortion

Initially painless bleeding in early pregnancy. There may be moderate abdominal pain associated. The cervical os remains closed and the pregnancy tests remain positive.

Inevitable abortion/Incomplete abortion

Progressive, intermittent low abdominal pain radiating to the back with dilation of the cervical os and negative pregnancy test.

Complete abortion

Spontaneous evacuation of all products of conception with closure of the cervical os and cessation of bleeding (this is not universally recognized as a clinical entity).

Septic abortion

When abortion is associated with infection and fever.

Missed abortion

When a threatened abortion is followed by no demonstrable uterine growth and pregnancy tests become negative.

Habitual abortion

When three successive pregnancies end in inevitable abortion.

Therapeutic abortion

When a pregnancy is terminated according to the requirements of the Abortion Act 1967.

Aetiology

Fetal – malformation or chromosomal abnormalities
Maternal
- fever or anaesthesia
- renal or cardiovascular disease
- trauma or stress (including illegal abortion)
- severe Rhesus isoimmunization

Placental – progestogen deficiency
Mechanical
- retroverted uterus
- septate uterus
- fibroids
- cervical incompetence

In the majority of cases the cause is unknown

Differential diagnosis

Ectopic pregnancy
Salpingitis
Ovarian cyst
Fibroids
Delayed period and pseudocyesis

History

Onset and degree of bleeding
Associated pain – before or after the onset of bleeding
Confirmation of the pregnancy
Dates and duration of menstruation
Contraceptive history
Recent history of
- intercourse
- trauma
- anaesthetic
- stress
- fever
- self-induced trauma to the uterus

Examination

Record
- Volume of blood loss
- BP
- Temperature

Check for
- Signs of shock or anaemia
- Signs of free fluid in abdomen with peritonism

Pelvic examination
- For cervical dilation
- Uterine position
- Pelvic masses

Emergency care

Clear retained products of conception from cervical os
Establish i.v. line
Ergometrine 0.5 mg i.v.
Urgent transfer to gynaecological unit

Threatened abortion
- Remove IUCD if present
- Bed rest until 12 hours after cessation of bleeding
- Consider sedation
- Review if the pain or the rate of blood loss increases
- Repeat pregnancy test and FBC

Inevitable or incomplete abortion

Refer to gynaecological unit for evacuation of uterus

Complications

Maternal death
Shock due to dilation of cervical os and blood loss
Infection
Persistent bleeding
- consider missed abortion
- hydatidiform mole
- blood dyscrasia
- incomplete evacuation

Habitual abortion

Referral

Emergency
Inevitable or incomplete abortion when patient is in shock for further stabilization, and evacuation of uterus.

Urgent
Inevitable, incomplete or septic abortion for evacuation of uterus and observation.

Routine
Missed or habitual or therapeutic abortion for specialist assessment and care.

Follow-up

Counselling during 'bereavement'
Contraception or sterilization advice
Check Rubella status
Give anti-D immunoglobulin in Rhesus negative patients
Discussion of future pregnancies

Polyhydramnios

Defective circulation and excess production of amniotic fluid occurs in 1:250 pregnancies and carries an increased risk of abortion, and post-partum haemorrhage.

Associated conditions

Maternal
- Multiparity
- PET
- Diabetes
- Congestive cardiac failure
- Rhesus isoimmunization

Fetal
- Twins
- Anencephaly
- Oesophageal atresia
- Spina bifida
- Hydrocephalus
- Chorioangioma

History Family history or symptoms of diabetes
Abdominal discomfort

Examination Weight gain
Oedema
Urinalysis
Inaudible fetal heart
Fluid thrill and ballotment of fetal parts

Referral All cases for investigation.

Oligohydramnois This is a rare condition of reduced amniotic fluid volume. It is associated with intra-uterine growth retardation, post-maturity and fetal renal agenesis.

Rhesus disease In the UK 17% of all women have Rhesus negative blood groups and this percentage represents a continuing risk in pregnancy. Other antibodies can cause isoimmunizations but will not be discussed here. The introduction of anti-D immunoglobulin has eliminated many of the complications but only by careful supervision will complications continue to be avoided.

Assessment History of
- previous stillbirth
- jaundiced baby
- previous transfusions

Maternal blood group determined at the first antenatal visit

Paternal blood group determined if mother is Rhesus negative

Screening of Rh antibodies at
- 12, 28, 32 and 36 weeks in Rh negative mothers
- 12 and 34/36 weeks in Rh positive mothers

Kleinhauer test if fetal/maternal bleed is suspected

Management Puerperium – if mother is Rh negative and baby is Rh positive give anti-D immunoglobulin 100 μg within 72 hours of birth

Abortion, termination or amniocentesis give anti-D immunoglobulin 50 μg within 72 of event.

Hydatidiform mole With an incidence of 1 in 2000–3000 this is a rare but premalignant condition of the placental trophoblast associated with chorioncarcinoma. Despite this sinister potential, in its mildest form a pregnancy may progress normally.

Patterns of presentation

History of previous abortions
Indefinite dates for uterine growth
Persistent vaginal bleeding in early pregnancy
Nausea and vomiting
Early onset of PET
Late onset of vomiting in association with PET

Assessment

Large for dates
No palpable fetal parts
No fetal movements or audible fetal heart
Anaemia
Vesicles in vaginal loss
Raised urine HCG estimation
Abnormal ultrasonic scan

Referral

All cases on suspicion of the diagnosis.

Follow-up

Urine and HCG levels every 3 months for 2 years
Delay further pregnancy for 2 years
Barrier methods of contraception for at least 1 year since oral and intra-uterine methods are contraindicated.

Ante-partum haemorrhage

By definition this is vaginal bleeding after the 28th week of gestation. APH occurs in 3% of pregnancies and is more common in first pregnancies. With the advances in neonatology there is now a tendency to manage cases of vaginal bleeding before 28 weeks as cases of APH. The bleeding can rapidly become life threatening.

Causes

Placental abruption
Placenta praevia
Cervical erosion, polyp or carcinoma
Vaginal varicosities or infection
Bleeding from rectum or urethra

History

Estimated volume of blood loss
Association of pain
Fetal movements
Previous blood loss
Recent trauma

Examination *No pelvic examination* (to avoid disturbing a possible placenta praevia)
Abdominal examination
BP
Temperature
Pulse
Urine analysis – oedema
Estimate blood loss – by inspection of clothes, bedding and surroundings
Fetal movements and heart rate

Emergency care Establish i.v. line
Maintain a circulating blood volume
Contact obstetric flying squad
Monitor fetal movements and heart rate

Referral All cases for hospital assessment which will include placental localization and fetal monitoring.

Complications Intra-uterine death
Maternal death
Coagulation defect

Follow-up Frequent antenatal care until term if mother is discharged from hospital with diagnosis of placental abruption.

See also:
Eclampsia (p. 520)
Vaginal bleeding in pregnancy (p. 544)

The fetus at risk

During pregnancy the fetus may be put at risk by certain infections, maternal disease or drugs. Though mothers are made aware of the potential hazards of drug taking it remains the responsibility of the doctor to record the LMP when prescribing for or immunizing a woman of reproductive age.

Infections **Rubella** – the maternal infection may be sub-clinical but the virus will damage the fetus in 60% of cases in the first month (this figure falls to 5% by the 16th week). All organs can be affected depending on the time of exposure.

Rubella antibody titre in all mothers must be established early in pregnancy or preferably before conception.

When titre is > 20 units the patient is rubella immune.

When titre is < 20 units vaccinate in puerperium.

When rubella contact is suspected paired blood samples should be taken 10 days apart. A rise in titre indicates current infection; consider termination.

Cytomegalovirus – causes several congenital malformations.

Herpes virus – only a primary infection is a risk and may cause brain damage. Chronic or recurrent infections are not a risk.

Hepatitis A antigen – is a suspected risk.

Syphilis – if untreated will result in the classical syndrome of congenital syphilis.

Toxoplasmosis – glandular fever-like illness in the mother but hydrocephalus and choroidoretinitis and sometimes stillbirth occur in the fetus.

Maternal disease

Diabetes mellitus – (see p. 457)

Thrombocytopenia

Thyrotoxicosis – careful monitoring of maternal thyroid function to ensure euthyroid fetal state

Hyperparathyroidism – is very rare but can result in neonatal hypocalcaemia and tetany

Myasthenia gravis – 25% of neonates will have the disease in a transient form.

Drugs in pregnancy

It is best to avoid the use of drugs in pregnancy and the following list is included only as a guide. The doctor should refer to drug information, supplied by the manufacturer, if there is any doubt.

Early pregnancy

Antiemetics

Following thalidomide and the recent doubt over Debendox drugs should be the last resort in management of vomiting in pregnancy. (See p. 352)

Anticonvulsants

Risk to the fetus is probably worse if epilepsy is left untreated. Folic acid antagonistic effect may be mitigated by folic acid supplements. Neonates can demonstrate barbiturate withdrawal and clotting defects. Carbamazepine and sodium valproate may be safest.

Antibiotics

Both co-trimoxazole and sulphamethoxazole are folate

antagonists and are a theoretical risk to the fetus. In practice 'Septrin' has been widely used with no recorded complications.

Tetracycline

Causes yellow staining and delay in the basic development of teeth. It is contraindicated.

Chloramphenicol

Causes aplastic anaemia.

Aminoglycosides

May cause VIII nerve damage and should be avoided.

Metronidazole

Has an effect on purine synthesis and is therefore a potential teratogen and should be avoided before the 12th week.

Podophylline

May be absorbed and cause fetal damage. It is contraindicated.

Hormonal preparation

Oestrogen/progesterone in high dose combination causes abnormalities in CVS, limbs and neural canal. In the dosage of the oral contraceptive pills they are not a risk.

Anticoagulants

Warfarin – may be teratogenic in early pregnancy and should be avoided.

Nicotinamide

Present in many vitamin preparations and is associated with an increased incidence of malformations and should be avoided.

Chloroquine

May cause cochlear and retinal damage.

Salicylates

In high dosage are associated with increased incidence of malformation and should be avoided.

Folic acid antagonists

Contraindicated because of high risk of malformation.

Alcohol

Fetal alcohol syndrome occurs only with excessive alcohol intake and is usually associated with low socio-economic grouping, poor diet and smoking.

Smoking

The nicotine, cyanide and carbon monoxide components of smoke have an adverse effect on birthweight, perinatal mortality, PET and fetal abnormality.

Drugs in late pregnancy

Antihypertensives

Reserpine – adverse effect on neonates.

Thiazides – theoretical risk of thrombocytopenia, also raises uric acid level affecting monitoring of renal function in pregnancy – best avoided.

Beta-blockers delay intra-uteric growth and cause fetal distress in labour then neonatal hypoglycaemia – not recommended.

Thyroid drugs

Radioiodine ablates fetal thyroid – absolute contraindication.

Carbimazole can cause neonatal hypothyroidism.

Anticoagulants

Warfarin – stop 3/52 before term to avoid neonatal haemorrhage.

Heparin is the drug of choice.

Steroids

May be associated with placental insufficiency but not contraindicated. Use as in the non-pregnant state.

Sedatives

May supress neonatal respiration and should be avoided during labour.

There is no known adverse effect in pregnancy.

Tricyclic antidepressants

Not contraindicated in pregnancy but neonate may demonstrate withdrawal symptoms.

Sulphonylureas

Have no advantage over insulin for diabetic control.

Tolbutamide – short half-life – should be used in labour to avoid neonatal hypoglycaemia.

Lithium

Fetal goitre associated.

Chlorpromazine

Retinal damage.

Chloramphenicol

Aplastic anaemia and 'Grey syndrome' in the neonate – it is contraindicated.

Maternal disease in pregnancy

Cardiovascular disease

The cardiovascular changes in pregnancy include an increase in blood volume, a reduction of peripheral resistance and a rise in cardiac output and renal blood flow.

These changes adversely affect the efficiency of the heart in patients who have previously been at risk – up to 2% of all mothers.

The management of such cases should be carried out in consultation with a cardiologist.

History

Cardiovascular symptoms
Past history of
- cardiac disease
- rheumatic fever
- anaemia
- hypertension
- thyroid disease
- heart disease

Examination

Record BP
Auscultation of the heart
Systolic murmur of Grade III/VI or more is significant
Diastolic murmurs are always significant
Check for signs of cardiac failure

Complications

Pulmonary oedema and haemoptysis
Complicating factors are
- anaemia
- stress
- infection
- anxiety

Referral

For full cardiological assessment
For shared care between obstetrician and cardiologist.

Deep vein thrombosis

(See p. 62).

Anaemia in pregnancy

With the increased circulating volume of blood and the increased demands on iron and folic acid reserves the haemoglobin concentration falls during pregnancy (Fig. 2.1).

Maternal anaemia does not have an adverse effect on fetal growth but it becomes an obstetric risk factor if anaemia is present at delivery.

Prior to the WHO recommendations it was standard practice to prescribe prophylactic iron and folic acid preparations from the 12th week onwards and into the puerperium. Now it would seem more logical to

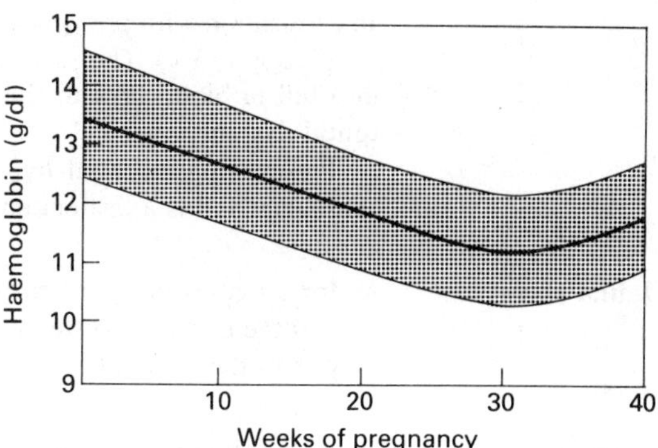

Fig. 2.1. Average pattern of the fall of whole-blood haemoglobin concentration during normal pregnancy

prescribe haematinics only if anaemia is proven on investigation, or prophylactically if the diet is obviously deficient.

Presentation

Routine pre-conception or antenatal checks
Pallor
Breathlessness
Fainting
Poor diet
Abnormal bleeding
Multiple pregnancy

Investigation

Protocols vary in different centres and the following is only a suggested routine

First visit at 12 weeks

Hb
MCV
Haemoglobin electrophoresis in susceptible groups

Subsequent visits at 28, 32, and 36 weeks

Hb
MCV

Consider

Iron and TIBC
Folate and B_{12} if no response to oral iron and folate

Options

Iron and/or folate preparations if Hb falls below the normal range.

Iron, e.g. 'Jectofer' i.m. if Hb is below the normal range in the final 10 weeks of pregnancy.

Hypertension

Elevation in the diastolic blood pressure during pregnancy is directly related to a rise in fetal mortality. There is also an association with pre-eclampsia (30%) and abruption of the placenta (5%). The elevation of blood pressure results in a fall in blood flow to the uterus and subsequent placental dysfunction.

Pre-existing essential hypertension is exacerbated by pregnancy and is a distinct entity from pre-eclampsia.

Initial assessment As for all cases of hypertension (see p. 475) taking care that the mother is rested preferably sitting and not subject to the supine hypotensive syndrome.

Options Frequent attendance at antenatal clinic to check
- BP
- fundi
- proteinuria
- oedema
- weight gain
- urea and uric acid
- fetal growth

Bed rest

Hypotensive medication – in consultation with the specialist.

Complications Hypotensive drug side effects

Hypotension is directly related to
- intra-uterine death
- prematurity
- small for dates infants

Follow-up BP – check throughout the puerperium and at three months post-natal

Renal disease This occurs in 0.2% of pregnancies but in 5% of cases of PET and is directly related to an increase in perinatal mortality.

Acute renal disease is caused by acute pyelonephritis or glomerulonephritis.

The risk of infection is increased by the relative stasis of the compressed and dilated ureters.

History Presence of urinary symptoms (but there may be no symptoms)

Previous renal disease

Examination Check BP
Excessive oedema

Investigation MSU
Urea and uric acid

Referral All cases for shared care between nephrologist and obstetrician.

Urinary tract infection 1–2% of mothers have urinary tract infection during pregnancy, 70% of cases are asymptomatic. Since it is the asymptomatic cases that are associated with the increased risk of developing pyelonephritis, an MSU should be taken at the first visit and after detection of proteinuria at any time subsequently.

Initial assessment As for urinary symptoms in non-pregnant state
MSU should always follow the detection of proteinuria

Management Advice on toilet hygiene
Increased fluid intake
Appropriate antibiotic therapy (avoiding Septrin, other sulphonamides and tetracycline)

Complications Anaemia
Hypertension
Small for dates babies
Pyelonephritis
PET
Prematurity

Follow-up Antenatal – regular MSU examination
Post-natal – IVP in puerperium

Hyperthyroidism in pregnancy These conditions seldom coexist since relative infertility is a complication of hyperthyroidism although adequate treatment does improve fertility. The physiological changes of pregnancy affect the laboratory investigations of thyroid function.

The clinical diagnosis of hyperthyroidism during pregnancy is described on p. 479. It should be noted that raised cardiac output, tachycardia, sweating and emotional lability are features of both conditions.

Options Referral to an endocrinologist
Bed rest

β-blockade, e.g. propranolol 40 mg 6 hourly
Carbimazole initially 30 mg daily.

Complications

Maternal myocarditis
Increased incidence of
- abortion
- intra-uterine death
- premature labour

Obstetric risk with fetal goitre
Neonatal hypothyroidism with carbimazole
Neonatal hypoglycaemia and bradycardia with β-blockers

Diabetes

The WHO recognizes several types of 'diabetes.'

'**Clinical diabetes**' with symptoms and complications of the disease, a raised fasting or random blood glucose estimation or an abnormal GTT.

'**Asymptomatic, subclinical** or **chemical diabetes**' with no clinical evidence of the disease but an abnormal GTT response.

'**Latent diabetes**' in which the symptoms, complications and abnormal laboratory tests become evident only under the stress of infection, obesity, steroids, or pregnancy (gestational diabetes).

'**Prediabetes**' is a retrospective diagnosis which has little practical value in the management of diabetes in pregnancy.

Complications

Diabetes in pregnancy

Mother
- subfertility
- UTI
- PET (20%)
- abortion if diabetes is poorly controlled
- vaginal infection
- renal disease

Placenta
- placental insufficiency
- placental abruption

Fetus
- hydramnios
- malformation
- large babies
- malpresentation
- cephalo-pelvic disproportion

Neonate
- respiratory distress syndrome

jaundice
hypoglycaemia
hypocalcaemia

Pregnancy in diabetics

Insulin requirements increased and are very labile
Glucose tolerance is reduced
Renal threshold for glucose is reduced
Diabetic complications are exacerbated

History

Symptoms of diabetes (see p. 000)
Family history of clinical or latent diabetes
Obstetric history of
gestational diabetes
stillbirth
large babies (in excess of 4 kg)

Examination

Check for complications

Investigation

Urinalysis is a poor indicator of diabetic control
Blood glucose estimations e.g. 'BM Stix' preferably with spectrophotometer for greater accuracy
24 hour serial blood glucose profile – requires hospital admission

GTT

Repeated glycosuria
Family history of diabetes
Obstetric history suggesting latent diabetes
Previous intra-uterine death
Previous heavy baby
Hydramnios

Referral

Early referral to joint obstetric and diabetic clinic.

Obstetric disorders of pregnancy

Small for dates

The description of 'small for dates' is preferable to the presumption of placental dysfunction. It is relative to the dating of the pregnancy, the size of the parents and any underlying pathology in the fetus, placenta or mother.

Causes

Microcephaly
Chromosome abnormalities
Congenital heart disease

Transplacental infection, e.g. Rubella
Placental insufficiency
Ante-partum haemorrhage
Essential hypertension
Renal disease
Maternal hypoxia, e.g. severe anaemia
Smoking and alcohol

Assessment

Confirmation of dates
Maternal weight gain
Height of fundus – measured
BP and oedema
Smoking and alcohol habits
Amount of liquor

Investigation

Ultrasound for successive BPD
Urinalysis for proteinuria
Urea and uric acid
FBC
Rubella titre
γGT and LFT
Urinary oestriols

Options

Referral for observation and investigation
Advice on
- rest
- diet
- smoking
- alcohol
- vitamin and iron supplements.

Cephalo-pelvic disproportion

Will present as obstructed labour unless the problem is anticipated by careful examination during the final weeks of pregnancy.

Fetal causes
- Large baby
- Position and extension of head
- Hydrocephalus
- Malformation
- Postmaturity

Maternal causes
- Maternal diabetes leading to large baby
- Pelvic mass
- Pelvic malformation
- Narrow pelvis

History Previous obstetric history including birth weight
Height of father
History of injury to the pelvis

Examination Height
Urinalysis
Pelvic examination for malpresentation or high head at term in primigravid mothers

Referral All cases to the obstetric unit for 'trial of labour'.

Follow-up Pelvimetry in the puerperium
Genetic studies if indicated

Fibroids Uterine fibroids are more common in multipara and should be detected by pelvic examination at the first antenatal visit. However, they may present later with complications.

Complications Subfertility
Torsion of pedunculated fibroids
'Red degeneration' – ischaemia due to rapid growth
Malpresentation
Obstructed labour

History Menstrual history
Abdominal pain with fever in early pregnancy

Examination Check for localized tenderness
Avoid confusion with examination of fetal parts especially in multiple pregnancy
Consider differential diagnosis e.g. appendicitis or abruption of placenta

Referral To exclude ectopic pregnancy or other pelvic mass (see p. 238).

Malpresentation Malpresentation is a problem of intra-partum rather than of antenatal care. Recognition of malpresentation however is important in the anticipation of problems in labour and for planning intra-partum care if other complications of pregnancy are present.

Breech presentation As pregnancy progresses the fetus tends to assume the cephalic presentation
at 22 weeks 36% (approx) are breech presentation
at 28 weeks 12% (approx) are breech presentation

at 34 weeks 6% are breech presentation
at term 3% are breech presentation

Recognition of a breech presentation is by finding a ballotable fetal head in the fundus, a fetal heart heard loudest above the umbilicus and by palpation of the breech on pelvic examination

Some obstetricians would consider external cephalic version at 32–36 weeks but it is now believed that a fetus which turns easily would probably turn spontaneously, while the use of force may lead to complications including
intra cranial haemorrhage
ante-partum haemorrhage
rise in neonatal mortality.

Persistent occipito-posterior presentation (POP)

Occurs in 10% of pregnancies at the onset of labour.

Recognition is by prominent anterior fetal parts, a relatively flat umbilicus, a high head at term and a fetal heart heard loudest in the loins.

Complications include caesarian section and forceps (1:4), and prolonged labour (the majority).

Transverse lie

Associated with placenta praevia, hydramnios, multiple pregnancy and uterine or pelvic malformation.

Refer during final weeks of pregnancy or urgently if there is spontaneous rupture of membranes.

Face presentation

1 in 500 pregnancies.

Brow presentation

1 in 1500 pregnancies

Face presentation may be suspected with palpation of an extended head during pregnancy.

Cord prolapse

1 in 200 pregnancies

An obstetric emergency that should be excluded in all cases of spontaneous rupture of membranes when associated with an unengaged head, prematurity or malpresentation.

Multiple pregnancy

Twins occur in 1:90 pregnancies, triplets occur in $1{:}90^2 = 8100$. Dizygotic (non-identical) twins are five times more common than monozygotic (identical) twins. Identical twins can be confirmed by demonstration of common aminion on placental inspection.

History

Age and parity
Family history of multiple pregnancies

Confirmation of dates
Fertility drugs

Examination

Large for dates
Three or more fetal poles on palpation
Two or more distinct fetal heart rates heard at the same time
Hydramnios
Check for maternal complications

Referral

Confirm diagnosis and assess growth by ultrasound
Consider bed rest at 28 weeks
Consider early confinement.

Complications

Maternal
- Anaemia
- PET (hypertension)
- Placenta praevia
- Hydramnios
- Premature labour
- Uterine infection
- Post-partum haemorrhage

Fetal
- Malpresentation
- Prematurity
- Cord complications
- 'Transfusion syndrome'

The puerperium

Post-natal care

The puerperium is a stressful time for a new mother. At a time of emotional lability she is faced with conflicting demands from her new baby, her husband and family and her medical attendants. It is therefore important that the visits by midwife, health visitor or doctor are regular and thorough, sympathetic and supportive and planned so that she has adequate time to herself and her baby.

Examination of the newborn

(See p. 392)

The birth

Date and place of birth
Gestation and mode of onset
Antenatal and perinatal complications
Sex and weight of baby
Neonatal complications

History

Maternal mood and fatigue
Post-natal exercises
Perineum, episiotomy, lochia
Micturition and bowel habit
Feeding and neonatal problems (see p. 417)

Examination

Record
- Pulse
- BP
- Temperature

Check
- Breasts
- Lochia
- Perineum

Uterine size

End of labour (fully contracted)	equivalent to 20 weeks size
6th day post-partum	equivalent to 16 weeks size
12th day post-partum	equivalent to 12 weeks size
6 weeks post-partum	full involution

Follow-up

Daily for the first 10 days after delivery (often shared with the midwife)
Frequency of visits is then determined by mother's support at home; or by complications of the puerperium
Final post-natal examination at 6 weeks post-partum

Infant feeding

An infant can usually be expected to regain birth weight within a week and then to increase in weight by 30 g a day for six months, Subsequently weight gain is 15–20 g a day. To achieve this the baby will require 170 ml of milk per kg per day. Solids are usually introduced at around 4–6 months of age.

The mode of feeding seems to be dictated by fashion and entrenched health beliefs since bottle feeding is still common despite health education to the contrary. The advantages of breast feeding far outweigh those of bottle feeding.

Breast feeding – advantages

Species specific – composition of fats, amino acids, minerals and low risk of hypernatraemia
Protection from infection (especially gastroenteritis) – IgA, antibodies, complement, white cells, interferon.
Protection from allergies
Obesity uncommon

Enhanced mother–infant bond
Convenience
Hygienic
Inexpensive

Bottle feeding – advantages

Milk composition and feeding regimens can be tailored to special needs
Pleasure of feeding can be shared with the whole family
Mother has more social freedom
Feeds required less frequently
Vitamin D content is assured

Assessment

Mother and family attitudes to feeding
Examination of breasts

Management

Breast feeding

- Supportive bra
- Preparation of nipples
- Adequate mixed diet
- Initial feed
- Demand feeding 10 mins each breast
- Supplement with expressed milk or water only
- Relaxed mother and baby during feed

Bottle feeding

- Milk preparation with low protein and mineral content
- Meticulous care in making up the feed
- Cool the boiled water before mixing
- Cool milk to body temperature to feed
- Meticulous care in sterilizing utensils
- Day 1:20 ml/kg/24 hours increase by 20ml/kg daily
- Day 7:150 ml/kg/24 hours

Follow-up

(Usually shared with midwife and health visitor)
Reassurance and encouragement
Monitor maternal health
Monitor accuracy and sterility of milk preparation
Monitor infant weight gain

Contraindications – breast feeding

Failure to thrive
Cleft palate or nasal obstruction
Neonatal enzyme deficiency states (e.g. PKU)
Renal or cardiac disease
Active thyroid disease or diabetes
Carcinoma of breast or ovary
TB
Drugs – e.g. tricyclic antidepressants

Complications of breast feeding

'No milk' – reassurance and perseverance for 2 weeks

'Too little' – increase food and drink and rest periods, persevere for 2 weeks before supplementing

'Too slow' – avoid interruptions or excessive 'winding', exclude neonatal infection, thoracic or neurological disease or nasal obstruction

'Vomiting' – anatomical causes are rare. Sudden onset suggests infection, so monitor weight gain. May be simple regurgitation

'Too much' – breast engorgement may be relieved by a good support bra and expressing remaining milk after feeds

'Cracked nipples' – advise on suckling technique. Consider nipple shields and antiseptic sprays or creams

'Painful breasts' – examine for signs of infection or abscess formation. Advise continued feeding or one-sided feeding with expression of the affected breast. Consider prescription of antibiotics

'Too demanding' – the baby that cries may be hungry. He or she may also be thirsty, wet, soiled, colicky, ill, in pain or just wanting company

'Sagging breast' – loss of contour in the breast may be helped by good bra support throughout pregnancy and feeding. The patient may request plastic surgery

Complications of bottle feeding

'Too demanding' – see above

'Vomiting' – see above

'Too slow' – as above but teat holes may be too small

'Too fat' –obesity or rapid weight gain may be due to an endocrine disease but the accuracy of milk preparation must be assessed

'Infection' – non-sterile milk preparation must be considered as a potential source of infection.

'Green stools' – a feature of certain milk preparations

'Constipation' – add soft brown sugar (one teaspoonful per bottle)

Referral

Blood stained discharge from the nipple
Recurrent breast abscess for incision
Persistent feeding problems (see p. 417)

Post-partum haemorrhage

Post-partum haemorrhage (PPH) is the commonest cause of collapse in the puerperium. Other causes are listed but their management is not described.

Primary PPH is a vaginal blood loss of more than 600 ml within the first 24 hours of delivery. It can constitute a major medical emergency but is seldom the direct responsibility of the doctor who shares care with an obstetrician.

Secondary PPH is any abnormal vaginal bleeding occurring within 6 weeks of delivery. It may occur in 3% of pregnancies.

Patients at risk

Anaemia
Previous PPH
Multiparity
Prolonged labour
Placenta praevia
Manual removal of placenta
Retained placenta
Infection
General anaesthesia
Clotting defect
Fibroids
Hydramnios
Twins
Diabetes

History

Bleeding in early pregnancy, APH or primary PPH
Complications of delivery or puerperium
Estimation of blood loss

Examination

Assess blood loss
BP
Pulse
Temperature
Pelvic examination to locate site of bleeding
Abdominal examination to assess uterine size

Emergency care

Establish i.v. line
Ergometrine 0.5 mg i.v.
Call obstetric flying squad
Clear cervical os
Bimanual compression of uterus
Catheterize the bladder
Manual removal of placenta – if death is imminent

Referral

All cases for hospital management, investigation, and observation.

Complications

Death
Anaemia
Clotting defects
Infection

Failure to control Consider alternative cause of collapse
DVT or pulmonary embolism
Eclampsia or epilepsy
Subarachnoid haemorrhage or coronary thrombosis
Diabetes or steroid crisis
Septic shock or uterine inversion
Amniotic fluid embolism

Follow-up Check Hb at post-natal examination
Vigilance in subsequent pregnancies

Deep vein thrombosis The puerperium is a period of high risk for this condition and preventive measures must be observed (see p. 62)

Puerperal fever This is defined (in law) as a fever of more than 38°C occurring within 14 days of delivery.

Causes Urinary tract infection and pyelonephritis
Infection in the birth canal
Breast infection
Wound infection
DVT or pulmonary embolism
Respiratory infection

History Urinary symptoms
Nature of vaginal loss
Chest, breast, abdominal or loin pains

Examination Full examination of all systems
Check for
- involution of uterus
- URTI
- chest infection
- signs of incipient breast infection
- signs of DVT

Investigation FBC and blood cultures
MSU
Swabs from vaginal vault, perineum and throat
CXR or lung scan
Consider need for LP

Management Infection – appropriate antibiotic
DVT – (see p. 62)

Failure to control

Consider alternative diagnosis
- Septicaemia
- SBE
- TB
- Pneumonia
- Malaria
- Typhoid

See also:
- Deep vein thrombosis
- Newborn babies
- Feeding problems
- Stillbirth
- Early post-natal death

Post-natal depression

This term is generally used to cover the gamut of mood changes that can affect a woman after a pregnancy. Symptoms and signs usually occur within ten days but may not be declared or demonstrated for some months after the pregnancy.

Patterns of presentation

Acute delirium in labour
Flattened affect
Restlessness
Anorexia
Hallucination
Psychotic confusion
Depression
Suicidal thought content and action

Mental examination

Symptoms and signs of depression
- No fun or laughter
- No future
- Sense of guilt
- Anxiety
- Panic
- Non-coping
- Sleep disturbance
- Sadness
- Crying
- Self-injury

History

Previous expectations of the puerperium
Relationships with family and friends
Premorbid personality and ability to cope with previous life events
Medication

Prevention

Anticipation of patient's needs if a previous history exists sufficient support by the immediate and extended family to allow adequate time for the mother and child to be together and also for mother's rest.
Helping agencies involvement to encourage mother's participation in all her usual activities after a pregnancy. Also to educate and be available as a sympathetic ear to the mother's attitudes.

Options

Social support by family and helping agencies
Rest
Psychotherapy – maintaining the mother in an active role
Sedatives, e.g. diazepam 5 mg 8 hourly
Antidepressants, e.g. amitriptyline 25 mg 8 hourly (but breast feeding shouls be discontinued)
Neuroleptics, e.g. haloperidol initially 1.5 mg 8 hourly.

Complications

Suicide or infanticide
Prolonged marital disharmony
Recurrence (20% in subsequent pregnancy)

Referral

Involve psychiatrist – while patient is still at home the mother may be a risk to herself or her baby if domiciliary support is inadequate.

Final post-natal examination

This is usually carried out 6 weeks after birth to establish that the mother, and in particular her pelvic organs have returned to the non-pregnant state.

History

Vaginal loss and/or menstruation
Symptoms in perineum
Feeding and breast problems
Micturition and bowel habit
Abdominal symptoms
Mental state

Social support
Mother–child bonding, and change in family dynamics

Examination Anaemia
BP
Weight
Breasts
Abdomen
Perineum
Vagina
Uterine size and appearance of cervix

Investigation Hb
Urinalysis
Cervical smear when idicated (see p. 438)
Pelvimetry (referral to hospital if indicated)

Management Medication
Rubella status
Family planning and contraception
Sexual intercourse
Post-natal exercises
Feeding and infant care
Child allowances, prescription exemption, etc.

See also: Feeding problems (p. 417)

3 Child Care

Accidents

Accidents are the commonest cause of death in children aged 1 to 15 years. Although individually they may be by definition unpredictable, many are preventable.

Prevention is the responsibility of society and legislation. Health education and vigilance can serve to minimize the risk of accidents.

Safety education is usually left to the school and health visitor. The doctor is ideally placed to advise parents both in the surgery and during home visits and by encouraging safety awareness in the local community.

To insist on avoidance of all dangers would limit the everyday activities of children so much that normal development would be disrupted. However, many accidents can be prevented by simply becoming more safety conscious. Children are great imitators and so will imitate the habits of their parents.

Children under 4 years of age have little awareness of safety and initially the parents must ensure that dangers are avoided. As a child matures an understanding of safety should form part of everyday activities.

A wider knowledge of first aid would improve secondary prevention of accidents.

Causes

Road traffic accidents	44%
Drowning	13%
Fires	8%
Falls	6%
Burns and cuts	4%
Suffocation	3%
Choking	3%
Accidental poisoning	2.5%
Electric shocks	1.5%
Other causes	15%
	100%

Prevention

Road traffic accidents

Children travelling in cars can be made safer by using carry cot harnesses, safety seats or belt restraints

Children under 12 years should not be allowed to sit in the front seat unless they are big enough to safely use the adult seat belt

Child proof locks should be used on the rear doors

Children under 10 years should not be allowed to cross major roads alone
All children should learn the 'Green Cross Code'
No children should ride bicycles on the open road until they are safe; preferably after taking the cycling proficiency test. Check bicycles regularly for safety.

Drowning

All children should be taught to swim as early as possible
Do not leave small children unattended in the bath or paddling pools
Keep garden ponds fenced or covered when children are young. Wear life-jackets on all boats.

Fires

It is a legal requirement that in homes with children under 12 years all fires should be guarded
Position all heaters where they cannot be knocked over
Keep matches out of the reach of children.

Falls

Use stair gates when children are very young
Open plan stairs should be avoided
Make upper floor windows safe
Avoid highly polished floors
Do not leave a ladder up against a wall unattended
Avoid dangerous paths around quarries, cliffs, etc.

Burns and cuts

Do not leave hot liquids where they can be pulled off a table or work surface
Do not leave small children unattended in a kitchen when cooking
Turn saucepan handles out of reach of small children
Do not use oil heaters in children's bedrooms
Use safety glass in glass doors
Keep knives, scissors, razor blades, pins and needles out of reach.

Suffocation and choking

Keep plastic bags out of children's reach
Check toys for loose buttons or beads, especially teddies
Do not let small children eat peanuts
Cover the baby's pram with a cat net when leaving it out in the garden.

Accidental poisoning

Keep medicines out of reach, preferably in a lockable cabinet
Use childproof medicine bottles

Keep disinfectants, cleaning fluids and weed killers out of reach of children

Teach children to recognize poisonous plants.

Electric shocks

Ensure electrical appliances are earthed and working properly

Replace worn cables immediately or do not use the appliance

Electric blankets should be switched off before putting the child to bed and should not be used if the child wets the bed

Unplug appliances when not in use. If this is not possible use a safety cover

Do not use electrical appliances in the bathroom.

See also:

Burns (p. 514)
Electrocution (p. 521)

Babies that cry excessively

Crying is the most immediate form of communication available to a baby. Just as adults vary in their verbosity so babies do in their crying. Parents vary in their tolerance of crying and an anxious, inexperienced mother is more likely to seek help from friends, relatives and professionals.

Usually crying is a signal of hunger, thirst, discomfort or need for more physical contact. Occasionally no obvious cause can be found. Providing the baby is feeding and gaining weight appropriately then the parents can be reassured that the problem will resolve spontaneously when the baby is 3 or 4 months old.

There are many reasons for a baby to cry but the following provides a simple guide to the more common causes.

Hunger

It is usual for the new born baby to cry when a feed is due.

Babies vary in their needs for frequency and volumes of feeds. Premature babies in particular may need larger volumes and at 2–3 hourly intervals.

Demand feeding is preferable if the baby gets hungry before the 'standard' 4 hourly interval.

Babies vary in the age at which they can sleep through the night without feeds but it commonly occurs when the weight has increased beyond 5 kg.

The best guide to adequate feeding is to regularly weigh the baby and to follow the progress on a growth chart.

Thirst

If the baby is feverish or the weather is hot the problem may be one of thirst rather than hunger, and so fluids should be offered between feeds if the baby appears restless or continues to cry. This may become more obvious if the baby becomes dehydrated with signs of depressed fontanelle, decreased skin turgor or sunken eyes.

Evening colic

This is a common problem seen in babies up to the age of 3 or 4 months. It characteristically occurs in the evening between 5 and 10 o'clock. The baby cries and draws up his legs at the same time as if in pain. He cannot be comforted by feeding, changing or cuddling. The cause is not known but is thought to be due to an irregular peristalsis.

Wind

'Trouble with wind' is a fashionable explanation for a restless baby. Some babies appear to be very windy, presumably due to air swallowing. It may be due to blocked teats on the feeding bottle or excessive secretion of breast milk in the first few minutes. In this case the mother should be advised to express some milk before starting the feed.

Nursing in the upright position after a feed or carrying the baby in a harness may help to expel the gas. The ritual of winding the baby is often carried to excess.

Need for physical contact

Babies will often stop crying when they are picked up or rocked. Many babies need physical contact particularly when they are wakeful between feeds after the first few weeks.

Carrying the baby around in a harness or keeping the baby nearby in a reclining canvas chair may pacify the child.

Failure of infant–mother bonding may result in crying and it is useful to observe the pair to see how the mother handles the baby. In particular the mother's mental state should be assessed to exclude puerperal depression.

As the baby gets older he may relate particularly to only a few adults and may be frightened by strangers. It is best to allow the baby to get used to new people before they are encouraged to pick him up.

Changing Babies seem to tolerate soiled nappies with little trouble but some babies cry when changed. This may be because they feel cold, because the nappy is too tight or because the skin has been scratched or punctured by the nappy pin!

Fatigue Babies who have been overstimulated by play may become tired and irritable.

Illness If the crying is unusually persistent or associated with other symptoms or signs then the baby should be examined to exclude organic disease. This is dealt with more fully on page 432 ('Very ill baby'). It is particularly important to check for fever, otitis media, intestinal obstruction, meningitis or urinary tract infection. It may be necessary to admit the child to hospital for observation.

See also:

Infant feeding (p. 378)
Post-natal depression (p. 383)
Very ill baby (p. 432)

Child abuse

Not all bruised children are maltreated, accidents will happen. Conversely, not all maltreated children are bruised since neglect and emotional deprivation can be just as damaging.

The prevalence of child abuse is not really known since only the tip of the iceberg is appreciated by those in authority to act. It is exceedingly difficult to define 'abuse' in a general sense. When does a cautionary smack become ill-treatment? Individual doctor's abilities to recognize possible cases and act confidently on suspicion are enormously variable.

Families at risk

Mother – not coping
- little support from father
- presents frequently with minor problems
- confesses to angry or agressive feelings
- ambivalence about pregnancy
- postnatal depression

Parents were abused as children
Alcohol or psychiatric illness
Co-existent marital problems
Past history of child abuse with a sibling
Poor housing conditions

History

Account of injuries vague, implausible and inconsistent
Delay in seeking help
Reluctance to allow examination
Multiple injuries or frequent presentation of separate injuries
History of unconsciousness
Presentation *by* someone other than the parent
Presentation *to* someone other than the usual doctor, e.g. a partner or casualty doctor
Parents often welcome the offer of help and support

Examination

Child's behaviour – frozen watchfulness.
Nature of injuries
- slap marks on face or buttocks
- grip marks on upper arm
- torn frenulum when bottle or dummy is forced into the mouth
- bites or cigarette burns on the hands and feet
- sub-dural haematoma from violent shaking
- sexual abuse

Investigation

X-ray suspected fractures
Skeletal survey
Blood clotting studies

Options

Consult with health visitor and social services, most areas have set protocols
Admission to a place of safety. Usually to a hospital in the event of a serious injury. Brief the hospital medical staff. Admission into care is not a decision for the GP alone and is the responsibility of the juvenile court
Record keeping should be comprehensive in the event of future litigation.

Prevention

Consider families at risk
Accessibility should be as open as possible in spite of the parent's demanding and often aggressive behaviour
Facilitate communication with the parents to allow and encourage open discussion of aggressive feelings
Involve the health visitor in discussion of 'at risk' children

See also:

Problem drinking (p. 261)
Post-natal depression (p. 383)

Child development

A systematic assessment of child development, medical examination and immunization programme are best combined in Child Welfare Clinics. The organization of such clinics is complex and important and is usually the responsibility of the health visitor. However the clinical responsibility of the developmental, medical and immunization check is shared between doctors and health visitor, and the degree of sharing must be decided by each team. Regular clinics, regular attendance and a follow-up for defaulters are essential.

Child welfare clinics provide an opportunity to discuss health education and child care with parents. There is also an opportunity to detect or anticipate child abuse.

All aspects of child development should be fully assessed at each of the routine checks. After 1 year of age these are better conducted at home, if possible. The 'toddler' will then be more relaxed and not distracted by unfamiliar surroundings.

All babies must be examined at birth. The initial examination is brief to assess viability, to exclude gross defects and to exclude any sign of birth trauma. The subsequent and fuller examination should be made when 'moulding' of the skull bones has settled (24–48 hours).

Medical examination in the newborn and in the older child should be confined to observations that might have significance for future health. Most physical abnormalities should be detectable by 8 months and the initial examinations are therefore the most critical.

The ages at which developmental checks are carried out varies. There follows a set of suggested protocols for

the newborn
six weeks
eight months
eighteen months
three years
five years.

The newborn

History

Record details of pregnancy and delivery
Family history – hereditary disease, health of siblings
History of convulsions or vomiting

Examination at birth

'APGAR' score at 1 minute and 5 minutes
Skull and spine
Limbs and gestation
Birth weight

Table 3.1. The 'APGAR' score

	0	1	2
Appearance	Blue	Pink body Blue extremities	Pink
Pulse	Absent	100	100
Grimace	No responce	Grimace	Cry
Activity	Limp	Flexion in extremities	Active
Respiration	Absent	Slow & irregular	Strong cry

Placenta – cord vessels, texture of cotyledons, membranes

Emergency care – rescusitation

Establish airway
- gentle suction
- O_2 stream directed over nose and mouth

Assess pulse and respiration

Consider intubation
- if pulse rate is <100 and falling
- if no spontaneous respiration at 1 minute
- O_2 at 52/min (30 cm H_2O pressure)

External cardiac massage (at 120/min if arrest occurs

Pethidine antagonist
- Naloxone (Narcan) 0.01 mg/kg i.v. or i.m. to reverse any respiratory depressant effect of pethidine

Monitor
- temperature
- pulse
- spontaneous respiration

Record time of each event

Examination – at 48 hours

Record
- Head circumference
- Height
- Weight
- Temperature
- Pulse
- Respiratory rates

Examine
- Facies
- Skull
- Palate
- Anterior fontanelle
- Eyes
- Ears
- Lung sounds

Heart sounds
Femoral pulses
Abdomen
Genitalia
Anus
Skeletal symmetry
Skin
Muscle tone
Reflexes

Check for

Gross skeletal or neurological abnormality
Hypothermia or fever
Jaundice
Cyanosis
Skin lesions
Patent airway
Idiopathic respiratory distress syndrome
Heart failure
Cardiac murmur
Hernia
Abdominal masses
Patent anus
Congenital dislocation of the hips

Investigation

All newborn

Guthrie test for PKU by heel prick at 7 days

When indicated

CXR
MSU
Cord blood (for haemoglobin, group, bilirubin)
Heel prick (for calcium, sodium, glucose, bilirubin, T_4 + TSH)

Six week check

Average baby at six weeks

Head level momentarily in ventral suspension
Quietens to a sound
Fixates and follows through 90° from midline (when supine)
Smiles at mother

Toys and equipment

Measuring tape
Percentile chart
Rattle and bell

History

Pregnancy and birthweight
Suspected abnormalities or medical history
Family history
Feeding

Examination

Reflexes and posture – prone and ventral suspension
Eye fixation – through 90° from the midline
Responsiveness – alert and smiling
Weight
Head circumference
Anterior fontanelle
Palate
Reflexes and squint
Skin
Heart sounds
Femoral pulses
Abdomen and herniae
Genitalia and hips

Follow-up

Abnormal head circumference
Abnormal growth rate
Squint
Failure to fixate
Poor head control
Undescended testis
Hydrocoele

Referral

Congenital dislocation of hip
Heart murmurs
Cataract
Persistent primitive reflexes
Failure to thrive.

Eight month check

Average baby at eight months

Sits unsupported – rolls supine to prone
Responds to more than four sounds (above the ears)
Grip is intermediate between palmar grasp and pincer
Eats biscuit unaided

Toys and equipment

Measuring tape
Percentile charts
1 inch cubes (×2)
Set of vision test balls
Hearing tests – bell, rattle, paper, cup and spoon

History

Pregnancy
Previous suspected or detected abnormality
Developmental milestones
Family history
Immunization status
Feeding – helping himself

Mobility – rolling, crawling, sitting
Sleep pattern

Examination

Posture and reflexes – sitting, prone, standing
Hearing – three tones test
Manipulation – pincer grip and transferring
Vision – distant vision and squint
Responsiveness – alert and happy
Weight
Head circumference
Anterior fontanelle
Skin
Reflexes
Heart sounds
Femoral pulses
Abdomen
Herniae
Hips
Genitalia

Follow-up

Abnormal head circumference
Abnormal growth rate
Suspect hearing
Minor orthopaedic deformity
Hydrocoele
Undescended testis

Referral

Clicking hips
Heart murmurs
Squint
Persistent primitive reflexes
Delayed smiling
Failure to fixate
Failure to transfer
Failure to thrive.

Eighteen month check

Average toddler at eighteen months

Runs, climbs into a chair, throws without falling
Uses jargon, three words
Scribbles, builds a tower of three cubes
Takes off socks, slow feeding, sphincter control

Toys and equipment

Measuring tape
Percentile charts
1 inch cubes

Set of vision test balls
Picture puzzles
Auroscope
Hearing tests – bell, rattle, paper, cup and spoon

History

Pregnancy
Previous suspected or detected abnormality
Developmental milestones
Family history
Immunization status
Feeding
Toilet training
Sleep pattern
Dressing
Walking
Speech
Play – mimicry, concentration
Mood – happy, tempers

Examination

When indicated

- Height
- Weight
- Head circumference
- 'Glue ears'
- Hearing
- Squint
- Nystagmus
- Distant vision
- Heart sounds
- Muscular tone
- Reflexes
- Hips

Referral

Persistent 'mouthing', 'drooling', or 'primitive reflexes'
Absent vocalization or constructive play
Abnormal grasp, stance or limp.

Three year check

Average child at three years

Jumps down one step, stands on one foot, rides a trike
Questions everything, knows surname, talks to himself
Copies a circle, builds a tower of nine cubes
Dresses himself, dry at night, recites nursery rhymes

Toys and equipment

Measuring tape
Percentile charts
1 inch cubes (× 12)

Set of vision test balls
Crayons and drawing pad
Auroscope
Hearing tests, bell, rattle, paper, cup and spoon

History

Pregnancy
Previous suspected or detected abnormality
Developmental milestones
Family history
Immunization status
Feeding
Toilet
Sleep pattern
Dressing
Speech
Play
Mood
Right- or left-handed

Examination

Height
Weight
Head circumference
Vision and squint
Hearing
Glue ears

Five year check

Average child at five years

Skips, dances and catches
Counts to 20, abstract words, knows age and birthday
Draws a house, copies a square
Ties a shoelace, uses knife and fork, has a 'best friend'

Equipment

Measuring tape
Percentile charts
Reading card
Writing pad and pencils
Auroscope

History

Previous suspected abnormality by doctor, parent or teacher
Developmental milestones
Family history
Immunization status
Food fads
Toilet training
Dressing

Knowledge of age, time of day, colours (4)
Behaviour
Emotional development
Right- or left-handed

Examination

Height
Weight
Head circumference
Hearing
Glue ears
Speech
Vision and squint
Follows three consecutive commands correctly
Heart sounds
Genitalia

Children that limp

Limping in children is an important physical sign that demands a full and careful assessment. The underlying problem is commonly postural and self-limiting but occasionally the cause is more serious and requires referral for specialist assessment and treatment.

Causes

Irritable hip
Congenital dislocation of hip
Slipped femoral epiphysis
Osteomyelitis
Septic arthritis
Juvenile rheumatoid arthritis
Neurological lesion
Rickets
Perthes' disease
Osgood-Schlatter disease
Funny feet (in and out toeing)
Crooked legs (bow legs and knock knees)
Trauma (including non-accidental injury)
Haemophilia
Sickle cell disease

History

Patient's age
Onset of symptoms (unilateral/bilateral)
Degree of disability
Associated fever or general malaise

Recent trauma (risk factors for NAIC)
Milestones of development
Family history of postural deformity
Social history – particularly diet and disruption of activities

Examination

Temperature
Anaemia
Gait
Standing posture
Lying posture
Muscle wasting
Measure leg length and gap between knees and ankles
Bone and joint tenderness and swelling
Range of movement of joints
Check lumbar spine
Neurological assessment of legs

Investigation

FBC
WBC
Calcium
Alkaline phosphatase
ANF
Rheumatoid factor (latex test)
X-rays

Options

Reassurance – postural deformities of the feet or crooked legs are usually benign and self-correcting, provided there is full passive mobility. Patients with simple soft tissue trauma can also be reassured
Rest – in the absence of a fracture children with traumatic limps should be advised to rest as far as possible
Analgesia – simple analgesic with paracetamol
Vitamin D supplement for rickets.

Referral

Suspected fracture
Unexplained limps with persistent pain
All arthritides
Non-accidental injury
Knock knees and bow legs where the gap between the limbs is greater than 10 cm when standing erect with legs together.

See also:

The hip (p. 146)
Child abuse (p. 390)
Rheumatoid arthritis (p. 493)

Clumsy children

The 'clumsy child' is often presented by an anxious parent or school teacher with inappropriate expectations. Strictly it refers to poor co-ordination of motor skills in the absence of demonstrable neuromuscular disease. The impairment may be either of fine movements such as writing, drawing and doing up buttons, or in gross motor activity such as climbing, running, throwing and catching.

It is not known whether clumsiness represents the lower end of normal distribution of skills or whether there is a definite, but as yet unidentified neurological abnormality.

Some organic causes of weakness and clumsiness are discussed on page 333.

History

Onset and full history of 'clumsiness'
Interference with daily living and acquisition of motor skills
- writing
- drawing
- dressing
- running
- climbing
- throwing and catching
- bat and ball games
- kicking
- riding a bicycle

Clinical course
- improving, deteriorating or relatively slow progress with skills
- loss of an acquired skill usually indicates a more serious underlying condition

Parents' and teachers' attitudes
Child's attitude
Birth history
Past history of neurological disease
Family history of mental handicap or neurological disorder
Psychological and social history to assess the level of stress and support at home and school

Examination

Careful observation of the child performing a variety of motor skills
Full neurological assessment with emphasis on motor co-ordination

Head circumference
Evidence of minor spina bifida

Investigation This is only necessary if underlying neurological disease is suspected (see p. 333)

Options Explanation and reassurance – in the absence of an identifiable neurological lesion it is probably kindest to explain that the clumsy child represents one extreme of normal motor development. It is important to stress that no neurological abnormality has been detected.

Occupational therapy – the more successful programmes concentrate efforts on the specific deficiencies rather than to attempt a general improvement in 'clumsiness'. Encourage the parents to get involved in teaching these activities.

Liaise with school teachers involved but avoid the label of 'specific handicap'.

Social skills – the clumsiness often leads to ridicule and ultimately withdrawal and loss of self-confidence. Everyone involved should be aware of this long lasting effect because although the clumsiness may improve with age the social effects are carried for life.

Common infectious diseases of children

These common diseases seldom appear in hospitals and can be neglected in medical school education. The patterns of presentation are characteristic and the complications, though infrequent, may have serious consequences. The appearances of these rashes are best learnt by clinical recognition.

Hand, foot and mouth disease, fifth disease and sixth disease are not common but the signs are quite distinct and they deserve wider recognition.

Mumps Incubation period 2–4 weeks
Infectious period 2 days before } parotid swelling
7 days after }

Spread Contact with saliva, or droplet spread
Epidemics 3–4 years

Pattern of presentation

Fever and malaise associated with pain and swelling of parotid glands, bilateral or unilateral. Testes, pancreas, other salivary glands and meninges may also have primary infection

Complications

Orchitis
Mastitis
Encephalitis
Polyneuritis
Labyrinthitis
Deafness
Myocarditis, thyroiditis and thrombocytopenia are rare

Options

Paracetamol
Cooling
Fluids
Bland diet
Mouth washes.

Measles

Incubation period 1–2 weeks
Infectious period 4 days before } appearance of rash
4 days after }

Spread Contact and droplet spread

Pattern of presentation

Fever malaise and cough for 4 days with associated red eyes, throat and ear drums. The fine white 'Koplik' spots on the buccal mucosa precede the rash.

The rash is blotchy, confluent and red, becoming a dirty brown. It starts around the ears and spreads to the face and then the trunk

Complications

Otitis media
Bronchopneumonia
Croup
Diarrhoea
Appendicitis
Febrile convulsions
Encephalitis (subacute sclerosing panencephalitis is rare)
Secondary staphylococcal infection

Options

Fluids
Cooling
Paracetamol

Antibiotic, e.g. amoxycillin or flucloxacillin, when indicated for secondary infections
Notify community physician (environmental).

Immunization

All children between 12 and 18 months
Except in
- failure to thrive
- acute febrile illness
- immunosuppression or radiation
- malignancy
- hypogammaglobulinaemia
- pregnancy (in adults)

Rubella

Incubation period 2–3 weeks

Infectious period 7 days before / 4 days after } appearance of rash

Spread Contact or droplet spread
Epidemics 6–9 years

Pattern of presentation

Mild illness with red eye, red throat, and occipital gland enlargement
The rash is of pale red fine spots affecting the ears, face and upper trunk

Complications

Transplacental spread resulting in congenital rubella syndrome
Arthritis
Glandular fever-like illness
Thrombocytopenia
Encephalitis is rare

Options

Termination of pregnancy if infection is confirmed by serology
Paracetamol
Cooling
Fluids.

Immunization

All girls in early puberty
Contraindicated if early pregnancy is suspected
Pregnancy should be avoided for 3 months after immunization

Chicken pox

Herpes zoster
Incubation period 2–3 weeks
Infectious period 2–5 days before / 5–7 days after } appearance of spots

Spread Droplet and contact with vesicles of chicken pox or shingles (the scabs are not infectious)

Pattern of presentation

Fever and malaise. Sore throat and abdominal pain. Spots appear in crops over 5 days on the trunk more than the limbs. The mucous membranes including the mouth and urethra are affected but the soles of the feet are spared. The macules become vesicles then pustules before crusting.

Complications

Latent shingles
Secondary staphylococcal or streptococcal infection
Pneumonia
Thrombocytopenia
Death in immunodeficient or immunosuppressed patients
Encephalitis
Meningitis
(Congenital malformations – evidence is inconclusive)

Options

Paracetamol
Cooling
Fluids
Calamine lotion
Antibiotics, e.g. flucloxacillin when indicated.

Hand, foot and mouth disease

Coxsackie A17 virus
Infectious period 2 days before } appearance of spots
7 days after }
Spread Droplet spread
Epidemics 3 yearly and predominantly in the summer months.

Pattern of presentation

Mild illness with fever and malaise. The rash of grey vesicles is characteristically found in the mouth, the fingers, palms, soles, heels and the buttocks.

Complications

Secondary bacterial infection can complicate the condition. The virus may cross the placental barrier.

Fifth disease

('Slapped-cheek' disease)
Parvovirus
Incubation period 4–14 days
Infectious period 7–10 days
Ages – more than 2 years

Pattern of presentation A fine macular rash appears on the cheeks but not around the mouth. The rash may later spread to the trunk. The disease is without complication and children can be managed with paracetamol, cooling and fluids.

Sixth disease (Roseola infantum)
Infectious period first five days of the illness
Ages – 1–2 years

Pattern of presentation Three days of high fever and irritability which subsides with the appearance of the fine, pink, macular rash on the trunk and limbs. The occipital, sub-mandibular and post-auricular glands might be enlarged. Probably viral in origin, it occurs in sporadic epidemics.

Complications Febrile convulsions

Options Paracetamol
Cooling
Fluids.

Scarletina (*Streptococcus pyogenes* Group A)
Scarletina is a euphemism for Scarlet fever which was previously a more severe and complicated disease.
Incubation period 1–5 days
Infectious period 24 hours after introduction of antibiotics
Rash 2–5 days
Spread Contact or droplet

Pattern of presentation Sudden onset of exudative tonsillitis with malaise, fever and headache. The tongue is furred and the cervical lymph nodes are enlarged. The rash starts on the face, sparing the lips – circumoral pallor – and spreads to the trunk and limbs. It is a find diffuse macular rash which blanches on pressure and may be followed by patchy desquamation during the following week.

Complications Peritonsillar abscess
Otitis media
Vulvovaginitis
Carditis, rheumatic fever and glomerulonephritis are now extremely rare

Options Throat swab to identify the bacterium
Phenoxymethyl penicillin for 10 days (erythromycin if penicillin sensitive)

Aspirin or paracetamol
Cooling
Fluids
Notify community physician (environmental).

Whooping cough

Pertussis bordatella
Incubation period 10–14 days
Infectious period 4 days before / 3 weeks after } start of paroxysmal cough

Spread Droplet and contact
Epidemics occur in 2–3 year cycles

Pattern of presentation

Initial cough and cold progressing over 2 weeks to paroxysmal coughing with 'whooping' and vomiting. Petechiae, epistaxis and low grade fever are often present. The illness lasts about 6 weeks. Paroxysmal coughing may persist and recur with subsequent URTI.

Complications

Anoxic fits in infants
Weight loss
Lobar pneumonia
Bronchopneumonia
Otitis media
Subconjunctival haemorrhages
Cerebral hypoxic damage

Options

Per nasal swab
CXR
Erythromycin or amoxycillin given early in the illness may moderate symptoms
Clinical review for complications, fortnightly until clear
Referral to hospital if complications occur
Notify the community physician (environmental).

Immunization

Recommended as part of routine immunization of all children in the UK
Except
Absolute contraindications
- Acute febrile illness
- Severe local or general reaction (including a neurological reaction) to a preceding dose
- Neonatal cerebral irritation or damage

Special considerations
- Parents or siblings who have idiopathic epilepsy

Developmental delay due to neurological defect
Neurological disease

Common surgical problems in children

There are numerous surgical procedures carried out on children and judging the appropriate age for surgery is often difficult. The indications for referral for some of the more common operations are discussed below.

Circumcision

Large numbers of boys are still circumcised for social rather than medical reasons.

Initially the foreskin is adherent to the glans penis but by the age of two years the foreskin is usually retractable. Patience is preferable to forceable retraction. There are three main indications for operation.

Phimosis

The foreskin cannot be retracted because of a narrowed orifice. This may be congenital or acquired through recurrent balanoposthitis. If this is combined with poor stream and ballooning foreskin on micturition then operation is indicated.

Paraphimosis

This is a more urgent condition when the tight foreskin gets stuck behind the corona of the glans. If it is not reduced quickly then the constriction leads to venous engorgement and oedema of the penile tip. The reduction should be accompanied by circumcision unless there is marked oedema in which case operation should be delayed.

Recurrent balanoposthitis

This is an infection between the glans and the foreskin. There is associated inflammation, purulent discharge and painful micturition. Initial treatment is with topical antiseptics. Recurrence is common and may lead to phimosis and so repeated attacks are an indication for surgery.

Inguinal hernia

These are always of the indirect type through a persistently patent processus vaginalis. The incidence is about 2% and it is far more common in boys. It may be noticed at birth but frequently is not seen until the child becomes ambulent.

The mother usually presents the child because she has noted a lump in the groin or scrotum. It rarely causes symptoms. The lump may be only intermittently noticeable and so the diagnosis is sometimes made on the history alone. Because of the risk of strangulation or damage to the testis it is best to refer these children as soon as the diagnosis is made. The referral becomes urgent if there is associated pain.

Hydrocele

This is usually noticed in the first few weeks of life. It is really a cyst of the tunica vaginalis or may be more localized along the spermatic cord. It is distinguished from a hernia by the fact that it is possible to palpate the vas above the swelling and it is also transilluminable.

The swelling is usually soft and causes no discomfort. Surgery is best delayed until after the first year since in many cases the hydrocele will resolve spontaneously.

Umbilical hernia

True umbilical hernias rarely cause any problems and can safely be left until after the age of 2 years since the majority will resolve spontaneously without any treatment by that age.

Paraumbilical hernias rarely resolve spontaneously unless very small and should be referred for repair. Since it rarely causes any problems surgery can be delayed until the age of 2–3 years.

Undescended testis

The majority of boys will have both testes in the scrotum at birth unless premature. Only 0.3% of boys continue to show undescended testes by the age of 1 year.

In many cases when a testis cannot be felt in the scrotum it is simply retracted by the action of the cremaster muscle. In these children the testis can be coaxed into the scrotum. If this is not possible or if the testis is not palpable in the line of descent then the child should be referred to a surgeon.

If left untreated spermatogenesis becomes irreversibly affected, malignancy is more common and the ectopic testis is more prone to torsion and trauma.

The optimum age for operation is 4–5 years.

Tonsillectomy

The indications for tonsillectomy are far from decided.

There are some serious drawbacks including

- mortality of 1 or 2 per 10,000 from post operative haemorrhage
- possibly increased risk of developing asthma

Children with chronically infected tonsils will benefit but it is difficult to identify them simply on clinical grounds.

As a general rule a child with six or more attacks of tonsillitis per year and requiring time off school is now the usual indication.

Recurrent quinsy is a less common reason for operation.

Adenoidectomy

The indications for adenoidectomy are clearer but the benefit is not definitely proven. The operation is usually recommended for the treatment of recurrent otitis media and secretory otitis media when the adenoids are enlarged and blocking the post nasal space. Symptomatic adenoidal hypertrophy is itself an indication for surgery.

Since there is usually spontaneous regression of adenoid and tonsillar lymphoid tissue after the age of 8 years it is wise to be conservative in treatment until then if possible.

Enuresis

Most children are dry at night by the age of 4 years. Beyond the age of 5 years anything other than very occasional wetting is considered as enuresis.

Prevalence	*Age*	% *wetting*
	5 yrs	11%
	10 yrs	5%
	15 yrs	2%

There is an equal distribution between the sexes at 6 years of age but boys predominate by 11 years of age.

It is a natural tendency to become dry at night even without training. However the acquisition of bladder control may be delayed by any of a variety of factors.

Causes

Stress – associated factors which are not necessarily causative
- Maternal separation
- Prolonged illness with hospital admission
- Broken home
- Birth of a sibling
- Maternal anxiety about dryness

Social – there is a higher incidence in social groups 4 and 5 and in children from overcrowded homes

Familial – there appears to be a genetic or familial link since bedwetting tends to run in families

Infection – urinary infection is four or five times more common in enuretic children

History

Daytime or night-time wetting
Primary or secondary
Frequency of micturition
Adequacy of stream of urine
Associated dysuria
Bowel function
Milestones of development
Physical or mental handicap
Psychological and social history of stress factors
Family history of enuresis
History of medication

Examination

Palpate abdomen for enlargement of bladder or kidneys
External genitalia for developmental defects
Neurological assessment for spinal lesions (e.g. minor forms of spina bifida)

Investigation

Urine for culture and glycosuria

Options

Explanation – most children acquire dryness in time.

Encouragement – diaries or 'star charts' help to analyse the extent of the problem and encourage the child by monitoring his progress and involving him in the management of the problem. One can use small rewards but avoid punishment.

Lifting – may be useful but avoid establishing it as routine.

Bladder training – children with small bladder capacities should be encouraged to delay passing urine if possible and to control the stream by stopping and restarting.

Fluid restriction – is of limited value.

Medication

Antibiotics when appropriate

Imipramine 10–25 mg at night for children over 5 years. The dose should be doubled if there is no response after 6 weeks. Continue for 3 to 6 months then gradually withdraw. Repeat courses may be necessary.

Buzzer alarms – these devices are available from local authority paediatric clinics. The health visitor can help with supervision. This method can achieve an 80% success rate in 4 months if used properly.

Referral

For investigation of recurrent urinary infection
If abnormality of the urinary tract or neurological control of the bladder is suspected.

Faecal soiling

Most children have control of bowel action by the age of 4 years. One to two per cent of children continue to soil their pants. Boys are more commonly affected than girls.

The ability to achieve control depends upon an adequate and sympathetic training from the parent and a reasonable IQ in the child. Very occasionally an underlying inflammatory bowel disease or short segment Hirschsprung's disease is discovered. Occasionally a severe psychological disability leads to a deliberate distribution of formed faeces in inappropriate places.

The vast majority of cases of soiling occurs in children who have chronic retention of faeces with overflow and leakage. The rectum becomes loaded with faeces and the colonic wall loses its tone. The stools then become hard and even more difficult to pass. Various factors predispose to the development of this condition.

These may include anal fissure, inappropriate punishment for soiling from fastidious and demanding parents, or environmental factors, e.g. limited access to the toilet at appropriate times.

History

Frequency of soiling
Adequacy of toilet facilities
Type and consistency of stools
Associated pain
History of toilet training and major life events
Child and parental attitudes to soiling

Examination

Palpate abdomen for masses
Rectal examination if possible to assess fullness of rectum and consistency of stool
Exclude anal fissures

Options

Explanation regarding the development of chronic retention of faeces with soiling and discussion of psychological factors.

Soothing creams will help to settle an anal fissure.

Laxatives – effort should be made to clear the bowel of retained faeces.

A combination of a bowel stimulant, such as senekot, with a stool softener, such as dioctyl, is usually sufficient. Gross retention may need enemas.

Behavioural training

Arrange easy access to toilet facilities
Reward successful defaecation rather than clean pants

Charting progress sometimes motivates the child and reassures the parents
Counsel parents to relax punative approach if appropriate.

Referral

For investigation and treatment of rare underlying organic disorders
- Inflammatory bowel disease
- Short segment Hirschsprung's disease

To a child psychiatrist if there is an underlying serious psychological problem with inappropriate defaecation as part of an antisocial behaviour
For enemas in gross retention.

See also:

Constipation (p. 55)

Failure to thrive

This is the cliché for inadequate weight gain and linear growth in infancy. Only a very small minority of children presenting in this way prove to have significant organic disease. The rarer causes are many and diverse so the dilemma is to sort out those situations requiring simple advice and support from those requiring referral for intensive investigations.

Causes

Incorrect weighing/measuring
Underfeeding
Wrongly constituted feeds
Genetically small size
Normal growth variation
Premature or small for dates
Maternal lack of confidence
Neglect
Child abuse
Malabsorption
- carbohydrate intolerance
- milk protein intolerance
- coeliac disease
- cystic fibrosis

Infection
Metabolic
- hypothyroidism
- hypopituitarism
- hypocalcaemia

Malformations
- renal

gastrointestinal
cardiac
CNS

History

Birth weight and gestational age
Previous measurements if available
Genetic factors – parental size and sibling growth patterns
Feeding history
Systematic history
Developmental history
Bonding (mother–child relationship)
Family dynamics

Examination

Weight, height, length and head circumference should be plotted as a centile chart. These measurements should be repeated over several months to obtain some idea of growth velocity

A full physical examination rarely reveals anything unexpected but can be a great reassurance for the parents.

Check for
- dehydration
- wasting
- delayed closure of fontanelles
- failure of teeth to erupt
- signs of infection
- congenital heart disease
- liver enlargement
- stigmata or congenital abnormality

Investigation

Repeated growth measurements
Urine for infection and renal disease
Stool for reducing substances (carbohydrate intolerance), pathogens
Hormone assays and jejunal biopsy should be left to the paediatricians

Options

Reassurance – when growth rate appears normal the parents should be confidently reassured and offered continued support perhaps through the health visitor. It is interesting how often apparent growth problems conceal unexpressed maternal anxiety about the baby or family.

Continued observation – may be appropriate to gather more information on repeated measurement. Parents vary in their ability to cope with this period of insecurity. They should be involved with the measurements and the growth charts explained. Even so the anxious parents may force an early referral for their own reassurance. In this case continued support through the health visitor is essential since there are frequently more unexpressed fears.

Advice about feeding – again the health visitor should be involved.

Referral

For investigation if the growth rate is falling or persistently below the 3rd centile.

For management of suspected underlying disease.

To reassure the parents.

If child abuse or neglect is suspected the family should be referred to social services and health visitor. (See p. 390)

See also:

Child abuse (p. 390)

The fat child

Fat babies tend to become fat children and the majority in turn become fat adults. The doctor is in an ideal position to encourage good eating habits early in the life of the child. Obesity should be completely preventable.

About one-fifth of all children under 1 year are more than 20% above the predicted average fat weight (i.e. obese by definition).

Common misconceptions

'Chubby babies look better and are healthier'

This is no longer true. In the past TB was less likely to affect fat babies. Attitudes and fears about health are often learnt from parents and grandparents, and inappropriate health beliefs can 'leap-frog' through generations. Fat children tend to walk later, have less energy, are more short of breath and are at more risk of developing various respiratory infections. They are also more likely to suffer the consequences of adult obesity.

'His glands aren't working properly'

Endocrine or metabolic disorders are extremely rare causes of obesity and in these cases the child is usually also of small stature. Children who are obese from overeating are at least of average height.

'Its only puppy fat and he will grow out of it'

This does not appear to be true. It is still fat and as such equally unhealthy. While the fat may be lost in adolescence it is soon replaced if the eating habits of childhood are not modified.

'Being fat delays puberty'

In fact the converse is true. Fat children start puberty on average 1 year earlier.

'He may be fat but he hardly eats anything'

This may be true when compared with his own family and friends but he is still eating in excess of his metabolic needs.

'He gets so upset if he doesn't have his food'

Food has long been the symbol of affection but if the baby needs comforting it is love and affection that is needed not food.

Causes of obesity

Genetic factors

7% of children with parents of normal weight become obese

40% of children with one parent overweight become obese

80% of children with both parents overweight become obese

Twin studies show that when reared separately the siblings follow similar weight patterns and do not correlate with the pattern of adoptive parents

Bottle feeding

80% of bottle fed babies gain weight faster, presumably because the mother is not satisfied until the bottle is finished

Breast fed babies are more likely to decide for themselves when their hunger is satisfied

Environmental factors

- Parental model
- Misplaced maternal caring and affection
- Excessive eating through boredom
- Lack of exercise
- Decreased ability to burn off extra calories (brown fat theory)

History

Duration of being overweight
Details of usual diet including extras between meals
Milestones of development, particularly walking
Level of energy and exercise
Comparison with parent's and sibling's weights
Parent's eating habits

Options **Inspection** – the best gauge of obesity is the ability to pick up rolls of fat especially over the scapulae and iliac crests.

Measurement – compare weight with height on standard development charts. Calipers are available to make objective measurements of skin folds.

Examination Prevention

encourage breast feeding
accurate mixing of bottle feeds
delay introducing solids until 4–6 months of age
resist using sweets if possible, e.g. as rewards
discourage eating between meals

Diet

The eating habits of the whole nuclear family should be considered and modified together

Modification of the existing diet and eating habits is more effective than the introduction of a new and strict regimen

Quantities should generally be reduced to a level at which weight is lost

Ideally the weight should remain static as the child gains in height.

A maximum weight loss of 1 kilo per week may be desirable in the very obese child

Crash dieting, while immediately rewarding is rarely successful. Original eating habits are reverted to more commonly after such diets.

Exercise

This helps to burn off some of the extra calories
It makes the child feel generally fitter
Unfortunately it tends to stimulate the appetite!

Follow-up Encouragement must be continued by regular, if infrequent, checks. Health visitors and nurses might share much of the follow-up support.

Referral Dietician – for more expert advice if available.

Paediatrician – for further investigation if the child is also of small stature in comparison with parents.

See also: Obesity (p. 224)

Feeding problems in babies

Many new and inexperienced mothers often worry that they are not feeding their baby properly. In the absence of a confiding relationship with an older relative or friend and with conflicting advice given in available books the anxious mother is likely to turn to the doctor or health visitor.

The problem may be presented in many ways but generally it falls into one of four categories.

The 'unhappy' baby

The 'unhappy baby' cries a lot, demanding attention and frequent feeding, settling for short periods, only to rouse again disturbed and unhappy. Obviously there may be an underlying illness which should be sought. In the presence of an afebrile and reasonably well baby consider:

Underfeeding
- failing breast milk
- insufficient feeds per day
- poor sucker or feeder (sleepy, premature)
- poor technique of feeding
- over engorgement of breasts
- sore nipples/inverted nipples
- oral thrush

Overfeeding
- too many feeds per day
- wrongly made up artificial feeds
- greedy baby
- cereal added to bottle

Colic
- three month colic
- air swallowing (windy baby)
- constipation
- teething

Gastrointestinal upset

In this category the symptoms of vomiting and diarrhoea predominate. Again an underlying illness may be present such as otitis media, gastroenteritis or pyloric stenosis and this should be excluded. Then consider
- overfeeding
- wrongly made up or imbalanced artifical feeds
- diet in breast feeding mothers
- milk intolerance
- air swallowing
- teething

Poor weight gain

See 'Failure to thrive' (p. 413)

Maternal problems

Failing breast milk
Post-natal depression

Domestic/career problems
Poor bonding
Lack of support
Interfering relative

History

Feeding schedule
- breast or bottle
- type and amount of artificial feed
- frequency of feeds
- plain fluid drinks between feeds

Weight gain – check on growth chart

Associated
- vomiting
- diarrhoea
- colic
- teething

Home circumstances
Maternal support

Examination

Baby
- Weight
- Distribution of weight
- Check mouth for thrush and teething
- Check palate for masses
- Check systems if underlying illness is suspected

Mother
- Nipples – inverted or sore
- Breasts – engorgement or infection
- Mental state

Investigation

Test feeding – observe the mother feeding to assess how she handles the baby and how she makes up artificial feeds.

Test weighing – before and after breast feeding to assess adequacy of milk.

Options

Health visitor – once illness or organic disease has been excluded the health visitor is the most appropriate team member to support the mother with a feeding problem and advise on feeding schedules and milk formulas

Oral thrush – e.g. Nystatin suspension 1 ml six hourly

Cracked nipples – e.g. Tinct. Benz. Co. in lanolin

Constipation – a traditional method is to add extra sugar to artificial feeds.

The feverish child

This is an extremely common presentation in primary care, and is usually due to self-limiting viral infection predominantly of the respiratory tract. However, since there are several more serious causes such as meningitis or occult causes such as UTI a careful history and examination should be undertaken with each child.

The mother will usually have taken the temperature in the older child but babies and toddlers present a problem. Skin and axillary temperatures are unreliable but may provide a useful guide. Temperature sensitive plastic strips are available which can be placed on the child's forehead – a much safer procedure than using a glass thermometer.

The oral or rectal temperature is slightly higher than the adult normal (usually about 37.5°C compared with 37°C in the adult).

Common causes

Viral upper respiratory infection
Otitis media
Tonsillitis
Common exanthemata (see p. 403)
Mumps (see p. 402)
Gastrointestinal infections
UTI
Appendicitis
Mesenteric adenoiditis
Pneumonia and bronchitis
Meningitis

History

Onset and duration of fever
Associated symptoms
- cough
- rhinitis
- earache
- sore throat
- rash
- wetting/frequency of micturition
- vomiting
- diarrhoea
- drowsiness
- joint swelling

Contact with infectious disease
Travel abroad
Pets

Examination

Record

Temperature
Pulse
Weight
Respiratory rate

Check for

Rashes
Lymphadenopathy
Ear infection
Throat infection
Jaundice
Joint swelling or inflammation
Localized signs in the chest
Abdominal tenderness and enlarged liver or spleen
Signs of meningism
State of fontanelle

Investigation

Usually not necessary in most cases but consider

throat swab
MSU (or bag urine in infants)
stool for pathogens
FBC
viral antibody screen and monospot
chest X-ray

Options

Antipyretics

Paracetamol – appropriate dose for age

Cooling

Facilitate heat loss by removing clothing, offering cold drinks or tepid sponging of the completely stripped child. This is particularly important in children who are prone to febrile convulsions

Antibiotics

The logical practice of withholding antibiotics until a bacterial infection is proven is quite feasible in hospitals. In primary care the decision is usually based on clinical impression with little recourse to investigations, the results of which are often delayed

There are several common clinical conditions in which antibiotics are considered and usually, but sometimes inappropriately, prescribed.

Tonsillitis

Most sore throats are caused by viral infections (when antibiotics are ineffective). There is also good evidence that antibiotics only reduce the duration of illness by less than a day in streptococcal infection. The serious streptococcal conditions of rheumatic fever and glomerulonephritis are very rare now and some children may receive some prolonged courses of penicillin unnecessarily

The commonly accepted indications for prescribing penicillin in tonsillitis are
severity of illness
prolonged high fever
marked cervical adenopathy
exudate on tonsils
positive culture of streptococcus on throat swab.

Otitis media

Amoxycillin is the drug of choice in children under 5 years, because *Haemophilus influenzae* is commonly involved. There is evidence that it is ineffective with the simple pink ear drum. In the older child penicillin V is probably sufficient

Accepted indications include
Severe earache
Bulging dull red ear drum
Perforation and discharge
Recurrent otitis media.

Croup

Most cases of croup are due to viral laryngotracheobronchitis which does not require antibiotic therapy. Very occasionally, *Haemophilus influenzae* causes epiglottitis; this is a very severe illness characterized by a rapid onset of high fever, drooling, stridor, respiratory distress and general debility which requires urgent hospital admission.

Asthma

Occasionally an asthmatic attack is induced by an infection. However, this is usually viral and antibiotics are inappropriate in most cases.

Persistent cough

Antibiotics are inappropriate in the case of a simple acute URTI. A problem occurs in young children when the cough has become a more prolonged distressing symptom. If it continues for more than 10 days many doctors would consider a trial of antibiotics. Since a fair proportion of these cases are due to a mycoplasma infection, erythromycin would be the antibiotic of choice.

Referral

Severe illness
Prolonged undiagnosed fever for more than 1 week
Suspicion of meningitis

Poor social circumstances
Associated dehydration or weight loss.

See also:

Fever (p. 106)
Common infectious diseases of children (p. 402)
Respiratory distress – croup (p. 537)

Fits and funny turns

As many as 1 in 10 children have one or more episodes of altered consciousness in their pre-school years. These are mostly simple faints, breath-holding attacks or benign febrile convulsions. While they are frightening, especially to the parents, the prognosis is usually excellent and the family can be confidently reassured. Only 1 in 200 children have a tendency to repeated epileptic fits. Very rarely, congenital heart disease can lead to unexpected syncope.

Faints

Usually occur in the older child often after a prolonged period of standing (e.g. school assemblies). The child may initially feel dizzy and sweaty prior to losing consciousness. Recovery is rapid and complete provided a recumbent or 'head down' posture is achieved.

Breath-holding attacks

These tend to occur in pre-school toddlers and are usually the result of a minor injury, punishment or temper tantrum. The child may start to cry but then holds its breath, goes blue in the face and subsequently becomes unconscious. The child starts to breathe again almost immediately, thus recovery is rapid and complete.

Febrile convulsions

These occur in children between 6 months and 3 years old – rarely after the age of 5 years. About one in 25 children may suffer a febrile fit; two-thirds never have another but 10% may go on to develop non-febrile epilepsy. These convulsions happen early in a febrile illness, and are most commonly due to an upper respiratory infection or the common exanthema. Very rarely they are due to an underlying meningitis.

Epilepsy

Of all children with epilepsy 75% are of idiopathic origin and tendency runs in families. See also p. 110.

Emergency management

Fits lasting more than 20 minutes may lead to permanent brain damage

Put the child into the recovery position

Check the airways (do *not* put objects in the mouth to prevent injury to the tongue)

Diazepam (i.v. or p.r.) 1 mg per year of age up to 5 years (0.1 – 0.2 mg/kg). Provided the child is not already on anticonvulsants this dose can be repeated in 15 minutes

Arrange transfer to hospital

Reassure and calm the parents – it can be a very frightening experience for all concerned

History

A careful history from the parents or those in attendance is the most important aspect of diagnosis

- exact timing and sequence of events
- duration of loss of consciousness
- associated involuntary movements, injury or incontinence
- warning signs or sensations (aura)
- sequelae – sleepiness, weakness or headache
- associated febrile illness
- previous history of fits or faints
- family history
- relevant developmental history

Examination

Temperature

Signs of infection

- ENT
- chest
- rashes
- neck stiffness
- LAP

CVS – pulse rate and rhythm

CNS

- level of consciousness
- head circumference
- unusual behaviour
- check fundi for papilloedema
- plantar reflexes
- meningism
- acute localized hemiplegia (Todd's paralysis)

Investigation

In primary care consider

- MSU for urinary infection
- CXR for chest infection
- 'Dextrostix' for hypoglycaemia

Options

Reassurance

For the majority of children the cause is benign and the family can be confidently reassured.

Control of fever

Remove excess clothing and blankets

Tepid sponging

Antipyretic drugs – paracetamol syrup

Encourage oral fluids or ice-lollies.

Drug management

Usually initiated and monitored in consultation with a paediatrician, e.g. sodium valproate 20 mg/kg

Occasionally for children with recurrent prolonged fits it may be helpful to teach the parents to give rectal diazepam.

Ketogenic diet

Occasionally an epileptic child who fails to respond to drug therapy may benefit from this diet. The diet can be unpleasant and requires skilled dietary advice.

Continued education and support

Families with an epileptic child may be more vulnerable and require careful support and advice about activities such as swimming and cycling. There may be a local supporting self-help group.

Referral

Acute

Prolonged fit lasting more than 20 minutes

Status epilepticus

Suspected meningitis

For an underlying acute cause such as head injury, blocked CSF drainage valve, etc.

Routine

For further investigation, diagnosis and drug management of non-febrile epilepsy

For parental reassurance

For dietary advice.

See also:

Fits (p. 110)

Convulsion (p. 518)

Heart murmurs in children

As many as 50% of children may be noted to have a heart murmur but only a very small proportion are associated with cardiac pathology.

Types of murmur

Minor clinical significance

Functional or flow murmurs
- soft short systolic murmur
- variable site
- accentuated by lying down
- no associated abnormal CVS signs or symptoms

Atrial septal defect
- often missed
- usually cause no harm
- due to increased flow through pulmonary valve
- characteristic fixed splitting of 2nd heart sound with no variation during respiration
- endocarditis is a very unusual cause

Small ventriculo-septal defect
- soft early systolic murmurs at left sternal edge
- usually have no effect on cardiac function
- endocarditis unlikely

Bicuspid aortic valve
- soft systolic murmur at the aortic area
- loud ejection click best heard at the apex with the patient sitting up
- little effect on cardiac function but may be prone to bacterial endocarditis and calcification in later life

Venous hum
- these are more continuous murmurs best heard at the root of the neck
- disappear if the child is tilted head down
- no clinical significance

Major clinical significance

Ventriculo-septal defect – loud murmur, more or less thrill. Maximal at 4th intercostal space at the left sternal edge

Pulmonary stenosis – loud systolic murmur in pulmonary area

Aortic stenosis – loud systolic murmur in the aortic area, may radiate to the neck

Mitral regurgitation – pansystolic murmur which may radiate to the axilla

History

Breathlessness
Cyanosis
Difficulty feeding
Failure to thrive

Examination

Record

Pallor and central cyanosis

Clubbing (usually after 6 months of age)
Pulse rate and rhythm
BP

Check for

Femoral pulses
Cardiac impulse
Character, site and radiation of murmur
Intercostal recession
Crepitations or pleural effusion on auscultation of lungs
Enlarged liver

Investigation

Only if a significant murmur is suspected
FBC
ECG
chest X-ray

Options

Reassurance if the murmur can be considered innocent
- systolic
- soft
- short
- site localized or variable
- variable loudness with posture
- no associated symptoms or signs of heart disease
- normal ECG and chest X-ray

Other or suspect murmurs should be referred for further investigations.

See also: Heart murmurs (p. 140)

Nappy rash

Nappy rash is a frequent problem in babies, one which often is first dealt with at home. The more severe or recalcitrant cases are presented to the doctor. The classifications of rashes, whilst well documented, tend to overlap, and most types become secondarily infected with *Candida* after 72 hours.

Ammonia dermatitis

This is an erythematous, desquamating rash in areas of contact avoiding the folds or creases.

It was thought to be due to the irritant effect of ammonia released when urea is split by bacterial organisms. However the principal factors are prolonged exposure to moisture, plus the use of tightly fitting plastic overpants in the presence of a sensitive or seborrhoeic skin.

Secondary infection is often present.

It may be associated with the use of irritant biological detergents left in inadequately rinsed nappies.

Options

Exposure
Frequent nappy changes (2 hourly)
Careful washing and rinsing of nappies
Nappy liners
Barrier creams (titanium dioxide – metanium)
Treatment of secondary infection.

Seborrhoeic dermatitis

This is a diffuse, red, shiny rash extending into the flexures.

It is also associated with other 'seborrhoeic features' such as cradle cap and lesions on the face and in other flexures.

Options

Exposure and frequent nappy change
Steroid creams (hydrocortisone or betamethasone)
Treatment of secondary infection (nystatin or clioquinol).

Thrush

This is a red, spotty rash affecting the flexures, scrotum or vulva, and perineum. There may be satellite spots outside the flexures.

Candida albicans is a common secondary invader of other nappy rashes.

If the rash is concentrated around the anus, oral thrush should be looked for.

It particularly affects breast-fed babies or those receiving antibiotics. Zinc and castor oil barrier ointment should be avoided.

Options

Exposure and frequent nappy changes
Nystatin ointment
Oral nystatin suspension if the gastrointestinal tract is involved or the rash recurrent
In breast-fed babies it may be wise to advise the mothers to use nystatin cream on the nipples.

Napkin psoriasis

This causes isolated, well demarcated, erythematous plaques extending out of the flexures. It may be associated with more classical scaly lesion on the limbs, face and scalp.

Options

Exposure

Steroid creams (hydrocortisones, betamethasone)
Treatment of secondary infection.

Diarrhoea

Frequent, loose, acidic stools may cause irritation of the perineal area if left in contact with the skin for prolonged periods. It may be associated with lactose intolerance.

Options

Frequent nappy changes
Barrier creams to the perineum (titanium dioxide)
Treat the diarrhoea with clear fluids for 24 hours before re-introducing milk feeds
Consider soya 'milk' for lactose intolerance.

Sleep disturbance in young children

Sleep disturbance presents very commonly to the family doctor, and perhaps, more often, to the health visitor. Epidemiological studies have yielded variable results. This suggests that the problem is probably more social and behavioural than physiological. What one family will tolerate another finds unacceptable. Cultural attitudes also vary. The prevalence of sleep disturbance in toddlers is estimated at around 30–50%. It is interesting that studies on children in institutions reveal a prevalence of only 3%.

There are essentially two phases of sleep: 'deep sleep' and 'active sleep'. Active sleep is related to periods with rapid eye movements. In this phase the child is more wakeful and indeed may wake several times during the night. Not all children demand attention on waking and may simply turn over and go back to sleep, as adults do.

Sleep disturbance falls into one of two categories
refusal to go to bed
night waking.

History

Pattern and duration of sleep – afternoon 'naps', and total number of hours asleep
Family dynamics and stresses
Father's involvement in child care
Maternal depression
Housing conditions – number of beds, rooms, neighbours

Examination

Usually not necessary

If illness is suspected, check appropriate symptoms

Options

Behavioural techniques

These are best if possible but require that the parents are motivated to adopt a fairly firm and consistent approach for a week or two to break the habit. It is essential that the child is not ill when the process is started.

Refusal to go to bed

Bring bed-time forward by 10 minutes each evening.

Avoid stimulating the child just before bed-time.

Leave the bedroom at the appropriate time and do not acceed to delaying tactics, e.g. another drink, story or cuddle.

If the child cries leave for 10 minutes then go in and gently but firmly put him back to bed again leaving as soon as the tears abate.

If the pattern is repeated leave the child crying for 15 minutes before returning or if possible the other parent should go in the second time.

This may go on for some hours but after a few hours the child usually gets the message.

Night waking

When the child wakes and demands attention, usually by crying, leave him for 5 to 10 minutes, then go in. The temptation is to cuddle the child or read stories until he goes to sleep leaving the child rewarded for his demanding behaviour and the parent wide awake and exhausted. Instead, gently calm the child until the crying stops then put him back to bed and leave without acceeding to delaying tactics.

If the crying starts again leave a little longer, 10–15 minutes, before returning and adopt the same gentle but firm approach. Each time the child wakes delay returning a little longer each time. Eventually the child will get this message too.

Sometimes the child gets out of bed on waking and goes downstairs or to the parent's bed. This can be a more difficult problem, but a similar firm approach should be adopted. If the child comes downstairs then he should be returned to bed gently but firmly and left after a very short time. If the pattern is repeated the other parent should try. Failing that another approach is to ignore the child, getting on with jobs as if the child wasn't there for a while before returning him to bed.

If the child goes to his parent's bed it may be more convenient to let him stay until he goes to sleep before returning him to bed. Those parents who find this unacceptable should not allow the habit to develop and adopt a firm approach from the start.

If the child continues to leave his bedroom there is another tougher tactic which some parents would find unacceptable. That is the bedroom door should be secured so that it opens but not wide enough for the child to get out. This will undoubtedly lead to frustrations and crying and the above approach of delaying going to the child for longer intervals should be tried. Eventually he gets the message.

Confounding problems

Difficult neighbours will have to be warned beforehand and are usually tolerant for the short time it takes to break the habit.

'*Light sleepers*' wake at the slightest noise. This can be very disruptive to the average household. They can be 'deconditioned' by putting a radio beside the bed and each night increasing the volume a little over a period of a couple of weeks until the child learns to tolerate the noise.

Delaying tactics to maintain the parent's attention is a common problem. The child pleads for a drink, a pee, a cuddle and so on. This can be endearing at first but should not be allowed to get out of hand. It can become a very unacceptable form of manipulation and needs more firm handling.

Some children wake early in the morning and are ready for the day. It would be inappropriate to try the above techniques here and instead the child should be encouraged to stay in his room and play with quiet toys or books. In this way the family may be afforded another hour or so of peace but unfortunately this is often a problem to be endured until the child is older and more self-sufficient.

In smaller homes the children often share bedrooms. This is often presented as an insurmountable problem for leaving the child to cry and delaying the comforting. However most siblings are tolerant for the short time it takes to break the habit. The only alternative is to alter the sleeping arrangement until the problem is solved.

Both parents must reach agreement on the methods used. A consistent approach is essential and a combined effort is preferable. All too often the father opts out of his responsibility and he should be encouraged to support his wife if they are to be successful.

Fear of the dark is a problem easily solved by leaving a low voltage light in the bedroom.

Nightmares and nocturnal screaming attacks are particularly anxiety provoking and not just for the child. It is usually easily distinguished from manipulative behaviour by the type of crying and response to the parent. A much more gentle approach should be adopted and he usually settles in 10 to 15 minutes if he can be reminded of the reality of familiar objects around his bedroom.

Night sedation

Many parents and doctors readily resort to sedation. It is best used for short courses with the following indications

In the short term during an intercurrent illness

To relieve family crisis when sleep disturbance is an added stress

To prepare the ground for the behavioural techniques by allowing the parents a brief respite from disturbed nights

Drugs, e.g. Promethazine 1–5 yrs – 15–20 mg at night
Trimeprazine 6–10 yrs – 20–25 mg at night

See also: Insomnia (p. 170)

The very ill baby

The very ill baby can provoke extreme anxiety in both parents and doctors. The medical care of very young babies is as much an art as a science. The doctor often relies on a 'sixth sense' to spot potentially serious disease at an early stage. Neonates are very vulnerable to infection and their condition may deteriorate rapidly. In particular pneumonia, meningitis, bronchitis and septicaemia can quickly prove fatal. And it must be remembered that acute abdomen, intracranial haemorrhage, gross anaemia, congenital heart disease, hypoglycaemia and renal failure can present non-specifically in an acutely ill baby.

This 'sixth sense' comes with experience and a clinical

sensitivity that is difficult to describe but it may be useful to outline a few cues that might alert the doctor to the fact that the baby is ill and needs more careful assessment.

History

Failure to feed
Fever
Vomiting and diarrhoea
Colic (drawing up of knees)
Excessive wetting of nappies
Difficult breathing
Noisy breathing
Abnormal cry
Non-acceptance of comforting
Responsiveness/alertness
Excessive sleeping/dopiness
Abnormal movements, twitching
Convulsions

Examination

It is essential to make a full examination with the baby undressed. Special attention should be paid to

Skin and colouring
- Pallor
- Jaundice
- Central cyanosis
- Purpuric rash

Hydration
- Sunken fontanelle
- Sunken eyes
- Reduced skin turgor
- Dry mouth

Muscle tone
- Floppiness
- Listlessness

Level of arousal
- Alertness
- Responsiveness
- Abnormal crying
- Acceptance of comforting

Breathing
- Rapid breathing >50/min in absence of crying
- Use of accessory muscles of respiration
- Subcostal recession
- Noisy respiration – crouping
- Too breathless to feed
- Localized signs in the chest

Abdomen

Abdominal distension
Enlarged liver or spleen
Visible peristalsis

Other

Convulsions
Bulging fontanelle
Neck stiffness (usually only seen in babies over 3 months)
Paralysis or favouring of a limb
Heart murmurs

Options

When the diagnosis is obvious the appropriate management should be instituted and may well necessitate referral to hospital

If on arrival the baby is not as ill as the parents would make you believe then reassurance and management of simple conditions may be all that is necessary. The mother herself may have perceived a subtle difference in her baby; the mother's fears must be carefully noted and assessed

Occasionally there may be nothing obviously wrong but your clinical suspicion may be aroused. In this case it is prudent to arrange to review the baby after a short interval and repeat a thorough examination.

4 Continuing Care

Care of the elderly

With the increasing number of over-65 year olds and the greater geriatric proportion in society there must be a re-allocation of resources both in finance and in manpower amongst the helping agencies. The care of the elderly will increasingly involve support from both the family and volunteer organizations who must in turn encourage a considerable degree of self-help by the individual.

The role of primary care continues to be prevention and anticipation of problems, and when problems do arise to provide prompt intervention and support.

A primary aim for care of the elderly, nicely epitomized in the motto of the British Geriatric Society, is to 'add life to years and not years to life.'

Prevention

Fitness

Maintain
- stamina
- suppleness
- strength
- skill
- sanity

Risk factors
- Extreme age
- Chronic illness
- Immobility
- Loneliness
- Bereavement
- Poverty

Anticipating change
- General health
- Mental state
- Social circumstances

Organization

Comprehenisve records
- data base
- repeat prescription systems
- Co-op cards
- 'at risk' registers
- disease registers

Surveillance clinics, 65 or 70 year assessments

Follow-up programme co-ordinated with other health workers

Self prescribing

Health education

Mobilize resources	Family support Accommodation Finance and allowances
Case finding and surveillance	**Record** BP Weight Urinalysis Teeth and dentures Sight and hearing Bowel and bladder function Memory and orientation Intellectual function Mobility and ADL Follow-up plan **Check for** Hypertension Carotid atherosclerosis Heart failure Heart block and arrhythmias Diabetes Thyroid status Osteoporosis Risk of hypothermia Tuberculosis Skin lesions Incontinence Rectal tumours Dementia Physical handicaps Depression Parkinsonism **Social factors** Rent, rates and maintenance Access and fire risks Stairs and alterations Heating and lighting Bathroom and toilets Housework and hygiene Laundry and shopping Cooking and diet TV and radio Pets and passtimes
Safe prescribing	Patient-held record of medication Consistent prescribing, dispensing and clinical review

Acceptable presentation, e.g. simple containers, adequate labelling, palatable taste, acceptable colouring
Recognize non-compliance, interactions, side-effects and toxicity
Monitor potential side effects, e.g. electrolyte disturbance with diuretics
Use appropriate dosage
Consider non-drug therapies
Rational medication at hospital discharge may need modification to *realistic* medication at home

Referral and co-operation

Responsible agencies

The patient's family
The primary health care team
Social services
Home help organization
Day hospital
Day centre
Part III accommodation
Private nursing homes
Laundry service

Other health workers

Geriatrician
Psychogeriatrician
Other hospital specialist
Community physician
Chiropodist
Dentist
Optician
Occupational therapist
Physiotherapist
Psychiatric nurse

Voluntary agencies

The Church
The Church Army
Age Concern
Help the Aged
Red Cross
St John Ambulance
WRVS
Meals on Wheels
Good Neighbour Schemes

Follow-up

Continuing medical or social difficulties
Friends' or relatives' opinions

Use of resources
social
financial
aids for ADL
Assess ADL
Exclude introgenic disease.

Cervical cancer screening

There is still a great debate concerning the effectiveness of the cervical cancer screening programme, including the respective roles of the doctor, the patient and the laboratory.

Screening is *associated* with a definite fall in mortality but other factors may also be involved in its reduction, such as the natural history of the disease and the different types of treatment.

A really intensive screening programme is required if it is to be effective.

Advantages of screening

Should detect cervical cancer at an earlier stage
Theoretically should produce a reduction in the incidence of and death from cervical cancer
The screening procedure may be reassuring to the patient with negative smears
The screening contact may provide an opportunity to detect other diseases such as breast lumps or pelvic pathology

Disadvantages of screening

An intensive programme is very expensive
The natural history of the disease may be changing and is, as yet, incompletely understood
Smear collection and processing technique is far from ideal in many cases
The rate of false negative and false positive cytology is too high
Evidence suggests that a large number of smear positive patients are inappropriately over-treated

Screening programme

The planning of a screening programme is affected by allocation of health care resources, high risk factors and the natural history of the disease, particularly with respect to age distribution

First smear

Within two years of becoming sexually active

Repeat

The current DHSS recommendation is for five yearly intervals. However there is growing concern that smears should be repeated every three years for more effective screening.

When to stop

At or after the age of 65 years if there have been three recent normal smears

Recall system

Many cytology laboratories run a local recall system for women aged over 35 years

Alternatively a practice age–sex register can be used to identify the population

After the first smear the patient's name is filed in order according to the month and year for future recall

A single letter can be sent to the patient when due for a first or repeat smear. If she fails to attend a note could be made in her medical records and the subject discussed at her next self-initiated attendance

If it is decided that the full screening programme is unrealistic at the present state of knowledge a more selective policy could be arranged

Smears could be taken from
- women at high risk – this group are least likely to attend without explicit invitation
- women with clinical signs and symptoms
- women attending contraceptive and antenatal clinics

Collecting samples

Insert an unlubricated bivalve speculum

Visually inspect the cervix and note irregularity and ulceration

Sweep the spatula around the whole circumference of the squamocolumnar junction including cells from the cervical canal

Spread the sample in a single thin layer along a microscope slide

Fix immediately with a 95% alcohol solution

If possible take the opportunity to perform a full vaginal examination, check for breast lumps and enquire about gynaecological symptoms

Cervical cancer
Natural history

$$\text{Normal} \underset{40\%}{\rightleftharpoons} \text{dysplasia} \underset{25\%}{\overset{10\%}{\rightleftharpoons}} \text{carcinoma in situ} \overset{20\%}{\rightleftharpoons} \text{invasive carcinoma}$$

Duration of disease in years	0	5	15

High risk factors

History of herpes genitalis or genital warts (advisable to have annual smears)
Age – peak incidence around 45 years (rare before 20)
Early intercourse – before aged 17 years
More than one male sexual partner
Lower socio-economic status
Patients with abnormal vaginal bleeding or discharge

Clinical presentation

Irregular bleeding especially post-coital or post-menopausal
Blood stained vaginal discharge
Visible changes on the cervix
Pain in sciatic nerve distribution
Ureteric complications
Pulmonary complications

Cytological staging

Class		*State*
I	Negative	
II	Atypical cells (metaplasia or infection)	Benign
III	Dysplasia	Suspicious
IV	Malignant cells seen	Cancerous

Options

Follow the cytologist's recommendation
Class I and II should be regarded as normal
Class III should be repeated after 6 months and referred for colposcopy, then annually until regression occurs or cancerous change is seen
Class IV should be repeated as soon as possible and if still positive referred to gynaecologist.

Chronic bronchitis

Chronic bronchitis can be defined as a daily cough productive of sputum for at least three months of the year in two or more consecutive years. Pathologically it is due to an increase in the number of mucus secreting glands and goblet cells in the airways. It is often associated with emphysema, but the linkage is not well understood. It may vary in severity from a simple disease to a disabling condition with poor exercise tolerance and cor pulmonale.

Associated factors

Incidence increases with age
Males more than females
More common in urban areas (atmospheric pollution)
Smoking
Family tendency
Lower socio-economic groups

History

Onset, duration and periodicity of symptoms
Presenting symptoms
- cough and sputum production
- haemoptysis
- dyspnoea
- exercise tolerance
- ankle swelling

Past history of chest disease
Family history
Occupational history
Environment
Smoking

Examination

Inspect for cyanosis and finger clubbing
Inspect the chest for position of trachea, expansion, hyperinflation
Auscultate to assess air entry and localizing signs
Check for signs of cor pulmonale
Record weight

Investigation

FBC (polycythaemia)
ESR
Sputum cytology when malignancy suspected
Chest X-ray
Peak expiratory flow

Options

Education
Regarding condition and avoidance of smoking
Consider occupation
Advise on breathing exercises
Co-existing infection
Should be treated with a broad spectrum antibiotic, e.g. amoxycillin 250 mg 8 hourly. Advise early presentation at the first sign of infection or give a supply of

antibiotics to start on the patient's own initiative and present later. Consider continuous antibiotic therapy in the winter months rotating three types of antibiotic every two weeks

Associated asthma

Should be treated appropriately (see p. 15). 'Atrovent' may be helpful in chronic bronchitics. There is evidence that a small proportion of these patients suffer a refractory form of asthma and some clinicians recommend a month long trial of oral steroids at high dosage

Influenza vaccinations

Should be considered in the autumn

Mucolytic medications

These have proved disappointing in practice but steam inhalation with Tinct. Benz. Co. may be helpful in association with physiotherapy

Domiciliary oxygen therapy

This may improve the patient's quality of life particularly when severely disabled by shortness of breath and by being house-bound. It should only be used with a 24% 'ventimask' or nasal catheters. Higher concentration may precipitate respiratory failure by inhibiting hypoxic drive

Sedatives and tranquillizers

Should be avoided because they depress respiration.

Follow-up

Patients should be checked at 3–6 monthly intervals or at times of acute exacerbations. The PEF should be monitored on each occasion

Failure to control

Continuing exposure to irritant fumes or tobacco smoke
Repeated uncontrolled infective episodes
Associated bronchiectasis
Misdiagnosis
- uncontrolled asthma
- cancer
- tuberculosis

Referral

Progressive respiratory failure with a falling PEF
For intensive physiotherapy and rehydration during acute exacerbations.

See also:

Asthma and wheezing (p. 15)
Shortness of breath (p. 281)

Chronic renal failure

Chronic renal failure is a condition of irreversible deterioration in renal function with the accumulation of waste products of metabolism. While not a common condition in primary care the patients will require prolonged and careful follow-up.

Causes

Chronic pyelonephritis
Chronic glomerulonephritis
Hypertension
Diabetes mellitus
Autoimmine disease
Congenital polycystic disease
Obstructive uropathy (including calculus disease)
Medication
Hypercalcaemia and hyperuricaemia

History

General ill health
- weakness
- polyuria
- nocturia
- anorexia
- thirst
- nausea
- vomiting
- hiccough
- cramps
- pruritis
- diarrhoea
- epistaxis
- bruising
- tremor
- fits
- symptoms of heart failure
- bone pain
- confusion

Past history of
- prostatism
- diabetes
- renal disease
- urinary infection
- hypertension

Family history of renal disease
Medication

Examination

Check for
- anaemia
- fluid overload
- bruising
- hypertension

Palpate for renal masses or tenderness
Rectal examination for pelvic masses or enlarged prostate
Mental examination

Investigation

FBC
U & E, Ca^{2+} + PO_4
Protein and albumin
Creatinine clearance
Uric acid
Blood sugar
Serum iron and TIBC
Serum B_{12} and folate
MSU
Abdominal X-ray
IVP

Options

Fluids

Increased fluid intake of 2–3 litres per day helps to eliminate toxic metabolites in high urine output

Diuretic e.g. frusemide 20 mg – 2 g/day if fluid retention develops

Potassium sparing diuretic, e.g. spironolactone may be added later

Fluid restriction may be necessary in terminal stages.

Drugs

Many drugs are excreted through the kidney so medication should be carefully controlled and dosages adjusted to the level of renal failure.

Diet

Reduced protein diets may be impalatable and should be planned with the help of a dietician; they may improve symptoms but not renal function

High carbohydrate calorie intake

Vitamin supplements may be necessary with restricted diets

Potassium intake should be reduced by avoiding fresh fruit juices, bananas, chocolate, soups

Sodium restriction and supplementation may be necessary according to plasma levels but may need careful supervision.

Infections

Should be treated vigorously. Both urinary and general infections can cause deterioration in renal function.

Hypertension

Must be treated appropriately since control of diastolic pressure below 95 mm Hg may improve or at least halt deterioration in function. In severe renal failure, control of hypertension may reduce renal blood flow and cause deterioration. Any antihypertensive therapy should be started at low dosage and renal function monitored regularly.

Anaemia

Is generally refractory to treatment unless due to intestinal blood loss

Transfusion may be necessary if Hb falls below 8.5 g/dl.

Pruritus

May respond to

Chlorpromazine 25 mg 8 hourly
Chlorpheniramine 4 mg 8 hourly
Aluminium hydroxide suspension 10 ml 6 hourly.

Referral

All new cases for assessment and consideration for dialysis or renal transplantation

In obstructive nephropathy relief of obstruction usually prevents deterioration of renal function

For dietary advice.

Follow-up

Should be arranged in conjunction with the hospital specialist

3 month check

Weight
BP
U & E
FBC
MSU

6 month check

Creatinine clearance

Indications for dialysis

Clinical deterioration with creatinine clearance less than 5 ml/min

New patients with rapidly progressive uraemia to allow time for full assessment.

See also:

Retinopathy (p. 274)
Maternal disease in pregnancy (p. 367)

Contraception

Contraception is a personal affair in which the doctor acts as an advisor.

Knowledge of the effectiveness, contraindications to and side-effects of the various methods is essential. It is also helpful to understand some of the techniques of sexual conselling (see p. 266).

Condom

The sheath is still widely used and second only to the Pill in popularity. It is particularly important in casual sex and when there is a risk of STD, AIDS or cervical dysplasia.

Effectiveness 5–20 failures per 100 women years. It may be more more effective if used with a spermicide

Contraindications Rubber sensitivity

Management **Patient**

The sheath should only be applied with the penis erect before penetration. After intercourse the penis should be withdrawn while still erect with the sheath held against the shaft.

The use of spermicidal creams and pessaries should be encouraged.

Vaginal diaphragm

The vaginal diaphragm is a useful alternative to the Pill and IUCD and is becoming increasingly popular. It requires some skill and good motivation for proper insertion. Most people use the soft spring vaginal diaphragm but vault and cervical caps are available. Effectiveness is enhanced by the use of spermicidal creams.

Effectiveness 2–3 failures per 100 women years if used carefully

Contraindications Vaginal prolapse
Vaginal abnormalities (septate vagina)
Rubber or spermicide sensitivity

Management **Doctor**

Using fitting rings select the largest size which is

comfortable and does not protrude through the introitus on straining down
It can be inserted either side up to cover the cervix
Check weight
Patient
Insert at any convenient time before intercourse
More effective if used with a spermicide
After insertion check it is covering the cervix
If sex occurs more than three hours after insertion use more spermicide (cream or pessaries)
Leave in place for six hours after last intercourse
Clean with warm soapy water after removal and dry carefully
Check periodically for perforation
Change in weight of more than seven pounds may require a refitting

Follow-up

Initially
Ask the patient to practise insertion and return in 1–2 weeks with cap *in situ* to check position
Subsequently
Annual checks including weight, renew the cap at least every 2 years

Side-effects

Hypersensitivity to rubber or spermicide

IUCD

The Intra-Uterine Contraceptive Device is a useful method as an alternative to the Pill in older, parous women and/or those who are less compliant with daily medication or barrier methods.
Two types are available
(i) plastic only (Lippes loop)
(ii) copper containing (copper 7, copper T or multiload)
The smaller copper devices have fewer side-effects but must be changed every 2 or 3 years.

Effectiveness

2–3 failures per 100 women years

Contraindications

Active pelvic inflammatory disease (PID)
Heavy or abnormal vaginal bleeding – particularly with anaemia

Abnormality of the uterine cavity (congenital, fibroids, scars)
Pregnancy
Valvular heart disease
Nulliparous women have increased risk of PID and subsequent infertility

Management

Doctor

The insertion should not be attempted without prior training

p.v. examination before insertion to assess uterine position and pelvic pathology plus routine cervical smear

The insertion is carried out at the time of or soon after menstruation, or 6/52 post partum, or after a termination

Keep the patient under observation for 15 minutes after fitting as a precaution in case of 'cervical shock'

Teach patient how to check for the threads

Patient

Expect some lower abdominal discomfort associated with insertion

Possibility of increased menstrual loss and intermenstrual bleeding (IMB)

The device may be expelled particularly at the time of periods

It is immediately effective as a contraceptive.

Ensure regular checks of the threads

Follow-up

Initial check

4 weeks or after next period
- p.v. examination to
  - check threads
  - pain in fornices
  - vaginal discharge.

Subsequent check

1 year and annually afterwards
- p.v. examination
- symptom review
- change copper devices at appropriate time.

Lost threads

Arrange ultrasound scan of the pelvis
Refer to gynaecologist if necessary

Side-effects

Pelvic infection (and subsequent infertility)
Menorrhagia and IMB
Increased chance of dysmenorrhoea

Increased risk of ectopic pregnancy
Risk of perforation or migration from uterine to peritoneal cavity

The Pill

The combined oestrogen/progestogen pill is the most effective reversible contraceptive available. It acts by inhibiting ovulation and altering the cervical mucus and the endometrial lining. The newer triphasic preparations such as Trinordiol or Logynon are thought to achieve better menstrual control; this is yet to be fully evaluated. Other preparations are listed in Fig. 4.1.

Effectiveness 0.36 failures per 100 women years

Contraindications

Absolute

Thromboembolism
Severe hypertension
Impaired liver function
Malignant disease of the breast or genital tract
Post splenectomy
Otosclerosis
Pituitary disorder
Porphyria

Relative

Women over 35 years
Mild to moderate hypertension
Epilepsy
Diabetes
Renal disease
Migraine
Valvular heart disease
Family history of cardiovascular or metabolic disease
Obesity
Oligomenorrhoea
Breast feeding
Contact lens wearer
Depression
Smoking
Varicose veins

Management

Doctor

Weight
BP

Urinalysis
Breast and pelvic examination
Rubella status and cervical cytology

Patient

Start first pill on

(*i*) 1st day of next cycle – effective from the start
(*ii*) 5th day of next cycle – other precautions for the first 14 days
(*iii*) 28 days post partum

If a single pill is missed take two the next day

After the 21 tablets take a 7 day break then restart the next packet

Vomiting and diarrhoea may interfere with pill absorption and effectiveness

Other medication e.g. anticonvulsants and some antibiotics may also interfere with effectiveness

Minor side-effects Change oestrogen or progestogen dosages of the Pill depending on the symptoms. See Figs 4.1 and 4.2

Follow-up **First check**

After 3 months
BP
Weight
Symptoms review

	Oestrogen	Progestogen
TOO MUCH	Mild hypertension	Depression
	Recurrent migraine	Loss of libido
	Premenstrual tension	Missed withdrawal bleed
	Breast discomfort	Breast discomfort
	Nausea and bloating	Acne
	Vaginal discharge	Hirsuitism
	Cyclical weight gain	Steady weight gain
		Recurrent thrush
TOO LITTLE	Break through bleeding	Break through bleeding
	Recurrent thrush	Heavy menstrual loss

Fig. 4.1. Indications for change in dosage of the combined pill

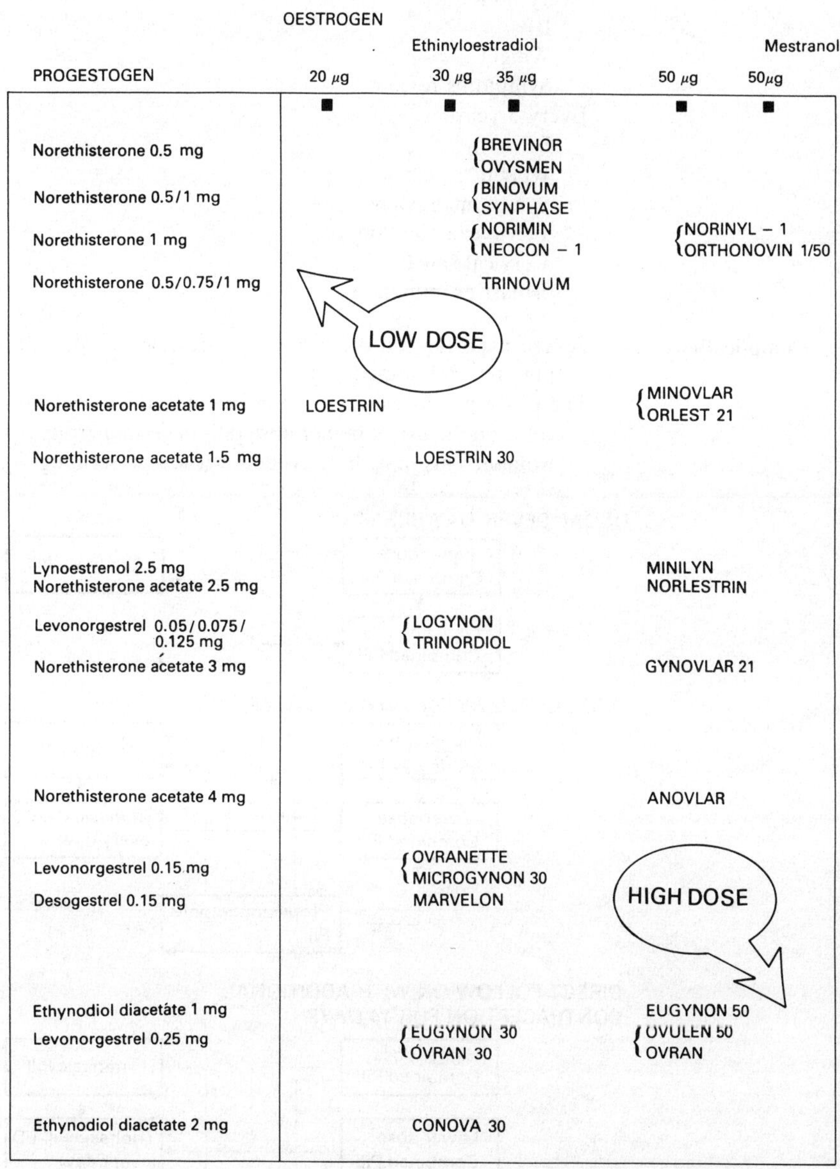

PROGESTOGEN	OESTROGEN: Ethinyloestradiol 20 μg	Ethinyloestradiol 30 μg	Ethinyloestradiol 35 μg	Ethinyloestradiol 50 μg	Mestranol 50μg
Norethisterone 0.5 mg			BREVINOR OVYSMEN		
Norethisterone 0.5/1 mg			BINOVUM SYNPHASE		
Norethisterone 1 mg			NORIMIN NEOCON – 1		NORINYL – 1 ORTHONOVIN 1/50
Norethisterone 0.5/0.75/1 mg			TRINOVUM		
Norethisterone acetate 1 mg	LOESTRIN			MINOVLAR ORLEST 21	
Norethisterone acetate 1.5 mg		LOESTRIN 30			
Lynoestrenol 2.5 mg				MINILYN	
Norethisterone acetate 2.5 mg				NORLESTRIN	
Levonorgestrel 0.05/0.075/0.125 mg		LOGYNON TRINORDIOL			
Norethisterone acetate 3 mg				GYNOVLAR 21	
Norethisterone acetate 4 mg				ANOVLAR	
Levonorgestrel 0.15 mg		OVRANETTE MICROGYNON 30			
Desogestrel 0.15 mg		MARVELON			
Ethynodiol diacetate 1 mg				EUGYNON 50	
Levonorgestrel 0.25 mg		EUGYNON 30 OVRAN 30		OVULEN 50 OVRAN	
Ethynodiol diacetate 2 mg		CONOVA 30			

Fig. 4.2. Oestrogen and progestogen levels in the combined dose contraceptive pill

Subsequent checks
Every 6 months
- BP
- Weight
- Symptoms review

Every 3 years
- BP
- Weight
- Symptoms review
- Pelvic examination
- Cervical smear
- Breast examination

Complications

Severe hypertension or thrombosis are reasons for stopping the Pill immediately

There is a possible link between breast and cervical cancers and the use of higher dose pills in certain groups of women. This must be considered when prescribing

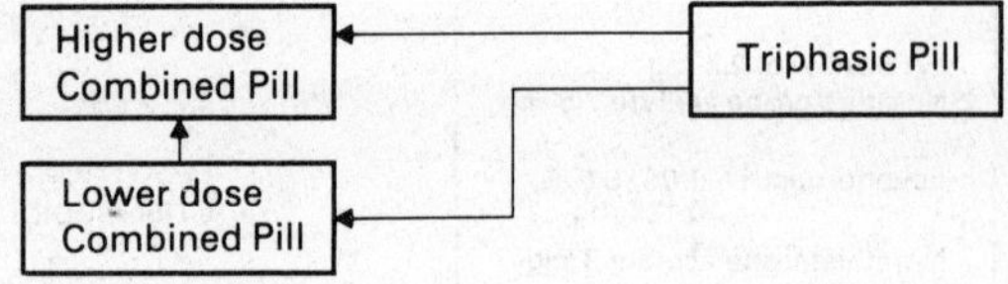

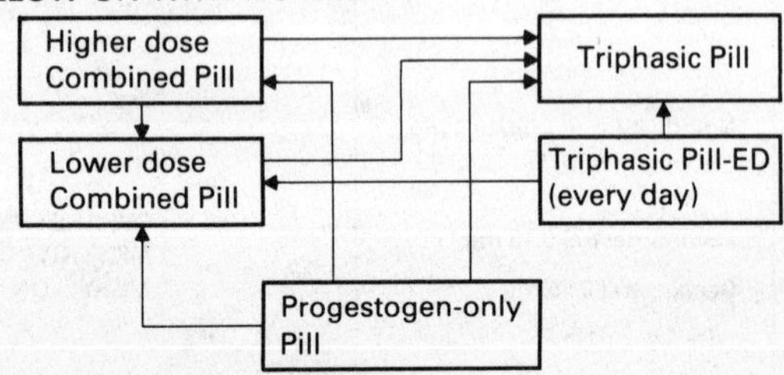

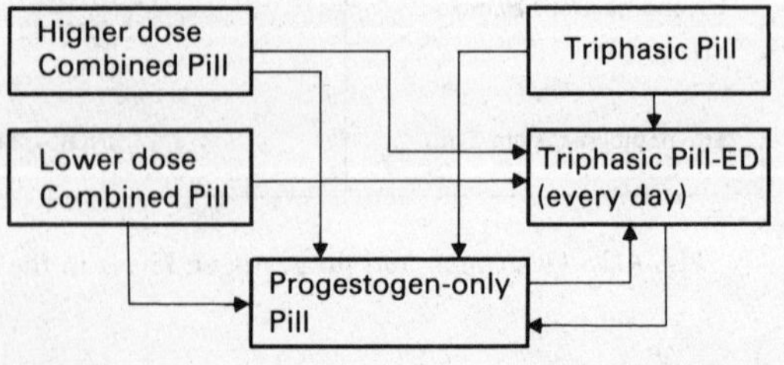

Fig. 4.3. Changing the Pill

Changing the Pill There are many ways of changing the Pill. Instructions to the patient are one of the following
usual 7 day break
direct follow-on (no break)
direct follow-on (with additional contraception for 14 days)

Progestogen-only pill (the 'mini-pill')

The progestogen-only pill is a useful and relatively safe alternative to the combined pill for women over 35 years or those breast feeding. However, there is less margin for error in compliance.

It acts by altering the cervical mucus and endometrial lining without inhibiting ovulation.

Progestogen-only contraceptives

Name	Progestogen	
Femulen	Ethynodiol diacetate	500 μg
Micronor/Noriday	Norethisterone	350 μg
Neogest	Levonorgestrel	75 μg
Microval/Norgeston	Levonorgestrel	30 μg

Effectiveness 2 failures per 100 women years

Contraindications These are subject to much debate; many doctors would consider the following as contraindications
those similar to the combined pill
ectopic pregnancy
poor compliance

Management

Doctor
As for the combined pill
Patient
Start pill on first day of next cycle
Take one pill not later than 27 hours after the previous pill
Use other precautions for the first 14 days
Vomiting and diarrhoea may affect absorption and effectiveness
If a pill is missed take it when remembered but use other precautions for 14 days
Periods may become unpredictable and erratic

Follow-up As for the combined pill

Minor side-effects As for the progestogen effects of the combined pill (see p. 450)

The rhythm method

This is an alternative method of contraception which poses no ethical or religious dilemma. It is more successful in women with a regular menstrual cycle and real motivation.

Effectiveness Approximately 20 failures per 100 women years

Contraindications If there is more than 10 days difference between the longest and shortest menstrual cycle in the preceding year

Management Record the duration of the previous 12 cycles

Irregular cycles

The unsafe period is calculated by deducting 18 days from the shortest and 11 days from the longest menstrual cycles:

i.e. shortest cycle 25 days (25 − 18 = 7)
longest cycle 30 days (30 − 11 = 19)

The unsafe period is the 7th to the 19th days of the cycle.

Regular 28 day cycles

The unsafe period is day 14 ± 4 (i.e. 10th to 18th days of the cycle)

A temperature chart is a particularly useful adjunct to establish the pattern of ovulation.

Older methods of contraception

Coitus interruptus, douching, intravaginal sponges, coitus reservatus and even coitus saxonicus are legacies of the days (and nights!) before effective contraception. None are entirely effective, some could have significant side effects and most detract from sexual satisfaction.

Advice and education should be directed towards the use of more effective methods.

Female sterilization

Tubal occlusion is a more complicated procedure than vasectomy.

Sterilization usually requires a general anaesthetic and an overnight stay in hospital (may be longer if laparotomy is performed). It is rarely reversible but success may be more

likely if the tubes are simply occluded with clips or 'fallope rings' rather than tubal destruction
It is immediately effective.

Types of operation

Laparoscopy – most commonly used
Laparotomy – when pelvic pathology, previous lower abdominal surgery or obesity may preclude laparoscopy
Culdoscopy – rarely used

Effectiveness

0.2 to 1.0 failures per 100 women years
Depends on the technique used and skill of the operator

Relative contraindications

Indecision regarding irreversibility
Unstable marital relationship
Doubts about subsequent libido
Careful counselling is necessary with young women or those of low parity
When hysterectomy may be more appropriate for menstrual disorders
Laparoscopy may be precluded by pelvic pathology or gross obesity limiting laparoscopic access
Active pelvic inflammatory disease

Management

Doctor
Discuss adequacy of present contraception
Consider male sterilization
Explain procedure and irreversible nature of the operation
Explore attitude towards the operation
Menstrual history – consider hysterectomy in the presence of severe menorrhagia or cervical or uterine pathology
Check cervical smear
Vaginal examination to exclude pelvic pathology
Obtain consent in writing (husband's consent is ethically recommended but not legally required)

Patient
Allow 1–2 weeks for post-operative recovery
Continue present contraception until the operation is performed
Immediately effective
Intercourse can be resumed when the patient feels ready

Follow-up Check wounds on the 2nd and 7th post-operative days and remove skin sutures when necessary

Complications Anaesthetic risk
Bleeding
Infection
Perforation of the bowel or uterus during the procedure
Air embolus from pneumoperitoneum in laparoscopic procedure
Pregnancy due to failure to identify fallopian tubes, incomplete occlusion or recanalization

Male sterilization

Vasectomy is technically easier, quicker and safer than female sterilization, and fertility can be easily checked post-operatively with a sperm count. There is, however, a delay after operation before sterility can be assured.

Sterilization is usually carried out as an outpatient procedure under local anaesthetic.

Effectiveness 0.15 failures per 100 women years
Failure usually occurs when the patient fails to obtain clear sperm samples before abandoning other contraception

Relative contraindications Indecision regarding irreversibility
Unstable marital relationship
Fear of subsequent impotence
Local genital pathology – varicocoele, large hydrocoele, local hernia or scar tissue, genital tract infections
General medical state – diabetes, recent myocardial infarction
If the wife is likely to need a hysterectomy or a laparotomy for any reason the vasectomy may be unnecessary

Instructions **Doctor**
Discuss adequacy of present contraception
Consider female sterilization
Explain procedure and irreversible nature
Explore patient's attitute to sterilization
Examine to exclude local and medical contraindications

Obtain consent in writing (obtaining the wife's consent is ethically recommended but not legally required)

Patient

Arrange for a few days off work after the operation

Intercourse can be resumed when the partners feel ready (from 3 days post-operatively)

Allow 4–5 months to clear the system of remaining sperm

Two consecutive clear sperm samples *must* be obtained before other contraception is abandoned

Follow-up

Obtain two consecutive sperm-free samples after approximately 4–5 months

Repeat operation may be necessary if sperm persist in the ejaculate

Complications

Pain when a haematoma develops

Bruising of the scrotum

Haematoma

Infection including tetanus

Recanalization

Granuloma formation in the scrotal wound or stump of the vas deferens

Diabetes

Case finding and control of diabetes are most appropriately carried out in primary care. This does, however, require effective recall, systematic clinical review and good co-operation with diabetic specialists in the management of any complications of the disease.

There are two diagnostic categories for patients with diabetes mellitus

Type I – juvenile onset, insulin dependent

Type II – maturity onset, non-insulin dependent

Type I occurs in a ratio of 1:4 with type II

The aetiology appears to be multifactorial including genetic, autoimmune and infective factors. Histocompatibility antigens (B8, BW15, BW18) may prove to be 'markers' of the disease.

2% of the UK population are estimated to be diabetic but only half of these will be known to the doctor. They may present with symptoms of the disease or be 'discovered' on routine urine testing or in the course of a deliberate screening programme.

Causes

Primary
- idiopathic

Secondary
- pancreatic disease or surgery
- pregnancy
- Cushing's disease
- acromegaly
- hyperthyroidism
- phaeochromocytoma
- steroids
- thiazide drugs
- advanced liver disease

History

Onset and duration of symptoms
- Change in weight or appetite
- Thirst, polyuria, fatigue
- Pruritis vulvae or balanitis

Symptoms of complications

CVS
- Angina
- MI
- Claudication
- Gangrene

CNS
- numbness and paraesthesiae of limbs
- failing vision
- TIA or strokes
- impotence
- persistent diarrhoea

Chest
- cough with chronic bronchitis

Renal
- polyuria, frequency and dysuria with associated infection

Skin
- recurrent boils and *Candida* infections

Family history of diabetes
Past history of pancreatic surgery
Obstetric history of large babies or stillbirths
Drug history of steroids, or thiazide diuretics
History of smoking

Examination

Record
- Height
- Weight
- BP

Check
- Urine for sugar and ketones

Thyroid disorder
Peripheral pulses
Neuropathy
Reduced visual acuity, cataracts, retinopathy
Trophic skin changes (necrobiosis lipoidica)

Glycosuria is only suggestive and not diagnostic of diabetes mellitus. It is necessary to proceed to blood sugar estimation. The diagnosis can be made on one or more of the following criteria:

random blood sugar	>11 mmol/litre
fasting blood sugar	>8 mmol/litre

If the levels are less than these but greater than 6 mmol/litre (fasting) then a formal glucose tolerance test should be undertaken.

Other investigations

FBC
ESR
Electrolytes
Urea and creatinine if biguanides are prescribed
LFT
MSU
CXR
ECG
Cholesterol and triglycerides

Emergency care

(See p. 525)

Options

Diet in consultation with a dietician

The aim should be to achieve and maintain an ideal body weight with a minimum of hunger and minimal drug treatment.

Simple diet sheets can be given to the patient with a daily calorie content of 1–2,000 according to the weight change, hunger and blood sugar balance.

Carbohydrate should contribute 50% of these calories.

Recommend a diet high in leguminous fibre and low saturated fats content. Advise a moderate alcohol intake.

Oral agents

Helpful in maturity onset diabetes if diet has failed in the obese, or from the start in diabetics of normal or low weight

Contraindicated in patients presenting with ketosis

Stimulate insulin release

Sulphonyl ureas

Best to use short-acting agents in the elderly to avoid hypoglycaemia

Start with a small dose increasing over the weeks as required
Short-acting, e.g. tolbutamide 500 mg–2 g daily
Medium-acting, e.g. glibenclamide 5–20 mg daily
Long-acting, e.g. chlorpropamide 100–500 mg daily
Inhibit glucose absorption and oxidation
Biguanides
These are less favoured now because of associated lactic acidosis particularly with phenformin, in the presence of renal, liver or cardiac disease
Metformin 500–850 mg 12 hourly may be helpful in obese type II diabetics in whom sulphonylureas have failed.

Insulins
The new patient requiring insulin is usually admitted to hospital for initial supervised control and stabilization. Insulin may be given on a once or twice daily basis perhaps as a combination of short and longer acting preparations.

Table 4.1. Examples of different insulin preparations

	Insulin	Peak effect (hrs)	Duration of action (hrs)
Short-acting	Soluble Actrapid*	1–4	6–8
Intermediate	Semitard*	4–8	10–16
	Semilente	4–8	10–16
	Rapitard	4–12	14–20
Long-acting	Lente Monotard* Isophane	6–12	18–24

*The newer insulins are largely purified and mono-component. They cause less local reaction and promote less insulin antibody formation. The dose of these insulins may be less than the older types.

General discussion Self-monitoring with urine testing or blood glucose estimation at home
Explain hypoglycaemia symptoms and carrying sugar or glucose
Urine testing
Foot care – liaise with chiropodist
Avoid smoking

Try to encourage a normal life
Regular gentle exercise – avoiding aggressive bursts which tend to produce hypoglycaemia
Recommend British Diabetic Association
Carry diabetic card
Influenza vaccine
Regular dental treatment
Eye checks
Prescription charge exemption for replacement therapy
Pre-conception check (see p. 346)

Follow-up

The patient must be followed up on a regular basis initially every week until under control, then as required (at least once a year). This may be best organized in a diabetic 'mini-clinic'

Each visit

Weight
BP
Review diet
Blood sugar (random or fasting samples)
Complications and symptoms
Medication
Self-monitoring of urine and blood sugars

Annual check

Health education about diabetes
Feet
Peripheral nerves
Retinoscopy
Visual acuity
Skin
Urinalysis for proteinuria

A follow-up procedure can be made more effective if arranged in conjunction with a special diabetic card which allows easier retrieval of information and acts as a reminder for checks at routine visits

Referral

Urgent referral of the unwell dehydrated ketotic patient
For more careful control of the insulin dependent patient
For assessment of complications
Dietician for advice if simple diets fail to achieve ideal weight
Diabetes in pregnancy is probably best monitored under specialist care.

Complications

CVS

Ischaemic heart disease
Peripheral vascular disease
Cerebrovascular disease

Eye
Cataracts
Retinopathy – 'spots and blots', hard exudates and new vessel formation (see p. 325)
Glaucoma

Renal
Glomerulonephritis
Pyelonephritis
Papillary necrosis
Cystitis

CNS
Peripheral neuropathy
Mononeuritis
Autonomic neuropathy

Skin
Sepsis
Lipoatrophy at injection sites
Necrobiosis lipoidica diabeticorum

See also:
Retinopathy (p. 274)
Pre-conception check (p. 346)
Maternal diseases in pregnancy (p. 367)
Hyperglycaemia (p. 524)
Hypoglycaemia (p. 525)

Gout

This condition causes episodes of acute arthritis due to crystal deposits in one or more joints and is usually associated with hyperuricaemia. However, hyperuricaemia can occur without clinical evidence of gout.

Any joint may be affected but it most commonly starts in the first metatarsophalangeal joint of the foot.

Men are more often affected than women (ratio 6:1); it is rare in women before the menopause. There may be a family history of gout.

Causes

Increased production of uric acid
- primary metabolic
- myeloproliferative disorders
- carcinomatosis
- severe psoriasis

Decreased excretion of uric acid
- chronic renal failure
- hypertension

myxoedema
toxaemia of pregnancy
drugs (aspirin, diuretics, alcohol)

History

Age
Onset of discomfort
Joints affected
Previous attacks of arthritis or urinary calculi
Family history of gout
General health enquiry (to exclude the above causes)

Examination

Temperature
Weight
BP
Assess affected joints
Tophi around affected joints or ears
Enlargement of liver or spleen
Thyroid status

Investigation

FBC
ESR
Urea and creatinine
Uric acid
Urine for protein and crystaluria
X-ray affected joints
Synovial fluid aspirate from affected joints for crystal analysis and culture

Options

Acute

Rest and elevation
Indomethacin 25–50 mg 6 hourly until pain settles, then reduce the dose slowly over 1 week
Naproxen orally or indomethacin suppositories are useful alternatives
Colchicine 1 mg then 0.5 mg 2 hourly until pain subsides or gastrointestinal side effects occur
Avoid thiazide diuretics.

Long term

Await resolution of the acute attack
Allopurinol 300 mg once daily increasing to 8 hourly until serum uric acid level returns to normal then continue with maintenance dose of 100–300 mg daily
or Probenecid 0.5 mg–1 mg 12 hourly. It should be avoided in patients with renal failure or uric acid crystaluria
or Sulphinpyrazone 100 mg 8 hourly
The introduction of these drug regimens can be

covered with colchicine 0.5 mg 12 hourly to avoid the precipitation of an acute attack
Avoid obesity and starvation
Avoid alcohol or purine intake
Avoid thiazide diuretics.

Follow-up

When starting long-term drug treatment check uric acid levels monthly until within normal limits
Annual check
- weight
- BP
- uric acid and creatinine
- drug compliance

Referral

Failure to control acute attack
For assessment of renal complications
For orthopaedic assessment of joints for possible surgical correction if severely damaged.

Complications

Renal damage
Hypertension
Ureteric calculi
Secondary osteoarthritis
Gouty tophi

Differential diagnosis

Septic arthritis
Superficial cellulitis of skin over the joint
Trauma
Haemarthrosis
Rheumatoid arthritis
Rheumatic fever
Pseudogout

See also: The foot and ankle (p. 115)

Health checks

The concept of regular health checks is becoming popular to the lay person. It can provide the 'bread and butter' of a private health service. In a cost conscious National Health Service, its effectiveness has yet to be proven.

Obstetric anticipatory care and paediatric surveillance are considered on pages 348 and 392.

Reasons for health checks

The patient
Reassurance
Covert reasons for consultation
Employment or insurance requirement

The doctor
Financial
For a third party (DHSS, Employer, Insurance)

To detect or even prevent disease (secondary prevention)

To alter behaviour in harmful habits (primary prevention)
Opportunity for health education

Several of these reasons would appear dubious and open to criticism. However, the early detection of disease and the opportunity for health education and correction of harmful habits would appear to be attractive.

On current medical evidence only a few conditions justify early detection in terms of cost effectiveness and availability of suitable treatment. The detection can be carried out by screening or case finding techniques.

Screening

This is a doctor-initiated programme to detect patients at risk of a particular disease in an apparently healthy population that would otherwise not present for medical advice. It is the responsibility of the doctor to detect early disease and it is essential that an appropriate treatment is available and beneficial.

To be effective the condition must be a recognized medical problem with a known natural history that includes a latent or pre-symptomatic phase which can be detected by a simple, acceptable and reliable diagnostic test. There should be a cost effective and acceptable treatment. The screening programme should be continuous.

There are only a few conditions which may be amenable to this technique but, apart from hypertension, proof is difficult to obtain, e.g.
hypertension
breast cancer
cervical cancer
colorectal cancer.

Case finding

In this process the patient initiates the consultation and the doctor offers additional investigations to detect disease. There is less responsibility on the doctor to provide a 'cure' although even this is a dubious concept.

The selection of patients can be at the doctor's discretion and is therefore more flexible.

Because of the increased selectivity it is possible that a few more conditions in addition to the above are appropriate to this technique, e.g.

anaemia
thyroid disease
glaucoma
visual failure
alcoholism
deafness
lung cancer
diabetes
kidney disease
occupational disease

The effectiveness assumes that most patients in a practice will present for some reason or another over a given period of time. Studies have shown that 60% of patients present at least once a year and 90–95% over 5 years.

To limit the size of the remaining 'at-risk' population an effective level of organization is necessary, with easy recording and access to relevant patient data in the medical records.

See also: Antenatal visits (p. 348)
Final post-natal examination (p. 384)
Child development (p. 392)

Health education

A primary role of the doctor is the promotion of good health. Health, as defined by the WHO in 1948, is 'a state of complete physical, mental and social well being and not merely the absence of disease and infirmity'. The concept of health is influenced by culture, family, folk-lore, educational experience and fear.

By contrast, it is the recognition of ill health that has been the traditional basis for medical education and, not surprisingly, it is usually through ill health that a patient enlists the help of a doctor.

The word 'Doctor' is taken from the Latin 'Docere' –

'to teach' – and increasingly one can recognize the crucial role of the doctor as teacher in health education. In particular, the doctor can encourage an individual's autonomy in the maintenance of good health. He can also reconcile the often perverse demands of the patient for health care with his own professional perception of health needs.

Aims

Promotion of a useful and relevant concept of health
Recognition and practice of a healthy life-style
Avoidance of adverse factors in health
Effective use of health resources
Effective action in primary, secondary and tertiary prevention

Prevention

The doctor in primary care has an important role to play in the prevention of ill health. Besides his symbolic role as teacher and healer he has contact with a given population and can recognize those at risk.

Primary prevention

Intervention before disease develops.

Education to avoid adverse factors and to promote a healthy life-style.

Secondary prevention

Prevention of complications of disease by effective management.

Education to recognize early symptoms and signs, to use medical services appropriately and to change life-styles accordingly.

Tertiary prevention

Prevention of avoidable disability from unavoidable disease.

Education in rehabilitation, availability of resources, compliance with professional advice and support.

Resources

Health workers

All members of the primary health care team, including receptionists
All hospital, medical and nursing staff
Health education units

Potential health promoters

Schools
Food industry

Sport and leisure industry
The media (books, newspapers, radio and television)

The population

Cultural factors – may help or hinder education
Self-help groups and organizations
Family and friends (folk remedies and 'old wives tales' are often misleading or inaccurate)

Finance

State funding
Commercial sponsorship

Opportunities

Consultation

The consultation enables the doctor or other health workers to discuss the aims of health education and to influence a change in attitude or behaviour. In contrast the inappropriate expectations of care from a patient can be reinforced by complying with every request without considering its basis.

Clinics

Immunization
Well Woman
Cervical screening
School
Obesity
Hypertension
Infant welfare
Antenatal
Family planning
Hospital out-patients
Diabetic
Geriatric

Reception

Information and explanation of the aims and limitations of the services offered.
Minor illness – instructions on self-help
Pamphlets and information sheets – most effective when presented by the doctor
Self-help groups – initiation and continuing support.
Patient participation groups
Health education displays – posters, audio visual, videos

Referral

Referral to other agencies – e.g. Citizens Advice Bureau or local council departments (e.g. Housing).

Referral to 'complementary medicine'

Acupuncture
Osteopathy
Chiropractice
Homeopathy
Hypnosis
Yoga
Meditation
Alexander technique
Bio-feedback
Music therapy
Herbal medicine.

Heart failure

This is largely a condition of the elderly but 10% of cases occur in those under 60 years of age. The classical symptoms and signs may be absent in the early stages.

It is conventional to classify heart failure into three types.

Left ventricular failure – insidious or acute in onset, resulting in increased pulmonary venous pressure and clinically detectable pulmonary oedema.

Right ventricular failure – can occur in isolation but is usually precipitated by left-sided failure. This is characterized by raised jugular venous pressure, enlarged liver and peripheral oedema.

Congestive cardiac failure – this is a combination of both left and right ventricular failure.

Causes

Pressure overload
- valvular stenosis
- pulmonary hypertension
- systemic hypertension

Volume overload
- valvular disease

- congenital heart disease
- fluid retaining drugs

Work overload

- anaemia
- thyroid disorder
- pulmonary embolism
- pneumonia and other infections

Myocardial disease

- ischaemic heart disease
- alcoholic and other cardiomyopathies
- heart block
- pericardial disease

History

Onset, duration and time of symptoms

Classical symptoms

- dyspnoea
- orthopnoea
- paroxysmal nocturnal dyspnoea
- peripheral oedema

Associated symptoms

- chest pain
- palpitations
- cough
- frothy sputum
- weight gain
- oliguria
- abdominal pain
- confusion
- lethargy
- weakness
- disturbed sleep
- general debility
- reduced exercise tolerance

Previous history

- heart disease
- lung disease
- kidney disease

Medication

Social and emotional factors

Examination

General

- pallor
- weight
- cyanosis
- oedema

Cardiovascular

- pulse

BP
JVP
heart size
heart sounds and murmurs

Respiratory
basal crepitations
wheezing
pleural effusions

Abdominal
enlarged liver
ascites

Investigation

FBC
ESR
U & E
LFT
Thyroid function tests
ECG
CXR (consider barium swallow)
Urinalysis (for protein and glucose)

Options

Emergency care (see p. 535)
Diet – salt restriction
Life-style – advise on exercise levels
Treat underlying conditions, e.g.
hyperthyroidism
anaemia
dysrhythmias

Diuretics – drug of first choice
Thiazide, e.g. cyclopenthiazide 500–1000 μg daily initially
Loop diuretic, e.g. frusemide 40 mg daily initially (beware hypokalaemia, especially if combined with digoxin)

Digoxin – drug of first choice in AF induced failure; dosage dependent on age and size (beware toxic effects)

Isosorbide dinitrate – used as a 3rd line drug or as an alternative to digoxin
Effective in reducing preload
Initially 40–80 mg daily gradually increasing the dose

Hydralazine e.g. apresoline 25 mg 12 hourly. Used to reduce after load but not appropriate if the patient is hypotensive. It may induce an SLE-like condition.

Follow-up

Regular weighing and clinical assessment to monitor initial diuretic therapy

Review symptoms and signs and potassium levels every 6 months
Monitor digoxin levels

Referral

Valvular disease
Congenital heart disease
Uncontrolled dysrhythmia for advice on further combination therapy.

See also:

Asthma and wheezing (p. 15)
Pleural effusions (p. 251)
Respiratory distress – LVF (p. 535)

Hyperlipidaemia

The management of hyperlipidaemia is still a contentious area of clinical practice. There is strong evidence that it is associated with an increased risk of coronary heart disease (CHD) but the efficiency of current treatment in reducing mortality is equivocal.

Hyperlipidaemia is defined as the elevation of serum cholesterol or triglyceride, or both, above the upper limits of normal. Statistically this is 6.5 mmol/l for cholesterol and 2 mmol/l for triglyceride.

Serum lipids are transported on protein carriers and are composed of a combination of

Very low density lipoproteins (VLDL) = mainly triglyceride

Low density lipoproteins (LDL) = major carrier of cholesterol

High density lipoproteins (HDL) = smaller portion of cholesterol (seems to have a beneficial effect as far as coronary heart disease is concerned).

Classification

There are five major types of hyperlipoproteinaemia but for practical purposes it is easier to consider the levels of cholesterol and triglyceride.

Raised cholesterol

An elevation of cholesterol with normal triglyceride may be found secondary to myxoedema and nephrotic syndrome. Occasionally it is familial and carries a much worse prognosis.

Raised triglyceride

This may be secondary to diabetes, liver disease, chronic

renal failure and alcohol excess. The majority of affected patients are overweight. Very high levels (>20 mmol/l) may lead to pancreatitis.

Combined hyperlipidaemia

Even modest elevation of cholesterol and triglyceride carries a much greater risk of CHD.

Indications for case findings

It would be inappropriate to screen the whole population and so a more selective approach should be considered in relation to other risk factors

- Strong family history of hypercholesterolaemia or early CHD in first degree relatives
- Hypertension
- Diabetes
- Associated physical signs – xanthelasma, xanthoma or premature arcus senilis
- Early development of coronary, cerebral or peripheral vascular disease (before 55 years)

History

Symptoms of ischaemic vascular disease
Past history of
- diabetes
- hypertension
- myxoedema
- pancreatitis

Family history of CHD or hypercholesterolaemia
Alcohol intake and smoking

Examination

Cutaneous stigmata
- xanthelasma or xanthoma

Arcus senilis
Pulse
BP
Peripheral pulses
Arterial bruits
Signs of cerebrovascular disease
Fundoscopy

Investigation

Fasting cholesterol
Fasting triglyceride
Fasting blood glucose
Urine protein
Plasma protein
Thyroid function
Urea, creatinine and amylase
LFT
MCV (may be helpful in indicating possible alcoholism)

HDL cholesterol may help to determine the relative risk and need for treatment (if available)

Considerations before treatment

The benefit of treating hyperlipidaemia with currently available techniques is equivocal. Each patient must be considered according to their risks including hypertension and smoking

Before undertaking treatment consider

- pre-menopausal women have a lower risk of CHD than men with equivalent cholesterol levels
- in the older patient (>55 years) the benefits aare less obvious according to currently available data
- if both cholesterol and triglycerides are raised the risk of CHD is greater
- results of cholesterol levels may be misleading if taken with 3 months of myocardial infarction

Options

General measures

Recommend regular exercise – this increases the level of HDL and improves general cardiovascular fitness

Treat co-existing risk factors such as hypertension, diabetes and smoking

Raised cholesterol

Exclude hypothyroidism and nephrotic syndrome

Reduce weight to achieve ideal body weight

Modify fat intake

- avoid fatty meats
- suggest alternative protein – chicken, turkey, veal and fish
- restrict dairy produce – milk, cream, cheese and eggs
- increase content of polyunsaturated fats – margarine from vegetable oils
- suggest grilling, rather than frying foods

Drug treatment if dieting measures fail after three months, e.g. cholestyramine 8 g twice daily with food and/or nicotinic acid 1 g three times a day.

Raised triglycerides

Exclude

- diabetes
- alcoholism
- liver disease
- chronic renal failure

Reduce weight to achieve ideal body weight

Modify fat intake (see above)

Drug treatment if dieting measures fail after 3 months and

triglyceride level is greater than 4 mmol/l, e.g. nicotinic acid 1 g 3 times a day. (The use of clofibrate should be restricted in view of possible long term effects.)

Referral

Failure to control hyperlipidaemia
Further investigations of CHD and underlying conditions.

Hypertension

Effective management of hypertension significantly reduces the incidence of hypertensive renal disease, strokes and cardiac failure; the evidence for a reduction in incidence of myocardial infarction is still wanting. It is therefore important to detect those patients at risk and maintain them at a safe level blood pressure for the rest of their lives. It is also important to inform the patient about the nature and risks of hypertension and to encourage their co-operation in the management.

A screening programme is the most complete way to detect hypertensives, but it requires careful organization and good motivation. Case finding is more simple. It is based on the observation that 95% of patients present to their doctor at least once every 5 years. Every patient contact should be considered as an opportunity to check that a recent BP has been recorded for patients aged over 35 years and particularly in those with associated risk factors.

Causes

Primary or essential hypertension
Accounts for more than 95% in general practice

Secondary hypertension
Renal
- Glomerulonephritis
- Pyelonephritis
- Renal artery stenosis
- Polycystic kidneys
- Polyartertis nodosum

Endocrine
- Conn's syndrome
- Phaeochromocytoma
- Cushing's syndrome
- Acromegaly

Coarctation of the aorta
Eclampsia in pregnancy
Medication
- oestrogen preparations
- steroids
- monoamine oxidase inhibitors

Risk factors

Raised systolic and diastolic pressures
Family history of hypertension or premature cardiovascular death
Raised cholesterol
Ischaemic heart disease
Diabetes mellitus
Renal disease
Smoking
Age <40 years

Complications

Premature death
Ischaemic heart disease
Stroke
Cardiac failure
Renal failure
Retinopathy
Encephalopathy

Measurements of BP

Avoid stress, anxiety and discomfort
Use appropriate cuff size and accurately calibrated sphygmomanometer
Measure BP in the right arm at the level of the heart with patient sitting
Allow mercury column to fall slowly
Record systolic and (phase V) diastolic pressures
Repeat recording later in the examination if the first BP is raised. Clinical intervention should be based on the average of at least 3 readings taken weekly (see Table 4.2)

Table 4.2

Age (years)	Investigate and treat (5% of patients)	Investigate and observe (35% of patients)	Normal (65% of patients)
40–64	>180/105	155/90 – 180/105	<155/90
<40	>165/100	140/85 – 165/100	<140/85
	Check 3 monthly	Check annually	Check 5 yearly

Case findings

Opportunistic measurements in all patients between 30 and 70 years old

Without evidence of end-organ damage there is no reason to treat hypertension in those over 65 since the disadvantages outweigh the benefits

History

Hypertension is usually asymptomatic but may be associated with
- chest pain
- shortness of breath
- ankle swelling
- claudication
- TIA
- visual changes

Past medical history of renal disease, diabetes, or hypertension in pregnancy

Family history of hypertension, cardiovascular or renal disease

Smoking

Drugs and alcohol

Diet

Social factors of occupation, driving and exercise

Examination

Weight

CVS
- BP in both arms
- peripheral pulses
- heart size and systolic murmur

Abdomen
- renal mass or bruit

CNS
- localizing signs
- check for hypertensive retinopathy

Grade		
	I	Arterial narrowing
	II	A/V nipping
	III	Haemorrhages and exudates
	IV	Papilloedema

Investigation

Urine – protein, glucose and microscopy

Urea and creatinine – renal functions

Electrolytes – endocrine disfunctions

CXR – cardiomegaly and rib notching

ECG – baseline for ischaemia and LV strain

Optional investigation

Serum lipids
Uric acid and glucose
Urine VMA
IVP
Haemoglobin

Options

Diet and life-style

- Weight reduction to ideal weight
- Consider a reduced salt intake
- Low fat/high fibre diet
- Moderate life-style and exercise
- Relaxation
- Meditation, bio-feedback, etc.
- Moderate alcohol intake
- Stop smoking.

Drug therapy

- β-blockers, e.g. atenolol 50–100 mg daily – the most common firstline drug
- Diuretic, e.g. chlorthalidone 50 mg daily – especially if associated with heart failure
- Combination of β-blocker with thiazide
- Calcium antagonists, e.g. nifedipine 10 mg 8 hourly initially – particularly in the elderly
- Vasodilators as a supplement to the above, e.g. hydralazine 25 mg 12 hourly
- Central hypotensives as an alternative to vasodilators, e.g. methyldopa 250 mg 8 hourly
- ACE inhibitors, e.g. captoprile 25 mg 8 hourly – usually in consultation with the cardiologist.

Follow-up

6–12 monthly when stabilized

Record

- BP
- Weight
- Pulse (if on β-blockade)

Check

- Electrolytes (if on diuretics)
- Proteinuria
- Retinopathy
- Cardiovascular status
- Drug side effects

Discuss

- Smoking
- Diet
- Drug compliance
- Reason for BP control and complications

Referral

Accelerated or 'malignant' hypertension, severe left ventricular failure or hypertensive encephalopathy for urgent therapy

Full assessment of renal functions if indicated
Treatment of correctable causes
Failure to control BP
Failure to control complications in the eyes, kidneys or CVS.

See also:

Retinopathy (p. 274)
Maternal disease in pregnancy (p. 367)

Hyperthyroidism

There is a well recognized pattern of presentation in thyrotoxicosis but the diagnosis can easily be missed especially when the patient is elderly, when cardiac signs predominate, or in 'apathetic hyperthyroidism'. There is a strong genetic factor, and thyroid stimulating immunoglobulins are know to be involved, yet the pathology is not fully understood. There are several rare causes but the most common causes are

- diffuse toxic goitre (Graves' disease)
- nodular toxic goitre (Plummer's disease).

Patterns of presentation

General
- heat intolerance
- excess sweating
- tiredness
- weight loss with increase in appetite

Goitre
- diffuse or nodular

Hands
- tremor
- sweating
- hot
- nail dystrophy
- clubbing

Eyes
- proptosis
- lid retraction
- lid lag

Cardiovascular
- atrial fibrillation
- tachycardia
- palpitations
- heart failure

Musculoskeletal
- proximal myopathy
- osteoporosis

Mental function
- mania

psychosis
agitation
overactivity
Gynaecological
amenorrhoea or menorrhagia

Examination — **Check for** the above presenting signs
Record
Neck circumference
Pulse rate
Weight
Cardiovascular status – including thyroid bruits

Investigation — T3, T4, and T3 uptake
ECG
Consider TRH tests

Options — Start antithyroid treatment
Initially carbimazole 10 mg 6 hourly (for 3 weeks)
Maintenance dose (for 12–18 months)
Carbimazole 5 mg 6–8 hourly
Start β-blockade if sympathetic symptoms are dominant, e.g. propranolol 40 mg 6 hourly (a regular dosage must be maintained).

Follow-up — Plan regular appointments
Record
Neck circumference
Pulse rate
Weight
Clinical assessment of thyroid status
thyroid function tests (e.g. T3) at intervals
Review drug therapy when euthyroid

Referral — For surgery
failure of medical treatment after 12–18 months
severe thyrotoxicosis
large goitre with or without symptoms of compression
For radio-iodine
post-menopausal hyperthyroidism
recurrent disease
surgery contraindicated.

Failure to control — Repeat thyroid function tests and include T3 concentration and/or TRH
Review the diagnosis
excessive thyroid stimulation
excessive thyroid hormone – ingested or secreted
excessive iodine
thyroiditis

Complications

Relapse (of hyperthyroidism) after medical treatment
Side effects of β-blockade
Hypothyroidism
Hypothyroidism in neonates if mother was treated in pregnancy
Hyperthyroidism in neonates if mother was not treated in pregnancy
Thyrotoxic crisis

See also:

Goitre (enlarged thyroid) (p. 93)
Maternal disease in pregnancy (p. 367)

Hypothyroidism

The classical pattern of presentation for advanced myxoedema should be easily recognized. With vigilance and clinical skill the patient need not suffer the early changes of the disease which are easily missed. Hypothyroidism is more common than hyperthyroidism. It is more common in women (10:1) and occurs in the older age groups.

Causes

Autoimmune disease (Hashimoto's disease)
Antithyroid drugs
Thyroidectomy
Irradiation
Iodine deficiency
Tumours

Patterns of presentation

General
- hypothermia and cold intolerance
- weight gain, fatigue

Goitre – usually diffuse

Mental function
- coma
- psychosis
- depression

Skin
- myxoedema
- dry skin
- hair loss

Eyes – puffiness

ENT
- hoarse voice
- hearing loss

Cardiovascular
- heart failure
- angina
- slow pulse

Digestive system – constipation

Gynaecological – amenorrhoea or menorrhagia
Neurological
- polyneuritis
- cerebellar features

Musculoskeletal
- arthritis
- aches
- carpal tunnel syndrome

Examination

Check for the above presenting signs
Record
- Temperature
- Neck circumference
- Pulse rate
- Weight
- BP
- Cardiovascular status

CNS examination – especially the reflexes

Investigation

TSH
T_4
Thyroid antibodies
Hb
MCV
Cholesterol
ECG
CXR

Options

Education on condition and need for continuing therapy
Thyroxine (50–300 μg daily) graduating the dosage by 50 μg every 2 weeks – with particular caution in the elderly
Iodine supplements
Treat any associated anaemia.

Follow-up

Every 2 weeks until euthyroid
Every 6 months when euthyroid
Record
- Neck circumference
- Pulse
- Weight

Clinical assessment of thyroid status
Thyroid function tests at intervals
Check for signs of hyperthyroidism from overdosage (see p. 479)

Failure to control

Review diagnosis, including
- enzyme defects
- pituitary failure

thyroid agenesis
thyroid atrophy (complication of Hashimoto's disease)
B_{12} deficiency anaemia (may be associated with hypothyroidism)

Review drug regimen especially in the elderly and in those with previous heart failure

Referral

Profound hypothermia
For initial therapy if frail and elderly or if known to have severe ischaemic heart disease
For investigation of suspected pituitary failure.

See also:

Depression (p. 63)
Enlarged thyroid (p. 93)
Hypothermia (p. 154)
Lethargy (p. 183)

Multiple sclerosis

Multiple sclerosis is a chronic and usually progressive disease with exacerbations and remissions. It affects 1:1000 patients; women more commonly than men (3:2). The onset usually occurs between 20 and 40 years of age.

It is a disease of demyelination affecting any part of the CNS. Various factors have been incriminated in the underlying mechanism including autoimmunity, virus infection, nutritional and genetic factors.

The presentation of symptoms and signs is 'disseminated' in time and location and so demands full and repeated neurological assessment. The diagnosis is usually made retrospectively after two or more acute exacerbations.

History

A full neurological history should include an enquiry about the following
diplopia, blurring of vision or unilateral visual loss
motor or sensory changes in the limbs
inco-ordination of movement or stiffness
sphincter disturbance
mood changes
exacerbation of symptoms by fever or exhaustion

Examination

A full neurological examination to determine the site and size of the demyelinated areas should include the following
visual acuity
fundi – optic atrophy following retrobulbar neuritis
srabismus and nystagmus
motor disturbance and cerebellar signs are common

sensory changes are difficult to assess
bladder size

Investigation

Refer to neurologist for
lumbar puncture analysis
visual and auditory evoked potentials on EEG
brain scan
Consider
serum tests for syphilis

Options

Specific therapy

Acute exacerbations
ACTH 120 units twice weekly reducing over one month (or oral prednisolone 10–30 mg daily)
Muscle spasms
Baclofen 5–20 mg 8 hourly increasing slowly
Diazepam 6–60 mg per day in divided doses
Depression – careful counselling
Amitriptyline 75–150 mg per day in divided doses or at night
Pain – simple analgesia
Aspirin or paracetamol
Carbamazepine 100–200 mg 8 hourly for neuralgias
Urinary frequency and urgency
Propantheline 15–30 mg 6 hourly
Emepronium 200 mg 8 hourly
Urinary hesitancy or retention
Phenozybenzamine 10–20 mg daily or catheterization.

Team care

Physiotherapy – to maintain mobility and independence
Occupational therapy – to assess for aids to daily living
Speech therapy – may be helpful in individual cases
Home help and domiciliary nurses – may be required in later stages
Health visitor – for general support particularly if the patient has small children.

General advice

Discuss with patient and family the diagnosis and prognosis according to individual circumstances
Diet – there is no specific dieting advice but there is some limited evidence that polyunsaturated fats high in linoleic acid may be helpful
MS society for information and support
Pregnancy is not precluded but may pose social problems and difficulties with future care.

Referral

To confirm or exclude the diagnosis of multiple sclerosis
Failure to control the symptoms

To exclude structural lesions in optic nerve or spinal cord
For specialist advice and support in rehabilitation.

Complications

Urinary symptoms – infection, retention, urgency and frequency
Depression
Psychosexual problems
Constipation
Epilepsy
Tremor
Trigeminal neuralgia
Contractures
Stasis ulcers
Obesity

See also:

Weakness and clumsiness (p. 333)

Osteoarthritis

Osteoarthritis is the commonest cause of arthropathy. It is a degenerative condition of joints with fibrillation and erosion of the articular cartilage, cystic destruction of the underlying bone and marginal osteophyte formation.

It may be primary, or otherwise is secondary to some other destructive arthropathy or to injury.

It occurs in any joint but primarily affects
hips
knees
lumbar spine
cervical spine
hands
feet
shoulders

The incidence increases with age, and women are more often affected than men. Females tend to suffer mostly in the hands and knees while men suffer more in the hips.

Obesity is said to be a predisposing factor in weight bearing joints. However, it is conspicuously less common in the ankle joint and symptoms are little improved after weight loss.

History

Distribution and duration of joint involvement
Pain at night
Morning stiffness (usually less than 15 minutes)
Degree of pain and disruption of activities of daily living
Occupation

Past history of
- trauma to joints
- peripheral neuropathy – syphilis or diabetes
- gout

Examination

Record
- Weight
- Leg length
- Swelling and deformity of affected joints
- Range of mobility and presence of crepitus

Check for
- Heberden's nodes on finger joints
- Associated muscle wasting
- Signs of nerve compression, e.g. cervical spine

Investigation

X-ray affected joints (assess loss of joint space, cystic degeneration and osteophyte formation)
ESR
FBC
Uric acid and biochemical screen
Rheumatoid factor and ANF

Options

Pain relief

There are many available drugs and it is often necessary to 'ring the changes' to find the most effective
Narcotic analgesia is not appropriate in osteoarthritis
Non-narcotic analgesia, e.g.
- Paracetamol 0.5–1 g 6 hourly
- Dextropropoxyphene 65–130 mg 6 hourly
- Nefopam 30–60 mg 6 hourly

NSAID enolic acids, e.g.
- Indomethacin 100 mg 6 hourly
- Piroxicam 20–40 mg daily

NSAID carboxylic acids
Acetic acids, e.g. diclofenac 25–50 mg 8 hourly; indomethacin 25 mg 8 hourly
Salicylic acids, e.g. aspirin 600–900 mg 4 hourly; benorylate 10 ml 12 hourly
Proprionic acids, e.g. naproxen 250 mg 8 hourly; ibuprofen 200–400 mg 8 hourly
Fenamic acids, e.g. mefenamic acid 500 mg 8 hourly.

Physiotherapy

Active exercise will improve muscle function. Heat treatment may improve pain and stiffness.

Domiciliary OT

Can help with practical aids and advice in the home and to

provide walking sticks and other aids helpful in hip disease.

Weight reduction

Seems reasonable when weight bearing joints are affected but efficiency in symptom relief has yet to be proven.

Exercise

To the limit of pain to maintain and maximize the function of the joint.

Referral

For surgical assessment in the presence of intractable pain
For special aids such as footwear, corsets or built-up shoes.

See also:

Rheumatoid arthritis (p. 493)

Parkinsonism

Parkinsonism is a condition characterized by tremor, rigidity and hypokinesia. It is a common finding, especially in the elderly and there are several causes.

Parkinson's disease was first described in 1817 by Parkinson, as 'Paralysis agitans'. It is a distinct entity and is only one of the causes of parkinsonism.

The doctor's observation of the classical signs may precede the patient's perception of the symptoms.

Causes

Paralysis agitans – idiopathic classical Parkinson's disease. Progressive type starting in 50–60 years age group. More common in males. There may be a familial tendency

Atherosclerotic – occurs in a slightly older age group and is usually associated with other signs of cerebrovascular disease such as upper motor neurone lesions, pseudobulbar palsy and dementia. It responds poorly to anti-parkinsonian therapy

Toxic – parkinsonism may be precipitated by phenothiazines, butyrophenones or poisoning with carbon monoxide, manganese or copper

Post-encephalitic – this was more common after the First World War but is still occasionally seen after encephalitis lethargica

History

Duration of symptoms
Difficulty rising, or initiating movements
Tremor
Poor balance and falls
Mood changes
Writing becoming smaller

Change in voice
Increased salivation
Drug history and exposure to toxins
Past history of encephalitis

Examination

Full neurological examination including
- tremor
- poor facial expression
- poor balance
- glabellar tap
- mental state
- rigidity (lead pipe and cogwheels)
- slow monotonous speech
- shuffling gait, leaning forward
- test writing

CVS – BP
Skin – seborrhoeic changes

Investigation

FBC
ESR
Serum tests for syphilis

Options

Levodopa
Improves hypokinesia
Most effective in idiopathic variety of classical Parkinson's disease
Is best used in combination with carbidopa (as Sinemet) to reduce extracerebral side effects of nausea, anorexia, cardiac arrythmias and postural hypotension
Dosage should be increased by small increments every 3 days until full benefit is evident or side effects supervene.

Anticholinergic agents
- Benzhexol 6–10 mg per day (in divided doses)
- Benztropine 1–2 mg per day
- Orphenadrine 150–300 mg per day (in divided doses)

These are most useful for rigidity
Side effects include blurred vision, dry mouth, urinary retention and glaucoma.

Other agents
Amantadine }
Bromocriptine } have a limited usefulness.

Antidepressants
- Tricyclics: amitriptyline 75–150 mg per day
- Tetracyclics: mianserin 30–90 mg per day

MAOI antidepressants should be avoided.
Physiotherapy may be helpful for rigidity.
Supportive counselling for the sufferer and his family.

Referral

Failure to control symptoms
For stereotactic surgery (particularly useful for tremor)
Poor medical control
Severe side effects of drug treatment.

See also:

Lethargy (p. 183)
Tremor (p. 315)

Prevention

The opportunities for effective prevention of illness are not exclusive to primary medical care. Historically, social reforms and public health measures have had more success than medical services in the eradication of disease. Education, local and central government, the media and the individual all have a part to play in prevention.

If the resources of manpower, expertise and knowledge within primary care could be mobilized and organized much avoidable suffering and many unnecessary premature deaths might be prevented.

Primary prevention

Intervention before a disease develops by removing the cause of that disease

Scope

Smoking related diseases
Alcohol related diseases
Occupational diseases
Accidents
- home
- work
- RTA
- leisure

NAIC and family violence
Affective disorders
Obesity and malnutrition
Dental disease
Hypothermia
Genetic disorders
Infectious diseases

Options

Medical practice
Advice on smoking and alcohol
Recognition of 'vulnerability factors' in personalities
Recognition of risk factors in family dynamics

Immunizations of children, adults and travellers
Genetic counselling

Health education

Diet and exercise
Accident prevention
Home management
Personal and dental hygiene

Legislation

Measures to promote good health, e.g.
- fostering orders
- food controls

Measures to prevent ill health, e.g.
- smoking laws
- alcohol controls.

Secondary prevention The prevention of complications, or even the development of a disease by early detection and appropriate intervention

Scope

Screening
- Cervical cancer
- Hypertension
- Occupational health, e.g. rubber workers

Case finding
- Diabetes
- Glaucoma
- Hypertension
- Rectal or colonic cancers
- Breast cancer
- Pelvic cancers
- Anaemia
- Developmental delay
- Adolescent problems

Options Clinical protocols for opportunistic or planned clinic intervention can be developed with manual or computerized 'call and recall' to serve the target population
- Cervical cytology
- Immunizations (e.g. tetanus)
- CVS risk factors (including BP, weight, smoking and lipids)
- Hypertension
- 'Well woman clinics'
- Infant welfare clinics
- Pre-school and school medical services (including audiometry).

Tertiary prevention The prevention or limitation of avoidable complications and disability in avoidable disease

Scope

Diabetes
Thyroid disorders
Asthma
Arthritis
Ischaemic heart disease
Cerebrovascular accidents
Old age
Personality disorders
Alcoholism
food allergy

Options

Early diagnosis
- glaucoma, alcoholism

Opportunistic case finding
- food allergy

Planned care
- 'mini-clinics' – asthma, diabetes
- 'protocols' – thyroid disorders, hypertension

Continuing care
- careful prescribing
- crisis intervention in vunerable personalities

Surveillance of social psychological and physical status
- housework, anxiety, incontinence in the elderly
- mobility, loneliness, pain in arthritis.

Co-operation

Hospital services
Health visitors
District nurses
Occupational therapists and physiotherapists
Families
Friends
Chiropodists
Dieticians
Dentists
Opticians
Counsellers

See also: Health education (p. 466)

Pulmonary tuberculosis

TB is now relatively uncommon in the UK but it must be included in the differential diagnosis of many presenting symptoms and signs.

Pulmonary TB is most commonly detected on routine chest X-rays but the diagnosis should always be considered in the clinical assessment of chest disease.

Differential diagnosis

Chronic bronchitis
Pneumonia
Bronchiectasis
Congestive cardiac failure
Bronchogenic carcinoma
Diabetes mellitus

Vulnerable groups

The elderly over 65 years
Asian immigrants
Vagrants and alcoholics
Diabetics
Patients after gastric surgery
Patients on steroids

History

Persistent cough – resistant to antibiotics
Weight loss
Night sweats and fever
Haemoptysis
Lethargy
Recent TB contact

Examination

Weight
Temperature
Finger clubbing
Enlarged lymph nodes
Erythema nodosum
Auscultate for localizing signs or pleural effusion

Investigation

FBC
ESR
Mantoux test (0.1 ml of 1:10,000 followed by 0.1 ml of 1:1000 if negative)
Tine test may be a more convenient alternative
Examination of sputum (three samples) for microscopy and culture
Early morning urine (three samples) for microscopy and culture
Chest X-ray

Referral

Refer all suspected or confirmed cases to chest clinic for chemotherapy and case contact.

Follow-up

In co-operation with chest clinic
- restrict contact until sputum cultures are negative
- continue supervision for several years after chemotherapy has stopped with 6 monthly or annual chest X-rays
- contacts should also be investigated.

Prevention

BCG
- for tuberculin-negative children aged 11–13 years
- for babies with suspected contact with an open case of TB

Rheumatoid arthritis

Rheumatoid arthritis may be caused by an autoimmune disorder. It affects connective tissue in general and synovial joints in particular, principally involving the peripheral joints in a characteristically symmetrical fashion.

The presentation and course of the disease are very variable. It tends to be chronically progressive perhaps with exacerbations and remissions leading to crippling destruction of the affected joints in over half the cases. The onset is often insidious with general aches and stiffness in the affected joints. It can be associated with a more acute febrile toxic state.

Females are more frequently affected than males (3:1)

It occurs at any age but more commonly between 25 and 55 years of age. There is a familial predisposition but genetic transmission has not been clearly defined.

Differential diagnosis

Rheumatoid factor positive
- Systemic lupus erythematosis
- Sjögren's syndrome
- Sub-acute bacterial endocarditis

Rheumatoid factor negative ('Sero-negative arthritis')
- Psoriasis
- Reiter's syndrome
- Ankylosing spondylitis
- TB
- Rubella
- Colitis and Crohn's disease

Polymyalgia rheumatica
Gout

History

Onset and duration of joint involvement
Associated symptoms
- weight loss
- fatigue and depression
- tenosynovitis
- carpal tunnel syndrome
- shortness of breath
- dry eyes

Disruption of activities of daily living and mobility
History of
- trauma
- previous arthritis
- fever
- enteritis
- gout
- psoriasis
- TB
- STD

Family history of arthritis

Examination

Note affected joints and assess for
- synovial thickening
- deformity
- instability
- subluxation
- range of movement and level of function
- subcutaneous nodules

Check for complications and associated features (see above)

Investigation

FBC
ESR
Uric acid and biochemical screen
Latex test or rheumatoid factor (not always helpful diagnostically since 25% are negative)
ANF
X-ray hands and feet and other affected joints for erosive changes
Viral screen (particularly rubella antibodies)
Protein electrophoresis

Options

Rest

Immobilization of individual joints or general recumbent rest can be beneficial in the acute phase.

Pain relief

There are many available drugs and it is sometimes necessary to 'ring the changes' to find the most effective.

Narcotic analgesia – seldom appropriate in rheumatoid arthritis.

Non-narcotic analgesia – e.g.

Paracetamol 0.5–1 g 6 hourly;
Dextropropoxyphene 65–130 mg 6 hourly;
Nefopam 30–60 mg 6 hourly.

NSAID–enolic acids, e.g.

Indomethacin 100 mg 6 hourly;
Piroxican 20–40 mg daily.

NSAID–carboxylic acids, e.g.

- Acetic acids, e.g.
  - Diclofenac 25–50 mg 8 hourly;
  - Indomethacin 25 mg 8 hourly
- Salicylic acids, e.g.
  - Aspirin 600–900 mg 4 hourly
  - Benorylate 10 ml 12 hourly
- Proprionic acids, e.g.
  - Naproxen 250 mg 8 hourly
  - Ibuprofen 200–400 mg 8 hourly
- Fenamic acids, e.g. mefenamic acid 500 mg 8 hourly.

Second line anti-rheumatoid drugs

Steroids – systemic or local injection
Penicillamine
Gold
Azathioprine
Chloroquine

Useful but very toxic and should be used only after consultation with a rheumatologist.

Physiotherapy

Should aim to maintain or improve muscle and joint function

Quadriceps exercises are particularly important in patients after prolonged bed rest

Until the acute arthritis is settled isometric exercises are best

Local heat or cold applications may ease the pain prior to exercising

Domiciliary OT

To advise on and provide practical aids for mobility, accommodation and activities of daily living (ADL).

Support groups

Family and friends
District nurse

Physiotherapist
Social worker
Home help
Clubs and church
British Rheumatism and Arthritis Association.

Referral

Failure to control symptoms with simple measures
To assess the use of long term second line drugs
For surgery to affected joints
For provision of special aids – walking splints, footwear, etc.

Follow-up

Response to analgesia
- pain
- stiffness
- mobility
- dexterity

Mobility
- ADL
- sticks or wheels
- car

Accommodation
- modification to house
- ramps and rails
- toilet and bath
- kitchen

DHSS benefits
Support group involvement

Complications

Joints
- fixed or deformed joints
- secondary osteoarthritis
- septic arthritis
- osteoporosis
- muscle wasting

Skin
- subcutaneous nodules and rashes

Eyes
- episcleritis,
- iritis and keratoconjunctivitis sicca

Heart
- myocarditis
- pericarditis
- valvulitis
- vasculitis

Blood
- anaemia (usually normochromic but may be iron deficient from GI blood loss with associated drugs)

Lungs
- pleurisy
- pleural effusions and fibrosing alveolitis

Nerves
- entrapment neuropathies
- peripheral neuropathies

Others
- amyloidosis of kidneys
- Sjögren's syndrome
- depression
- side effects of drugs

Indications of a poor prognosis

Older age at onset
Insidious onset
High titre of rheumatoid factor
Other systemic manifestations
Early appearance of bony erosions
Rheumatoid nodules
Polyarticular presentation
Vasculitis

See also: Osteoarthritis (p. 485)

Stroke

The incidence of strokes is 2 per 1000 patients per year and it increases with age. The mortality is 30% within the first month. However, another 30% will be back at work within six months. In the UK approximately 100,000 patients have a residual deficit from a stroke.

The initial assessment of a stroke is only one aspect of primary care; more importantly, the doctor must co-ordinate the rehabilitation and supporting agencies that become involved with stroke patients.

Causes

Infarction (80%)
- Cardiac embolism
- Atheroma
- The Pill
- Endoarteritis (TB, syphilis, SLE, PAN, giant cell arteritis)

Haemorrhage (20%)
- Aneurysm
- Anticoagulant drugs
- Hypertension

Patterns of presentation

Transient ischaemic attack (TIA)

Episode of focal neurological deficit of less than 24 hours duration due to disturbance of vascular supply to the brain

Symptoms include visual disturbance, weakness or loss of sensation in limbs, ataxia, dysarthria, dysphasia and vertigo.

Completed stroke

Episode of focal neurological deficit of more than 24 hours duration due to disturbance of vascular supply to the brain

The neurological deficit is usually persistent to some degree.

Sub-arachnoid haemorrhage (SAH)

Sudden onset of severe headache, 'like a kick in the head', with vomiting, unconsciousness, focal signs and neck stiffness.

History

Neurological deficit

Rate of onset

Associated symptoms
- Confusion
- Headache
- Fever
- Neck stiffness
- Fits
- Prodromal illness
- Vomiting
- Visual disturbance
- Level of consciousness
- Speech deficit

Past history
- Diabetes
- Migraine
- Stroke
- Vascular disease
- Hypertension
- Trauma
- TIA
- Contraceptive pill

Examination

Neurological
- Level of consciousness
- Neck stiffness
- Pupils
- Fundi
- Visual fields
- Localizing signs
- Speech
- Gait
- Power
- Co-ordination
- Reflexes

Cardiovascular
- Valve disease
- Bruits
- Pulses
- BP

Check for
- Fever
- Breast disease
- Liver enlargement
- Chest disease
- Metabolic disease

Functional assessment
- Mental function
- Hearing
- Balance
- Swallowing
- Sphincter control
- Speech
- Vision
- Power
- Sensation

Investigation

- FBC
- Platelets
- ESR
- U & E
- LFT
- Blood glucose
- Syphilis serology
- Chest X-ray
- ECG

Home care

Poor prognosis

Elderly, comatose, dense hemiplegia and conjugate deviation of the eyes

If the immediate prognosis is very poor then home care should only be undertaken with the consent of the family

Good prognosis

Elderly, mild disability and fully conscious

If the home circumstances are good and supportive then home care is indicated

Rehabilitation

Advise on
- bathing
- transferring
- lifting
- passive movements
- toilet
- dressing
- mobility aids
- pressure sores

Follow-up

Assess extent of deficit

Rehabilitation – regular co-ordinated visits by a member of a primary care team to detect complications and to check general health and morale

BP check if relevant

Referral

Hospital care
- SAH
- Coma
- Hypertension
- Incontinence
- Changing level of consciousness
- Bulbar palsy
- Poor home circumstances.

Neurological assessment
- TIA
- Young patients
- Cardiac embolism from vascular disease
- Consideration for angiography or CT scanning.
- Uncertain diagnosis

Rehabilitation
- Physiotherapy
- Occupational therapy
- Speech therapy
- Chest, Heart and Stroke Association.

Complications

Further stroke (30%)

Death in 5 years (50%)

Immobility resulting in DVT, pulmonary embolism, contractures, oedema, incontinence, pressure sores
Psychological effects, e.g. dementia, paranoia, apathy, depression, insomnia
Families of stroke patients may suffer depression, low morale and increased risk of physical illness.

See also:

Faints (p. 101)
Headaches (p. 133)
Numbness and tingling (p. 221)
Weakness and clumsiness (p. 333)

5 Terminal Care

Stillbirth

A stillbirth can provoke as profound a bereavement reaction as a death in later years. Sympathetic and well-informed advice given immediately after the birth may form the basis of subsequent counselling with the bereaved parents. Seeing and touching the stillborn child may be helpful in confirming the fact of death to the parents and they should be offered the opportunity to do so.

Abortion before 28 weeks' gestation requires no certification or notification to the Registrar provided the child has not breathed or shown other signs of life. Formal burial or cremation is at the discretion of the parents.

Stillbirth after 28 weeks' gestation or of a child which has shown signs of life irrespective of the gestational age must, by law, be certified by a doctor and midwife and notified to the Registrar of Births, Marriages and Deaths, within 42 days. He will then issue a certificate of burial or cremation. The funeral will be arranged privately or by the hospital.

Early neonatal death

Early neonatal death, within the first 28 days of life, must be certified on a neonatal death certificate and notified to the Registrar of Births, Marriages and Deaths. He will then issue a certificate of burial or cremation. The funeral will be arranged privately or by the hospital.

Cot death

Cot death, or 'Sudden Infant Death Syndrome' (SIDS) as it is more accurately described, accounts for half of all deaths before the age of 2 years. In the UK the incidence is 1:500 live births; it can occur between the ages of 1 week and 2 years, and has a maximum age incidence at 10 weeks.

With continuing research into the condition cot deaths are becoming better understood. The majority of cases occur in apparently healthy babies. In some cases sudden death occurs with co-existent minor illness, and in a minority an unrecognized abnormality or serious illness is discovered. Besides many other aspects of the condition certain epidemiological factors are becoming well recognized.

Factors associated with SIDS

Male:female ratio 5:4
Low birth weight
Young maternal age
Urban dwelling
Twins
Sleep related
Infection
Winter months (in older babies)
Siblings of SIDS babies

Patterns of presentation

The majority of cot deaths occur at home and the family doctor is often the first to be called

If the baby has been taken directly to a hospital the family doctor should make contact with the parents as soon as he has been informed

These families are in need of immediate, informed and sympathetic support

Action

Assess viability and resuscitate when possible
Confirm death and exclude non-accidental death
Contact parent or parents if absent
Discuss how to inform/explain to siblings
Enable parents to handle their baby, if they wish
Warn the parents and explain the reasons for subsequent events
Inform the coroner or his officer (police)

Report

For the coroner's information
Exact time and circumstances surrounding the discovery of the death including the position of the baby and attempts at resuscitation
Details of clothes, bedding and room temperature
History of pregnancy and neonatal period
History of recent illness
Family history if significant
Record observations of
- rectal temperature (and the time of measurement)
- rigor mortis
- skin colour
- signs of injury
- presence of blood or vomit

Other agencies

If the police are acting as the coroner's officer, they must exclude non-accidental death, supervise formal identification of the baby and arrange for the removal of the body.

The coroner may wish to call an inquest and will sign the death certificate

The hospital pathologist (or the coroner's pathologist) is responsible for the full investigation of the cause of death

Undertaker – arrangements are made by the family, the police or the hospital and the cost is met by the family

The health visitor who is already involved with the family is well established as a support and counsellor to the family

The hospital paediatrician may be called in to reassure the parents and to discuss any questions about the cot death and the investigations

A minister of religion (when appropriate) as a family support and comforter

The foundation for the Study of Infant Deaths are able to help and comfort bereaved parents by leaflets, telephone contact and direct counselling or support groups

Follow-up

Plan regular follow-up – co-ordinated when possible with the other helping agencies involved

Alleviate any sense of guilt

Discuss the 'normal'bereavement reactions

Suppress lactaction (e.g. bromocriptine 2.5 mg twice daily for 2 weeks)

Offer night sedation (e.g. temazepam 10 mg at night)

Encourage contact between the parents, their friends and the community

Discuss future pregnancies

Maintain contact with the family – the grief following a cot death may be profound and prolonged and can be exacerbated by the desertion of supportive counsellors ('the conspiracy of silence')

Complications

Sense of guilt

Loss of confidence in parenthood

Subfertility

Marital problems

Disturbed behaviour in the siblings

Extreme anxiety over future pregnancies

'Suspended grief' if the next pregnancy supervenes too soon.

Bereavement

The grief reaction of bereavement may start before the time of death and can continue for many years. Usually more than one person is bereaved after a death but often the grief of a family is projected onto one member. Grief can also follow abortion, stillbirth, cot death and death of pets. A dying person, too, may experience their grief of impending bereavement.

The grief reaction

Four phases are recognized but they do not necessarily follow consecutively and each phase may last a varying length of time

Numbness
Emotion (anger, guilt or protest)
Depression
Resolution

Assessment

Previous relationship with the deceased
Previous experience of death and bereavement
Previous personality and reaction of stress
Social support within and beyond the home
Arrangement of affairs, mourning and funeral
Assessment of domestic affairs
Mental state assessment of depressions or neurotic symptoms

Options

Before death – counselling the family and patient to anticipate the grief reaction and to recognize the need for mutual support.

At death – consider the opportunity for the bereaved to view the corpse especially in sudden death away from home or stillbirth in order to experience the reality which may be kinder than the fantasies that can develop later.

After death – honest discussion of the illness and bereavement. This also applies to children in the family.

Consider the use of sedatives and antidepressants.

Follow-up

Sympathetic assessment of the bereaved's grief reaction including their mental image of the deceased, their attitude to death and their own mortality.

Assessment of their new social role or degree of isolation

Review use of drugs and alcohol

Smoking and eating habits

Encourage any return to previous interests or adoption of new domestic skills

Complications

Mortality in the spouse increases up to tenfold in the first year of bereavement. This may be due to self-neglect, suicide, cardiac disease or a similar illness to that of the partner

Prolonged depression

Neurosis presenting as psychosomatic symptoms, obsessive behaviour patterns, fear of dying, hallucinations of the continued presence of the deceased

Delayed grief may only be experienced at the time of a later and less significant bereavement. Preoccupation with a pregnancy may postpone the grief reaction

Guilt and anger following death may be used as a potent emotional tool in disturbed family dynamics

Referral

Counselling by other members of the primary health care team, volunteers or the clergy

Association with Cruse, the Stillbirth and Cot Death societies, etc.

Psychotherapy

Psychiatric supervision if there is a danger of suicide or self-neglect.

Terminal care

This is the planned management during the final weeks or months when a patient is expected to die. When carried out comprehensively it is one of the most exacting and time consuming tasks the doctor has to undertake. The aim is to allow the patient to die in comfort and peace and with dignity, in the setting which is appropriate to his case. The process should also include the sympathetic handling of relatives involved in care of the patient.

Preparation

The setting

Hospital – the social trend in the UK has been towards terminal care in hospital. Most doctors and patients would prefer the death to occur at home in the company of caring relatives. Sadly, this is frequently not possible and many patients stay at home until the last few days when, because of social pressures, they are admitted to hospital. In a strange and busy ward the patient may feel rejected and lonely particularly when the terminal phase is only brief.

Hospice – the services of a hospice, if available, can be invaluable. Staff can be involved while the patient is still at home and if admission becomes necessary it can be into the care of trusted familiar and sympathetic 'friends'.

Home – Many patients wish to die at home. Whenever possible, the doctor should try to respect such wishes.

Counselling

Familiarity with the patient, his personality and social background is perhaps the doctor's greatest asset. It can give a good indication as to 'how, when and what' to tell the patient about his illness and prognosis, but it is important to let the patient progress at his own speed. Open ended questions about his understanding of the situation may give a clue as to when he is ready to discuss the subject. Some patients choose to remain in ignorance and this should be respected.

A sensitive and optimistically honest approach is preferable, otherwise trust may be lost. Regular and unhurried visiting is an important prerequisite to effective counselling by providing the opportunity for the patient to ask questions and it indicates the depth of personal support.

Relatives

It is important to involve the caring relatives. Where possible they should be included in discussions with the patient. This may help to overcome the 'conspiracy of silence' which can develop when the patient and his near relatives find discussion of the illness and the future difficult.

The relatives often have questions and fears which they may be too inhibited to bring up in front of the patient. They too may benefit from open discussion and it also sets the foundation for dealing with forthcoming bereavement. Arrangements for the funeral and possible financial affairs should also be considered.

Other helpers

Other helping agencies may be involved and the doctor has an important role as co-ordinator

- District nurses
- Health visitors
- Home help
- Domiciliary occupational therapists
- Marie-Curie Foundation

Ministers of religion
Social workers

Symptom control

Pain

As a general rule analgesics should be given prophylactically in adequate dosage and frequency and by the most convenient route (oral, suppository or injection). It is useful to have a protocol for preparations of increasing strength such as

Mild pain

Aspirin 300–900 mg 4–6 hourly orally
Paracetamol 500–1000 mg 4–6 hourly orally

Moderate pain

Dihydrocodeine 30–60 mg 4–6 hourly orally
Dextromoramide 5 mg 6 hourly orally

Severe pain

Morphine 10–20 mg 3–4 hourly orally or i.m.
Diamorphine 5–10 mg 3–4 hourly orally or i.m.

It is important to be familiar with the dosage and duration of action of the drugs. Ultimately they should be tailored to the needs of the patient without fear of addiction or tolerance

The opiates are often combined with cocaine but this is probably unhelpful and could be harmful. A better combination is with chlorpromazine for its tranquillizing and antiemetic effect. A laxative should also be considered with the long term use of opiates

Drugs should be given orally or by suppository as long as possible, saving the parenteral route until nearer the end

If these measures fail consider
nerve blocks
radiotherapy
cytotoxics
steroids.

Nausea and vomiting

Metoclopromide 10 mg 8 hourly – promotes gastric emptying

Chlorpromazine 25–100 mg 8 hourly – more sedating than metoclopromide

Prochlorperazine 5–25 mg 8 hourly – also useful in suppository form.

Anorexia

Loss of appetite and weight is often a distressing accompaniment of terminal illness. Patients may benefit from prednisolone 10–20 mg daily.

Shortness of breath

Treat associated heart failure with diuretics, e.g.

Frusemide 40 mg daily

Spironolactone 50–100 mg daily

Diamorphine 2.5–10 mg 3–6 hourly

Oxygen therapy

Consider aspiration of a pleural effusion if present.

Cough

For a dry irritating cough

Codeine linctus 5–10 ml

Methadone linctus 5–10 ml

For a 'death rattle' in the final stages

Hyoscine 0.4 mg by injection.

Anxiety/depression

These symptoms are commonly present in terminal illness and can enhance the effect of pain

Reassurance and regular attendance can often allay the development of these symptoms but consider the following drugs

Diazepam 2–10 mg 6 hourly

Chlorpromazine 25–100 mg 8 hourly

Amitriptyline 75–150 mg daily.

Insomnia

This frequent symptom is often not declared although a cause should be sought

Consider the following drugs

Nitrazepam 5–10 mg

Trichlofos 5–15 mg

Chlormethiazole 1–2 gm

Chlorpromazine 50–100 mg

Amitryptyline 75–100 mg.

Confusion

Increasing debility, anaemia, fever, electrolyte disturbance and cerebral metastases may all lead to a state of confusion. A drastic change in character sometimes with paranoid features can be very distressing to the relatives

Consider

Chlorpromazine 25–100 mg 8 hourly

Thioridazine 25–100 mg daily

Diamorphine 25–100 mg 3–6 hourly

Reconsider existing drug therapy which may be adding to confusion

Constipation see p. 55

Diarrhoea see p. 68

Incontinence see p. 190

Bereavement See p. 505

Management does not stop with the death of the patient. The relatives may still need support. A personal visit is helpful even if the patient died in hospital. It is essential to act as a sympathetic ear and to show a sensitive understanding of the guilt and anxiety sometimes associated with death.

See also:

Constipation (p. 55)
Diarrhoea (p. 68)
Loss of bladder control (p. 190)

6 Emergency Care

Anaphylactic shock

Assessment

Airway
- Stridor
- Bronchospasm
- Rhinitis

Circulation
- Hypotension
- Arrhythmia
- Tachycardia

Skin
- Angioneurotic oedema
- Urticaria
- Rash
- Pruritus

Gut
- Abdominal pain
- Vomiting
- Diarrhoea

History
- Allergies and exposure to allergens (Table 6.1)

Table 6.1. Common allergens

Antibiotics	Snake bites
Anti-inflammatory drugs	Insect bites and stings
Anti-arrythmic drugs	Various plants and pollens
Iron preparations	Nuts
Blood products	Eggs
Vaccinations	Milk
Desensitizing allergens	Shellfish

Action

Parenteral drugs
- Adrenaline (1:1000) 0.5 ml s.c. (repeated at 15 minute intervals if necessary)

Drugs
- Hydrocortisone 100–200 mg i.v.
- Chlorpheniramine 10 mg i.v. slowly

Circulatory collapse
- Establish i.v. line with electrolyte solution or plasma expander

Respiratory collapse
- Maintain airway and ventilation
- Oxygen
- Consider tracheostomy to relieve laryngeal obstruction.

Back injury

In any immobile casualty suspect a spinal injury until the diagnosis can be excluded.

Assessment

Establish the precise circumstances of the injury
Check for other injuries
Assess facilities for moving and transporting patient

Conscious patient

- May localize pain along the spine
- Sphincter control
- Check distribution of pain or anaesthesia
- Check the effect of cough impulse
- Observe movement of limbs and digits on request
- Check reflexes

Conscious or unconscious patient

- Palpate vertebral column
- Observe response to sensory stimuli – in *all* dermatomes

Action

Fractured vertebrae

Apply cervical collar on suspicion of spinal injury
Avoid patient slumping forward or changing position
Ensure adequate analgesia, e.g.

- Entonox
- Morphine 5 mg i.v./i.m.
- Prochlorperazine 12.5 mg i.v/i.m.

Move patient only when necessary

- in a fully supported position
- by a planned procedure
- gently
- with all available help

Transport in a supine position with padding to lumbar and cervical spine, and legs padded and bound
Accompany patient during transport especially if unconscious and supine to protect the airway

Acute back strain or prolapsed intervertebral disc

Ensure relaxed supportive position, e.g. supine on firm matress
Adequate analgesia
Muscle relaxants, e.g. diazepam 5 mg 8 hourly
Embrocation or warmth under the back
Refer to hospital if signs of nerve compression are present.

Bone injury

Assessment

Signs of a fracture

- Immobility or non-use (particularly in children)
- Pain and tenderness
- Deformity or shortening of the limb
- Instability
- Swelling
- Crepitus

Check for vascular or neurological complications
Exclude predisposing factors, e.g. osteoporosis or bony metastasis
Assess obvious and potential blood loss
Establish circumstances of the injury
Establish which bones are affected
Check for other injuries and/or shock.

Potential blood loss from fractured bones

Chest wall (closed injury)	2 litres
Pelvis (closed injury)	2 litres
Femur	1.5 litres
Other leg bones	1 litre
Arm bones	1 litre

Action

Establish i.v. line
- Normal saline, to maintain BP above 100 mm Hg systolic, or
- Haemacel 500 ml in 30 minutes

Immobilize the affected limb
- strap to adjacent limb
- inflatable splints
- Thomas splint or variant

Ensure adequate analgesia
- Morphine 5 mg i.v. with prochlorperazine 12.5 mg
- Entonox

Consider management of other injuries
Arrange referral for
- X-ray
- reduction of dislocation (and subsequent radiography)

Reduction of fractures and immobilization in plaster.

Burns

Assessment

Circumstances of burns
Distribution and extent of burns
'Rule of nines'
- Head 9%
- Trunk-front 2 × 9%
- Trunk-back 2 × 9%
- Upper limb 9%
- Lower limb 2 × 9%

Depth of burn
Associated shock (pulse and BP)
Check airway and respiratory involvement
Check for other injuries

Action

Immerse in water to
- reduce skin temperature
- reduce pain
- reduce severity
- dilute chemical burns

Leave blisters intact
Cover with sterile dressings
Resuscitate if necessary – i.v. fluids or plasma expander if available
Oxygen
Adequate analgesia

Home care

Small superficial burns
Cover with antiseptic dressings for 10 days – change when necessary.

Hospital care

Extensive burns
- 7% infant
- 10% child
- 15% adult

Burns to face, hands and perineum
Explosion injury or airway involvement
Large full thickness burns requiring skin grafting
Delayed healing of superficial burns.

Chest injury

Penetrating wounds and crush injuries, with or without 'flail-segments', are clinically obvious and require urgent action. The early changes of blunt injury are not clinically obvious but this too requires urgent action.

Assessment

Establish circumstances of the injury
Check for associated injuries
Check airway and degree of respiratory distress
Inspect skin for central and peripheral cyanosis
Inspect chest wall for
- deformity of ribs or sternum
- paradoxical movement
- penetrating wounds
- surgical emphysema
- trachea and mediastum – deviation from centre

Percuss and auscultate chest
Check for signs of internal haemorrhage
Aortic injury
Oesophageal injury
Diaphragmatic injury

Action

Cover any open chest wound
Maintain the airway
Ventilate if necessary
Arrange urgent transfer to hospital
Insert intercostal tube (with or without flutter valve) into second intercostal space anteriorly when a tension pneumothorax is present.

Coma

Assessment

Respiration
Establish that the airway is not obstructed
Note rate and rhythm of breathing

Circulation
Assess adequacy of pulse rate and rhythm; BP

Level of consciousness (record the time of examination)
Response to painful stimuli
Eye opening
Best verbal response

Other signs
Colour, hydration, skin changes
Evidence of injury – bleeding and fractures
Incontinence
Ketones or alcohol on breath
Pupils, fundi and reflexes
Neck stiffness
Rectal temperature
Evidence of overdose (drugs, vomit)

Witness report
Onset and duration of coma
History of injury
Patient's medical and drug history
Social circumstances

Differential diagnosis

Cerebral
Epilepsy
Stroke
Trauma
Infection

Metabolic
Diabetes
Hypoglycaemia
Biochemical imbalance (Na, Ca, P_{O_2}, P_{CO_2}, pH)
Respiratory failure
Hepatic failure
Hypothermia
Addison's disease
Uraemia

Toxic
Alcohol
Overdose

Circulatory
Low cardiac output (all causes)

Action

Resuscitation

- re-establish circulation and respiration
- i.v. drip and endotracheal intubation if possible
- control bleeding

Exclude spinal injury and major fractures

Do not move the casualty unnecessarily

Recovery position – in the absence of intubation consider nursing the casualty in the three quarters prone position

Establish diagnosis for further emergency treatment

Organize transport to hospital.

Convulsion

Assessment

Detailed description of convulsion – from a witness

Onset, duration, sequence of events and subsequent symptoms or signs

Medical history
- fever
- recent head injury
- epilepsy
- diabetes
- withdrawal of alcohol or drugs

Respiratory rate

Pulse

BP (sitting and standing)

Signs of
- injury
- incontinence
- fever
- focus of infection
- raised intracranial pressure (meningism)
- neurological deficit

Causes

Febrile convulsion

Hypoglycaemia (in neonates or diabetics)

Hypocalcaemia (in neonates)

Epilepsy

Tumour

Stroke

Syncope

Hyperventilation

Action

First aid

Maintain airway
Remove dentures
Three-quarter prone position
Avoid aggressive management
Cool the febrile child
Reassure attendants

Options

Anticonvulsants

Diazepam 5–10 mg i.v. or p.r. (0.2 mg/kg BW) repeat if necessary in adults

Paraldehyde 5 ml i.m. (0.1 ml/kg BW) repeat in opposite leg in adults if necessary

Brown paper pag in hyperventilation

Glucogan (i.m. or i.v.) 1 mg } hypoglycaemia in adult
50% Dextrose i.v. 20 ml } diabetic.

Referral

Immediate

Neonates
Persistent convulsion (>15 mins)
Incomplete recovery in 3 hours to exclude meningitis

Routine

Age <1 year or >75 years (for investigation of epilepsy)
Second febrile convulsion for investigation and prophylactic anticonvulsants
Signs of raised intracranial pressure
Management of stroke (see p. 497)

Eclampsia

Assessment

Confirm diagnosis – patient must be
- pregnant
- hypertensive
- convulsing

Obstetric history
Epileptic history
BP
Neurological examination
Fundal height
Fetal heart rate

Action

Control convulsion
- Diazepam 5 mg i.v. (repeat if necessary)

Control BP
- Diamorphine 5 mg i.v. (repeat if necessary)

Consult with obstetric flying squad
Continue to monitor
- pulse
- pupils
- BP
- reflexes
- conscious level
- fetal heart rate.

Electrocution

Assessment

Establish circumstance of the electrocution
- voltage, amps and duration of current
- source of the current
- points of entry and exit from the body

Do not approach patient until it has been confirmed that there is no continuing risk

Check
- Airway and respiration
- Cardiovascular status
- Level of consciousness and response

Assess
- Extent of burns
- Associated injuries
- Involvement of internal structures and organs

Action

Eliminate the source of electrocution
Ensure personal safety
Ventilate and/or resuscitate as necessary
Treat shock (see p. 540)
Treat burns (see p. 514)
Transfer to hospital.

Eye injury

Causes

Periorbital haematoma
Blunt injury
- 'blow out fracture' of orbit
- rupture of globe
- hyphaemia
- vitreous haemorrhage
- detached retina
- choroid rupture

Abrasions
Foreign body
Perforating injury
Burns
- toxic
- thermal

Assessment

Exact circumstances of injury
Associated symptoms (especially diplopia)
History of bleeding disorder or use of anticoagulants
Inspect cornea and conjunctiva (even when lids are closed by haematoma)
Inspect skin and eyelids
Examine visual acuity
Examine extra ocular muscle function to assess site and size of injury (see p. 300)
Avoid applying pressure to an injured globe

Action

Irrigate eye with water if there has been exposure to toxic material
Remove any foreign body under lid or in the cornea using 1% amethocaine drops and chloramphenicol drops or ointment for abrasions.

Referral

All other cases for hospital assessment
(nil by mouth in anticipation of general anaesthetic).

Head injury

Assessment

Check airway and respiration
Establish circumstances of the injury
Check for other injuries
Assess level of consciousness
Eye movements
Best verbal response
CNS examination particularly
- pupil response and size
- fundi

Check for
- CSF leakage from nose or ears
- skull fracture

If conscious assess the degree of pre- and post-traumatic amnesia

Action

Maintain airway if comatose
Organize transfer to hospital if there is
- loss of consciousness
- significant pre- or post-traumatic amnesia
- skull fracture

Monitor
- pulse
- BP
- respiratory rate
- pupil response
- limb movements
- level of consciousness.

Hyperglycaemia

Assessment

Known diabetic with
- inadequate control
- intercurrent infection

Undiagnosed diabetic

Recent history of
- Malaise
- Weight loss
- Infection
- Thirst
- Frequency of micturition
- Abdominal pain

Associated signs
- Gradual onset
- Flushed
- Bounding pulse
- Ketotic breath
- Dehydration
- Vomiting
- Confusion
- Coma

Urinalysis positive for glucose (+/−ketones)
Blood sugar >20 mmol/litre

Action

Blood samplc for glucose, urea and electrolytes
Soluble insulin 10 units s.c. or i.m.
i.v. fluids if dehydrated (normal saline 500 ml per 30 mins)
Organize immediate transfer to hospital.

Hypoglycaemia

Assessment

Known diabetic with oral agents or insulin

Recent history of

Excessive dosage
Excessive exercise
Delayed meals

Associated symptoms

Dizziness
Sweating
Hunger
Fainting
Nausea
Palpitations
Paraesthesia
Headache

Rapid onset of signs

Irrational or aggressive behaviour
Cold and clammy
Tachycardia
Coma
Incoordination
Pallor
Hypotension
Convulsions

Urinalysis negative to glucose
Blood sugar <2.4 mmol/litre

Action

Blood sugar for glucose
Conscious patient
Oral glucose or carbohydrate enriched meal
Unconscious or unco-operative patient
Glucagon 1 mg i.m.
Dextrose 50% 20 ml i.v. (repeat if necessary)
Urgent referral if no response
Review medication and diet.

Hypothermia

Assessment

Rectal temperature less than 35°C after 5 mins with a low reading thermometer
Cardiovascular state (particularly arrhythmia or bradycardia)
Level of consciousness
History of
- injury
- dementia
- drug abuse
- exposure
- hypothyroidism
- social problems

Action

Resuscitation
Attempt even after prolonged cardiac arrest
Refer to hospital
- rectal temperature less than 32°C
- home care inappropriate
- coma
- arrhythmia
- CCF
- stroke
- impaired respiration
- head injury
- overdose

Home care (see p. 154)
- Rectal temperature more than 32°C
- Room temperature 25–28°C
- Adequate supervision.

See also: Care of the elderly (p. 435)

Mental Health Act 1983 (England and Wales only) (Compulsory Admission to a Psychiatric Hospital)

Under this Act an application can be made for compulsory admission to a psychiatric hospital when the patient is suffering from a mental disorder warranting detention for their own health and safety or for the protection of others.

The following are the sections relevant to general practitioners.

Section 1 – Definition of mental disorder

Mental disorder
Means mental illness, arrested or incomplete development of mind, psychopathic disorder and any other disorder or disability of mind.

Mental impairment
Means a state of arrested or incomplete development of mind, which includes *significant* impairment of intelligence and social functioning and is associated with abnormally aggressive or seriously irresponsible conduct on the part of the person concerned.

Severe mental impairment
Means a state of arrested or incomplete development of mind, which includes *severe* impairment of intelligence and social functioning and is associated with abnormally aggressive or seriously irresponsible conduct on the part of the person concerned.

Psychopathic disorder
Means a persistent disorder or disability of mind (whether or not including significant impairment of intelligence), which results in abnormally aggressive or seriously irresponsible conduct on the part of the person concerned.

A person may not be regarded as suffering from mental disorder by reason only of promiscuity or other immoral conduct, sexual deviancy or dependence on alcohol or drugs.

Section 2 – Admission for assessment for up to 28 days

Application is made by the nearest relative or an approved social worker supported by two medical recommendations, one of them from an approved doctor, which states that the patient is suffering from a mental disorder which warrants his detention. The patient must be discharged after 28 days unless detained for further treatment.

Section 3 – Admission for treatment for up to 6 months

Application is made by the nearest relative or an approved social worker, supported by two medical recommendations, one of them from an approved doctor, which states that the patient is suffering from a mental disorder (severe) mental impairment or psychopathic disorder, that warrants his detention. In psychopathic disorders and mental impairment the treatment should be likely to alleviate the conditions or prevent deterioration. The two doctors must also indicate why other methods are inappropriate.

Section 4 – Admission for assessment in cases of emergency for up to 72 hours

Application is made by the nearest relative or an approved social worker, supported by one medical recommendation preferably from a doctor who knows the patient and examined him in the previous 24 hours. It must state that admission under Section 2 would involve undesirable delay. The grounds are those defined under Section 2. The patient must be discharged after 72 hours unless it is converted to Section 2.

Section 135 – Removing patients to hospital for up to 72 hours

A police constable or other authorized person on a magistrate's warrant may enter premises to remove a patient if he is considered to be suffering from a mental disorder, is being ill-treated, neglected, or is not under proper control, or that he is unable to care for himself and is living alone.

The patient is moved to a place of safety and detained for up to 72 hours until other arrangements can be made.

Section 136 – People in public places

A police constable who finds a person apparently suffering from mental disorder and in immediate need of care and control, can remove him to a place of safety for up to 72 hours for further assessment.

Relevant personnel

Nearest relative

In order

- Spouse
- Son or daughter
- Father
- Mother
- Sibling
- Grandparent
- Grandchild
- Uncle or aunt
- Nephew or niece

To the end of the list is added 'co-habitee' (who may be of the same sex), who has lived with the patient for five years or more.

Approved social worker Social worker approved by the local authority as having appropriate competence in dealing with mentally ill patients.

Approved doctor A doctor approved by the local health authority as having special experience in the diagnosis and treatment of mental disorder.

Action

Consult approved doctor (i.e. admitting psychiatrist)
Contact social worker who will supply documentation
Consider police and ambulance assistance
Complete documentation
Arrange transport to hospital
Make full notes for personal use in anticipation of any litigation.

Overdose and self-injury

Assessment

Establish circumstances of the event from patient or witnesses
- time and place
- sequence of events
- details of implements used
- degree of suicidal intent
- involvement of others
- quantity and nature of drugs used
- evidence of overdose
- evidence of alcohol abuse

General enquiry
- previous attempts
- recent mental state
- medical history
- psychiatric history
- social and environmental factors

Examination

Present mental state
Level of consciousness
Examination of injuries
General examination
Brief inspection of house for alcohol, drugs or toxic chemicals

Action

General supportive measures
Collect remaining drugs, containers, or implements
Contact poison centre (see p. 531)
Arrange transport to hospital
Arrange care for dependants.

Poisoning

Assessment

Poisons may be ingested, inhaled, injected or absorbed through the skin
Establish nature, quantity and time of poisoning
Symptoms and signs vary with the particular poison but consider
- nausea
- drowsiness
- headaches
- visual disturbance
- dyspnoea
- shock
- vomiting
- coma
- fits
- tinnitus
- failing respiration
- cardiac arrhythmias

Check for evidence of deliberate self-poisoning (see p. 530)

National poisons information service (24 hour cover)

Belfast 0232 30503
Cardiff 0222 492233
Dublin 0007 745588
Edinburgh 031 229 2477
London 01 407 7600

Action

Refer all cases if in doubt

Ingested poisons

Consider inducing vomiting with Ipecacuanha mixture, 15 ml with a glass of water. Do *not* induce vomiting if the patient has swallowed caustic chemicals or hydrocarbons or if the patient is comatose
Dilute the ingested poison with water or milk to drink if the chemical is caustic or a hydrocarbon.

Inhaled poison

Remove the patient from poisonous atmosphere as soon as possible
Clear the airway.

Transcutaneous absorption

Remove contaminated clothing with care
Wash the patient down.

General

Monitor pulse and respiration
Rescuscitate as necessary
Nurse comatose patients in the recovery position
Establish an i.v. line in shocked patients
Treat fits with intravenous diazepam (5–10 mg)
Try to send sample of poison or vomitus to the hospital with the patient.

Psychiatric emergencies

Causes

Confusion
Anxiety
Intoxication or withdrawal of drugs or alcohol
Personality disorders
Psychosis
Hypomania
Hypoglycaemia
Epilepsy
Suicidal depression

Assessment

Degree of social disturbance, embarrassment or threat to safety of self or others

History from witness

Onset and progress of disturbance
Preceding events
Previous psychiatric history
Drugs and alcohol

Examination

Pulse
BP
Temperature
Respiratory rate
Thyroid status
Focus of infection
Signs of trauma or intoxication
CNS especially tremor

Mental state

Clouding of consciousness
Orientation
Concentration
Restlessness
Paranoia
Fear
Mood – euphoria or depression
Memory
Attention span
Irritability
Psychotic thoughts
Panic

Action

Telephone advice as appropriate
Consider need for police or ambulance assistance
Reassure patient and family or attendants
Treat any underlying condition – at home or in hospital

- Diazepam 10–30 mg orally, i.m., i.v.
- Chlorpromazine 25–50 mg orally or initially 50–150 mg i.m.
- Chlormethiazole 1.5–2 g orally or i.v.
- Haloperidol 30 mg orally or i.m. (10 mg initially in elderly or patients with liver or heart disease)
- Propranolol 10–20 mg 6 hourly (in addition to diazepam for acute anxiety)

Rebreathing into a paper bag for hyperventilation

Discuss voluntary admission to hospital with patient and psychiatrist

Implementation of Mental Health Act 1983 (see p. 527)

Persuasion before coercion.

Respiratory distress – acute left ventricular failure

Assessment

Previous history
- Hypertension
- Myocardial infarction
- Valvular heart disease
- Paroxysmal cardiac arrhythmia
- Orthopnoea

Circulatory state
- Pallor
- Cyanosis
- Shock
- BP
- Pulse
- Heart murmurs
- Triple rhythm
- Signs of right heart failure

Respiratory state
- Bilateral basal crepitations
- Pleural effusions
- Frothy blood-stained sputum

Action

Frusemide 40–80 mg i.v. (further 40 mg if no response in 2 hours)
Diamorphine 5 mg i.v. or i.m. with prochlorperazine 12.5 mg if necessary after excluding chronic respiratory disease
Oxygen
Aminophylline 250–500 mg i.v. (slowly) if no response to above treatment or if asthma cannot be excluded
Nurse patient sitting up.

Referral

Failure to respond to therapy
Poor home circumstances
Suspected pulmonary embolism
Persistent arrhythmia.

Respiratory distress – asthma

Assessment

Previous history
Precipitating factors
- allergy
- stress
- infection
- environment

Current medication
Cyanosis and pallor
Pulse
BP
Signs of heart failure
Drowsiness
Expiratory wheeze
Hyperinflation
Peak flow assessment and respiratory rate

Action

Salbutamol – nebulized respirator fluid. 'Nebule' dosage depends on age
- Adult 250 μg i.v. or 500 μg i.m.
- Child 8 μg/kg i.m.

Hydrocortisone 100–200 mg i.v. or i.m. (of paramount importance in acute asthma)

Aminophylline – if it is difficult to differentiate between asthma and acute LVF use aminophylline 250–500 mg slowly i.v. (or 5 mg/kg in a child)

Monitor peak expiratory flow (PEF) before and after treatment.

Referral

Admit to hospital if
- Pulse >120/min
- PEF <100/min
- No response to treatment after 30 minutes
- Persisting cyanosis.

Respiratory distress – croup (laryngeal stridor)

The term croup is usually reserved for children under 3 years with infective laryngitis or epiglottitis and stridor. However, there are other causes which, although more rare, can occur in older patients.

Differential diagnosis

Laryngotracheobronchitis
Epiglottitis
Inhaled foreign body
Laryngeal trauma
Laryngeal oedema
Diphtheria
Whooping cough

Assessment

Onset of symptoms
Inspiratory stridor
Barking cough
History of inhaled foreign body
Fever, pallor, cyanosis
Pulse (tachycardia)
Respiratory rate
Respiratory effort (intercostal recession, use of accessory muscles)
Drooling saliva
Distress and level of consciousness
Avoid inspection of throat if epiglottitis is suspected

Action

For simple laryngitis sit the child up in a humid, steamy atmosphere
Consider antibiotics (amoxycillin or ampicillin as first choice)
Advise warm drinks
If condition settles quickly (within 30 minutes) reassess later.

Referral

No relief with initial management
Increasing respiratory distress or cyanosis
Inadequate social circumstances
Suspicion of epiglottitis, inhaled foreign body, laryngeal trauma or oedema, or diphtheria.

Assessment

Respiratory distress – pneumothorax

Chest pain of acute onset
Shortness of breath
Previous history of pneumothorax
Chest injury (puncture wounds, fractured ribs)
Asymmetrical chest expansion
Hyper-resonance to percussion (coin sound)
Decreased breath sounds
Deviated mediastinum (trachea and apex beat)

Action

Cover open chest wounds
Nurse in recumbent position on affected side
Oxygen
Organize transport to hospital
Tension pneumothorax – if there are signs of increasing respiratory embarrassment insert a wide bore needle through the second intercostal space on the affected side.

Road traffic accident

Approach

Ensure personal safety and wear reflective jacket
Park safely to
- protect casualties
- provide light
- warn other traffic

Co-operate with rescue services
Estimate the number and relative severity of casualties
Give clear instructions for any equipment or assistance required
Record relevant information and attach to patient

Assessment

Airway
Respiration
Circulation
Level of consciousness
Nature, degree and situation of injuries
Exclude or confirm spinal injuries

Action

Maintain the airway
Resuscitate
- stop any bleeding
- establish an i.v. line – N. saline or plasma expander

Ensure adequate analgesia
- Entonox
- Pethidine 100–200 mg i.v.
- Diamorphine 5–10 mg i.v.

Splint all suspected fractures
Avoid hypothermia
Monitor
- level of consciousness
- pupils and reflexes
- BP
- pulse.

Shock

Assessment

Airway
Respiratory rate
Skin colour
Level of consciousness
Restlessness
Stridor or bronchospasm
Pulse
BP
Temperature

History of

- Trauma or bleeding
- Chest pains
- Abdominal pain
- Vomiting or diarrhoea
- Allergen contact

Signs of

- External bleeding
- Internal bleeding
- Bone injury
- Crush injury
- Burns

Causes

Blood loss (external or internal)
Plasma loss (e.g. burns)
Electrolyte loss (e.g. dehydration)
Cardiogenic shock
Septic shock
Anaphylactic shock

Action

Maintain airway
Keep patient horizontal with legs elevated
Give oxygen
Monitor

- pulse
- BP
- respiratory rate
- skin colour
- level of consciousness

Fluid loss

Stop bleeding where possible
Take blood sample for cross matching
i.v. line N. Saline 1 litre (sufficient to maintain a BP of 100 mm Hg systolic)
Haemacel 500 ml in 15–30 minutes.

Cardiogenic shock
5% dextrose by slow i.v. infusion
Diuretic for CCF, e.g. frusemide 40–80 mg i.v.
Anti-arrhythmic drugs for arrhythmia (see p. 535)
Adequate analgesia
Splint any fractured bones
Ensure adequate analgesia, e.g.
  Morphine 5 mg i.v. (repeat after 15 minutes)
  Entonox (avoid in chest injuries)
Avoid hypothermia
Transfer to hospital without delay
Reassure patient and family.

Sudden loss of vision

Assessment

Onset and degree of visual loss
Preceding visual symptoms
Associated symptoms (e.g. pain)
Exact circumstances of any injury
Medication
History of diabetes or hypertension
Examine
- visual acuity
- visual fields
- cornea and conjunctiva
- retina, fundus and macula

Causes

Amaurosis fugax
Migraine
Glaucoma
Keratitis
Iritis
Central retinal artery occlusion
Central retinal vein occlusion
Vitreous haemorrhage
Retinal detachment
Retrobulbar neuritis
Giant cell cranial arteritis
Trauma including foreign body

Action

Refer for ophthalmological assessment.

Sudden unexpected death

Assessment

Confirm death has occurred
Establish circumstances from witness if possible
Confirm identity of deceased
Establish medical history from relatives or medical records if available
If unnatural death is suspected do not disturb the body or local environment until the police have been informed
Examine the body completely unclothed and particularly check for
- bruising
- injury
- wounds

Check the environment for evidence of possible suicide.

Action

Issue a certificate if the cause of death is known and the patient has received medical care in the last 14 days
Notify coroner's officer if
- the cause is uncertain
- there has been no medical care in the last 14 days
- the cause is suicide
- the cause is alcoholism or self-neglect
- the cause is the result of injury
- the cause is the result of medical treatment
- there are allegations of negligence
- the patient was receiving a war or disability pension
- the death occurs in prison or custody

Sympathetic support for the family in their bereavement
If the death is not reported to the coroner explain to the relatives the procedure for registering the death and offer the names of local undertakers
If there are no relatives arrange with an undertaker for the removal of the body
Arrange a post-mortem if it would help to confirm the cause of death.

See also:

Suicide
Cot death

Vaginal bleeding in pregnancy

Assessment

Blood loss
- rate and estimated volume
- fresh or altered
- noted products of conception

Associated pain before or after onset of bleeding
Progress in pregnancy
Obstetric history
Associated symptoms
BP and pulse
Abdominal tenderness
Shoulder tip pain
Fluid in abdomen
Fundal height
Fetal movements and heart rate
p.v. state of cervical os and adnexae (*avoid* after 28 weeks if patient is pregnant)

Differential diagnosis

Ectopic
Abortion
Abruptio placentae
Placenta praevia
APH (other causes see p. 363)
PPH

Action

Before 12 weeks
- reassurance and home management with bed rest if bleeding is minor and there is no associated pain
- otherwise arrange transfer to hospital
- if shocked – clear products from cervical os – i.v. fluid replacement

12–26 weeks
- for painless minor bleed arrange early antenatal assessment for ultrasound scan and cardiotocogram
- urgent admission for major bleed or associated uterine pain
- if shocked consider i.v. fluid replacement

After 26 weeks
- *avoid* pelvic examination
- consider placenta praevia
- consult with obstetric flying squad
- monitor fetal heart rate
- if shocked consider i.v. fluid replacement

After delivery
- major bleed > 500 ml
- contact obstetric flying squad
- i.v. line
- ergometrine 500 μg i.v.
- catheterize bladder
- bimanual compression of uterus.

7 Investigations

Biochemical investigations

Most doctors have open access to a biochemistry laboratory. The following is a simple guide to the causes of abnormal results in the biochemical blood tests most commonly requested. Normal values vary between laboratories and have not been included here.

	High	Low
Sodium	Dehydration Cushing's syndrome Conn's syndrome Post-traumatic Post-operative Intracranial lesions	Overhydration Fluid loss and then replacement low in sodium Inappropriate ADH secretion Addison's disease Burns Sodium-losing nephritis
Potassium	Addison's disease Excessive potassium therapy Haemolysis Renal failure Post-traumatic (early) Hypopituitarism	Diuretic therapy Vomiting Diarrhoea Potassium losing nephritis Diabetic ketoacidosis Cushing's syndrome Aldosteronism Steroid therapy Alkalosis
Bicarbonate	Excessive ingestion of bicarbonate Pyloric stenosis with vomiting	
Chloride		Pyloric stenosis with vomiting
Urea	Dehydration Renal failure Increased breakdown of blood protein (e.g. gastro-intestinal bleeding) Increased protein catabolism (e.g. fever, cachexia, post-operative)	Overhydration Normal pregnancy Hepatic necrosis
Creatinine	Renal failure	

	High	Low
Calcium	Cuffed sample with haemostasis Dehydration Hyperparathyroidism Vitamin D excess Sarcoidosis Milk–alkali syndrome	Hypoparathyroidism Osteomalacia and rickets Renal failure Protein deficiency Overhydration
Phosphate	Milk–alkali syndrome Hypoparathyroidism Renal failure	Hyperparathyroidism Osteomalacia Rickets
Albumin	Dehydration	Malnutrition Malabsorption Acute or chronic illness Severe burns Nephrotic syndrome Liver disease Protein losing enteropathy Thyrotoxicosis Cushing's syndrome Steroid treatment Pancreatitis
Bilirubin	Haemolysis Absorption of haematoma Cholestasis Liver cell disease Gilbert's disease Crigler–Najjar syndrome Dubin–Johnson syndrome	
Alkaline phosphate	Children (normal) Pregnancy Osteomalacia rickets Paget's disease Malignant bone secondaries Primary hyperparathyroidism Cholestasis, Hepatitis, Cirrhosis } with raised 5 NT	Vitamin C deficiency Cretinism Achondroplasia

	High	Low
Aspartate transaminase	Myocardial infarction Liver cell damage Severe haemolysis After trauma or surgery Muscle disease	
Lactic dehydrogenase	Myocardial infarction Haematological disorders Hepatitis Malignancy Pulmonary embolism Acute haemolysis After trauma	
Uric acid	Primary gout Thiazide diuretic Glomerular failure Pre-eclamptic toxaemia Increased nucleic acid turnover e.g. malignancy starvation pernicious anaemia myeloproliferative disorder	
Acid phosphatase	Prostatic cancer After rectal examination Acute retention of urine	
Amylase	Pancreatitis (more than 50–10 times normal) Acute abdomen Salivary gland disorders (smaller rise)	
Glucose	Diabetes mellitus Steroid therapy Myocardial infarction Cushing's syndrome Excess growth hormone Excess glucogen Excess thyroxine	Overdosage with insulin or oral hypoglycaemic agents Excess alcohol Insulinoma Liver failure Post-gastrectomy Glycogen storage disease

The blood count

Most doctors have access to a haematological laboratory. The following is a simple guide to the tests commonly performed. Sometimes the results may be abnormal due to a laboratory error and a repeat test might be considered before requesting more involved secondary investigations.

	High	Low
Haemoglobin Male 13–17 g/dl Female 12–16 g/dl Pregnancy 11.0 g/dl	Polycythaemia	Anaemia
Mean corpuscular volume 75–95 cu	Pernicious anaemia Folate deficiency Alcoholism	Iron deficiency Thalassaemia Sickle cell disease
Packed cell volume 40–54%	Dehydration Polycythaemia	Anaemia Over hydration
Mean corpuscular Hb concentration Lower limit 32%		Iron deficiency anaemia Anaemia of chronic disease Thalassaemia
Reticulocyte count Upper limit 2%	Newly treated anaemias responding to treatment Haemolytic states	
White blood cell count (total) 4,000–11,000/μl		
Polymorphs	Infection (particularly pyogenic) Polycythaemia vera Leukaemia	Virus infections B12 and folate deficiency Bone marrow deficiency Recent transfusions SLE
Eosinophils	Asthma Parasitic infection Polyarteritis nodosum Loeffler's syndrome Skin disorders pemphigus dermatitis herpetiformis eczema Medication	

	High	Low
Lymphocytes	Virus infection Pertussis Brucellosis Tuberculosis Salmonella Syphilis	
Monocytes High 400/μl	Infectious mononucleosis	
Platelets 150,000–400,000/μl	Post-splenectomy Polycythaemia vera Myeloproliferative disorders	Idiopathic thrombocytopaenia purpura Marrow depression drugs irradiation malignant infiltration Hypersplenism Infections (usually viral) SLE
Bleeding time 1–7 mins	*Prolonged* Platelet deficiency Platelet dysfunction	
Prothrombin time 10–14 secs	*Prolonged* Vitamin K deficiency Liver disease Anticoagulant drugs (Warfarin, phenindone)	
Kaolin cephalin time	*Prolonged* Factor VIII deficiency (Haemophilia) Factor IX deficiency (Christmas disease)	

Examination of urine

Routine examination of the urine is usually limited to simple tests for sugar and protein. This occasionally reveals unsuspected disease.

Other tests are readily available to the doctor. The most commonly requested tests are discussed below.

Protein

The 'labstix' test will detect a protein concentration of 150 mg/l or more. This is the upper limit of normal and so healthy patients with concentrated urine may produce trace positive results.

False positive

Can occur in very alkaline urine

True positive

Urinary infection
Postural proteinuria
Glomerulonephritis
Pyelonephritis
Multiple myelomiatosis
Toxaemia of pregnancy
Hypertensive nephropathy

The test is insensitive to Bence–Jones protein and so a salicyl sulphonic acid test should be ordered if myelomatosis is suspected.

Sugar

'Clinistix' – specific to glucose and very sensitive

'Clinitest' – partially quantifies the concentration of glucose according to the intensity of the reaction. It is less specific and will give a positive reaction to other reducing substances and salicylate derivatives.

True positive

Diabetes mellitus
Low renal threshold – particularly in young men and pregnant women
Lag storage response to glucose load (e.g. after partial gastrectomy)
Other sugars (with the 'clinites

Blood

'Haemastix' test reacts to free haemoglobin (and myoglobin) and relies on lysis of some of the red cells present in the urine. It should be checked against a microscopic examination.

Causes of blood in the urine

Renal tract
infection
trauma

stones
neoplasm
severe hypertension
acute nephritis
papillary necrosis
renal infarction
congenital cystic kidney
nephrotoxic drugs
prostatic hypertrophy or carcinoma
post prostatectomy

Bleeding diathesis
haemorrhagic states (e.g. haemophilia)
thrombocytopaenia
anticoagulant medication

Acute fevers
malaria
yellow fever

After prolonged exercise

Contamination from genital tract (menstruation)

Subacute bacterial endocarditis.

Ketones

The 'Acetest' reacts strongly to acetoacetic acid, weakly to acetone and is insensitive to β-hydroxybutyric acid.

True positive

Diabetic ketosis
Starvation
Acute illness (e.g. pneumonia or myocardial infarction)
Vomiting

Microscopy of urine

Cells

Red cells may be seen in any of the above conditions causing haematuria. More than a few pus cells per high power field indicates infection of the renal tract. Pyuria in the absence of bacterial growth on culture may indicate underlying glomerulonephritis, tuberculosis or partially treated infection.

Casts

Hyaline casts are not considered to indicate pathology
Granular casts tend to occur in renal parenchymal disease.

Crystals

May be found in normal urine and are rarely of diagnostic importance.

Culture

To be signficant the culture should demonstrate more than 10^5 organisms per millilitre. It should be associated with pyuria (i.e. >10 white cells per ml)

Reading the ECG

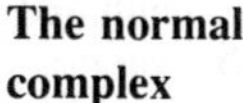

The normal complex

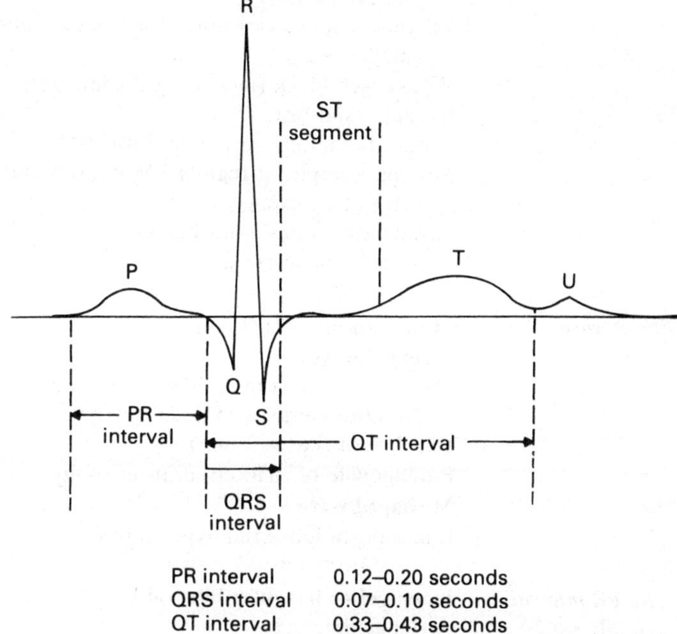

PR and QT intervals vary with the heart rate

Fig. 7.1. Normal electrocardiogram complex

Calibration

Large square = 0.2 sec or 5 mv
Small square = 0.04 sec or 1 mv

Rate

Ventricular rate/min = 300/No. of large squares between adjacent R waves

Rhythm

Regular and slow
Sinus bradycardia (normal complexes)
Complete heart block (P waves and QRS dissociated)
Myxoedema (small complexes)
Hypothermia (J waves at junction of QRS and ST segment)
Regular and fast
Sinus tachycardia (usually less than 120/min)
Paroxysmal atrial tachycardia (usually less than 150/min)
Ventricular tachycardia (140–220/min)

Irregular and slow
Sinus arrhythmia (rate varies with respiration and can be fast)
Varying heart block (more P waves than QRS complexes)
Wenkebach block (increasing PR interval)
Irregular and fast
Atrial fibrillation (no visible P waves)
Multiple ectopics (irregular RR interval and different QRS complexes)
Atrial flutter and varying blocks ('saw-tooth' base line)
Ventricular tachycardia

The P wave

(Best seen in leads II and V_2)
Absent P waves
The P wave is lost in atrial fibrillation and may be lost in the QRS complex in nodal rhythm.
Tall P wave (i.e. > 3 mm)
P pulmonale of right atrial hypertrophy
M-shaped wave
P mitralis of left atrial hypertrophy

The PR interval (usually <0.2 sec)

Increased or irregular interval
Atrial ectopic beats
Heart block of varying degree
Very short interval
Wolff–Parkinson–White syndrome

The Q wave

Amplitude or duration > 1 mm
This is pathological and on its own may indicate an old myocardial infarction

QRS complex

Duration > 0.12 secs
Bundle branch block (BBB)
M-shaped QRS in V_1–V_2 = Right BBB
M-shaped QRS in V_5–V_6 = Left BBB
Amplitude of RS waves increased
Ventricular hypertrophy
S in V1 + R in V5 = > 35 mm – left ventricular hypertrophy
R in V1 + S in V5 = > 17 mm – right ventricular hypertrophy
Usually associated with ventricular strain i.e. ST depression and T wave inversion in the appropriate chest leads

ST segment (normally flat on the base or isoelectric line)	**ST segment below the base line** (> 1 mm) Myocardial ischaemia Digoxin therapy (reversed 'tick' shape) Ventricular strain (associated hypertrophy) Bundle branch block (wide QRS complexes) Hypokalaemia (prominent U wave) **ST segment above the base line** (> 1 mm) Myocardial infarction (dome shaped) Pericarditis (U shaped)
T wave	**T wave inverted** Bundle branch block (wide QRS complex) Ischaemia Digoxin effect (reversed 'tick' shape ST + T complex) Ventricular strain (associated hypertrophy) Resolving myocardial infarction (associated Q waves) **Tall peaked T waves** Hyperkalaemia (also small P wave and wide QRS) **U wave** (may be normal: best seen in $V_3 + V_4$) Hypokalaemia (depressed ST segment) U wave prominent and merging with next P wave
Some common pathological conditions	**Myocardial infarction** Look for pathological Q waves ST elevation T wave inversion Inferior infarction: leads, II, III and AVF Anterior infarction: chest leads (V_{1-4}) Lateral infarction: chest leads (V_{4-6}) **Pericarditis** – U shaped ST elevation in most leads except AVR **Acute pulmonary embolism** Lead I–S wave Lead III–Q wave and inverted T wave **Cor pulmonale** Tall peaked P waves Signs of right ventricular hypertrophy **Ectopic beats** Supraventricular or atrial ectopic have normal QRS complexes Ventrical ectopics have abnormal or wide QRS complexes.

Index